Uncommon Malignant Tumors

John Antoniades, M.D.

Professor of Radiation Therapy and Nuclear Medicine
The Hahnemann Medical College and Hospital
Philadelphia, Pennsylvania
and
Associate Radiation Therapy and Nuclear Medicine
The Lankenau Hospital
Philadelphia, Pennsylvania

RC262
A67
1982

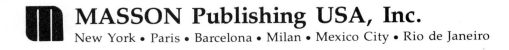 **MASSON Publishing USA, Inc.**
New York • Paris • Barcelona • Milan • Mexico City • Rio de Janeiro

Library of Congress Cataloging in Publication Data

Antoniades, John.
  Uncommon malignant tumors.

  (Cancer management)
  Bibliography: p.
  Includes index.
  1. Cancer. I. Title. II. Series. [DNLM:
1. Neoplasms. QZ 200 A625]
RC262.A67   616.99'4   82-6610
ISBN 0-89352-046-2   AACR2

ISBN 0-89352-046-2

Library of Congress Catalog Card Number: 82-6610

Printed in the United States of America

CANCER MANAGEMENT

Luther W. Brady and Vincent T. DeVita, Jr., Series Editors

PROLOGUE

The number of recognizable individual tumor types has increased considerably during the last three decades. The manual on International Classification of Diseases for Oncology (ICD-O), published by the World Health Organization, reveals a list of over 400 morphologically different neoplasms. This figure can be greatly expanded, considering the fact that histologically individual types may occur in various sites, thus creating separate and distinct oncological entities. In spite of the large variety of human neoplasias, the extremely high incidence of some overshadows the remainder, and demands most of the attention and efforts of the clinical oncologist. According to the Cancer Statistics for 1980, as published by the American Cancer Society, 53% of male malignancies originated in the lung, colon, and prostate, while cancer of the breast, colon, and genital tract constitutes 57% of all neoplasms seen in females. Current medical literature reflects this preponderance by focusing especially in primary growths of the breast, lung, and colon. Similarly, review of the standard textbooks on pathology and clinical medicine demonstrates the great emphasis placed on common tumors, while a cursory notation, or, in many instances, a complete omission, is reserved for the very many primary uncommon malignancies.

In our belief that the maturing specialties of oncology are presently in need of a more detailed, clearer understanding of all diseases involved, we undertook the preparation of the present manual during the last few years.

The precise definition of an uncommon tumor is difficult. Generally, it can be stated that a tumor is uncommon when it is infrequently encountered by oncological surgeons, radiotherapists, and medical oncologists. Keeping in mind this subjective definition, we have identified three main categories of such neoplasms. In the first, we have included tumors of usual histology such as squamous cell carcinomas, adenocarcinomas, melanomas, etc., that, when occurring in an unexpected site, create distinct uncommon entities. In the second category, we have placed those neoplasms whose microscopic appearance is distinct and separates them from those of a more common pattern. Finally, the third group deals with neoplasms which are site-specific. Many of them have individual histology, but unlike the previous subdivision, they are organ or system related. Such a tumor, for example, is the cloacogenic carcinoma of the anorectal junction. Excluded from this presentation are entities that may be uncommon for the general oncologist, but are nevertheless often seen by the specialists treating them. Such are the ophthalmological and pediatric malignancies. We have also refrained from describing the various manifestations of malignant lymphomas. As a whole, they constitute a major oncologic subject involving several disciplines while undergoing a continuous histopathological and clinical evaluation. A good number of soft tissue sarcomas have also been excluded. These are by no means common neoplasms, however their natural history, treatment, and prognosis are well defined and readily available in existing textbooks.

It is our hope that the detailed clinical presentation of the several "colorful" oncological entities will contribute toward a sharper identification of the diseases we are dealing with, and will broaden in a more tangible way the spectrum of our interest.

I wish to thank Dr. Luther W. Brady, professor and chairman of the Department of Radiation Therapy and Nuclear Medicine at Hahnemann Medical College and Hospital for his longstanding support.

Our thanks also go to Drs. George T. Wohl, chairman of the Department of Diagnostic Radiology at Lankenau Hospital, and Marvin E. Haskin, professor and chairman of the Department of Diagnostic Radiology at Hahnemann Medical College and Hospital for allowing us to review their teaching files and select appropriate radiographs for illustration. My good wife, Dr. Kristina Antoniades, has reviewed the pathology passages and coordinated the histopathological illustrations, and I thank her from this point too.

Finally, to our cheerful and eager secretary, Mrs. Sheila J. Cook, we express our appreciation and thanks once more.

John Antoniades, M.D.
Philadelphia, Pennsylvania

CONTENTS

Part 3: Uncommon Tumors Site-Specific   271

PART I

TUMORS OF
UNCOMMON LOCATION

1

Squamous Cell Carcinoma of the Thyroid

SQUAMOUS CELL carcinoma of the thyroid gland is a rare neoplasm and comprises approximately 1% of all primary thyroid malignancies.[1] The tumor represents a clinical oddity, since squamous epithelium is not normally found in the thyroid. In earlier years several theories regarding the genesis of this tumor were expressed; however, at the present time the most prevalent hypothesis is that squamous cell thyroid carcinomas arise in areas of squamous metaplasia.[3,4] Most cases have occurred in patients during their fifth and sixth decades of life, and there is no sex predisposition.[1]

PATHOLOGY

Characteristically, some form of chronic thyroid disease associated with goiter has been present in the majority of the patients prior to the development of squamous cell carcinoma.[1] Under certain conditions benign squamous cells do develop in the thyroid gland. Thus, in struma lymphomatosa (Hashimoto's disease), as well as in areas of scar formation in patients with involuting thyroids and especially in patients with chronic nonspecific thyroiditis, squamous metaplasias are observed. Microsopically, there is no doubt about these cells being squamous because well-defined intercellular bridges are to be seen.[3,4]

The gross appearance of the tumor is that of a firm, irregular mass that infiltrates the surrounding tissues. It usually measures 5–10 cm in its greatest diameter.[1-3]

Histologically, infiltrating strands and nests of squamous cells are observed. Often, they are well differentiated because foci of keratinization and pearl formation are present[1,2] (Fig. 1-1).

CLINICAL

As mentioned earlier, squamous cell carcinoma of the thyroid develops on a background of chronic thyroid disease. Usually the patients have a history of goiter of several years' duration. Suddenly, an accelerated growth is noted. This is associated with pain originally and subsequently with dysphagia, hoarseness, and shortness of breath. Generally, a rapid growth of the neoplasm takes place, with quick invasion of adjacent structures. This despite the fact that more often than not the histology is that of a well-differentiated tumor.[1-3] Radiographically, deviation of the trachea is a common finding and on thyroid scanning a defect corresponding to the mass is to be found. The tumors occur in the lobes of the thyroid rather than in the midline. For this reason the theory of origin from remnants of the thyroglossal duct is not considered very probable.[3]

TREATMENT AND RESULTS

The treatment of choice is radical surgical resection. Unfortunately, the tumor

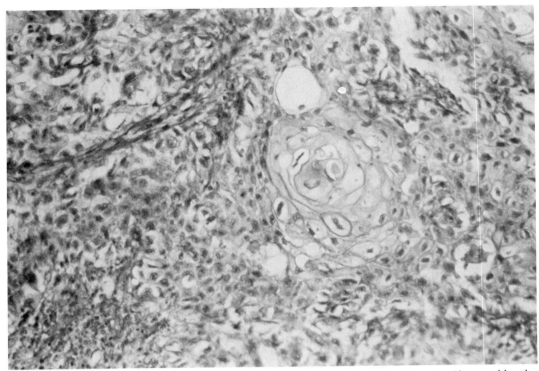

FIG. 1-1.   Squamous cell carcinoma of the thyroid with central area of pearl formation, in a 60-year-old male.

behaves in a manner similar to that of anaplastic carcinoma of the thyroid by infiltrating the surrounding skeletal muscles and invading the lymphatics and therefore has an extremely high tendency for local recurrence. In addition it is a radioresistant neoplasm. Even at relatively high dosage—5000 rad in five weeks—no appreciable effect was shown with regard to the growth or to the rate of local recurrence.[2]

Generally, therefore, the prognosis is extremely poor. No patient has been reported surviving for any significant length of time. Actually, several patients died during the immediate postoperative period.[2,3] Distant metastases also occur; however, the main problem is local, persistent, infiltrating disease.

REFERENCES

1. Goldman, R.L.: Primary squamous cell carcinoma of the thyroid gland: Report of a case and review of the literature. *Am Surg* **30**:247, 1964.
2. Huang, T.Y., and Assor, D.: Primary squamous cell carcinoma of the thyroid gland. A report of four cases. *Am J Clin Pathol* **55**:93, 1971.
3. Kampsen, E.B., Jager, N., and Max, M.H.: Squamous cell carcinoma of the thyroid: A report of two cases. *J Surg Oncol* **9**:567, 1977.
4. Saxén, E.: Squamous metaplasia in the thyroid gland and histogenesis of epidermoid carcinoma of the thyroid. *Acta Pathol Microbiol Scand* **28**:55, 1951.

2

Squamous Cell Carcinoma of the Breast

SQUAMOUS METAPLASIA may accompany the various histological patterns with which breast carcinoma appears. It represents the most common form of metaplasia. Although focal areas of squamous cell carcinoma may be found in association with several forms of breast cancer, pure squamous cell carcinoma of the breast is a distinct rarity.[1,3] Cornog et al.[1] reported on 24 cases of carcinoma of the breast in which squamous differentiation was a prominent histological feature. Of these only two were pure squamous cell carcinomas. There were 15 patients with adenocarcinoma containing squamous cell elements, five with anaplastic carcinoma, one with medullary carcinoma, and one with cystosarcoma phyllodes.[1]

The exact incidence of pure squamous cell carcinoma of the breast escapes determination. It is considered to be less than 0.1%.[2] Hasleton et al.[2] in a recent

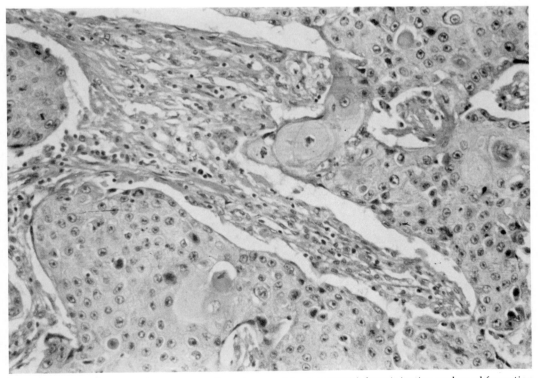

FIG. 2-1.   Well-differentiated squamous cell carcinoma of the breast with keratinization and pearl formation in a 54-year-old female.

5

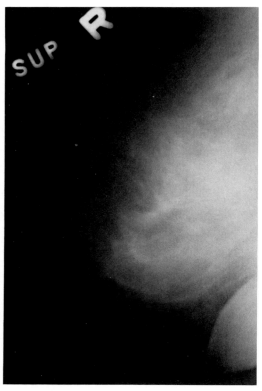

FIG. 2-2.   Squamous cell carcinoma of the breast in a
44-year-old female. Mammography, lateral view,
shows the tumor to lie deep within the central part of
the breast. The mass is dense and has ill-defined
borders.

viously existing benign epidermoid cyst.[2]
McDivitt et al.[3] on the other hand, are of
the opinion that the majority of these
neoplasms develop on the basis of squamous metaplasia. They support their view
by the fact that further metaplastic
changes toward the direction of a sarcomatous pattern are common.

Squamous cell carcinoma of the breast
exhibits the characteristics of this particular histological type, namely keratin production and intercellular bridges between
the cells[1,2] (Fig. 2-1). Coexistence of
squamous cell elements with elements exhibiting sarcomatoid pattern is also observed.[3]

CLINICAL

As is the case for all breast carcinomas, a
lump associated with nipple and skin
changes in the more advanced cases has
been the common presenting symptom.
The involvement of axillary lymph nodes
is not adequately documented in all the
reported cases; however, it appears that
there is no difference in behavior between
squamous cell carcinomas and the remainder of the breast tumors (Fig. 2-2).
When the disease has been present for a
certain length of time, the axillary lymph
nodes do become involved. Metastasis of
the squamous elements in tumors containing both adenocarcinoma and squamous
cell carcinoma has been observed. Of 11
cases reported in the series by Cornog
et al.[1] in which confirmation of axillary
lymph node metastasis was established,
six had squamous differentiation in the
metastatic deposits and five did not.
Along the same lines, distant metastases
composed of squamous cell carcinoma are
known to occur.

literature review on the subject encountered 26 cases of pure squamous cell carcinoma of the breast and added two of
their own. The average age of the patients
at the time of the diagnosis was 54.5 years.

PATHOLOGY

The tumors, grossly, have been found to
be approximately 5.0 cm in their greatest
diameter. There is a preference for the development of squamous cell carcinoma in
the left breast as compared to the right, a
preference that is known to exist for carcinoma of the breast in general.[2] Often in
the center of the tumor a cystic cavity is to
be found.[1] The presence of this cystic cavity has raised the question of the possible
role of malignant transformation of a pre-

TREATMENT AND RESULTS

Surgical therapy in the form of radical or
simple mastectomy has been the procedure of choice. Since the number of the

reported cases extends over half a century, no homogeneous method of treatment can be expected.[2]

The follow-up data in a number of cases are incomplete or the follow-up period covers a relatively short span of time. In reviewing the literature on the subject, we have found the three-year-survival rate to be in the range of 30%. Most of the studied patients were seen and treated prior to 1960.

REFERENCES

1. Cornog, J.L., Mobini, J., Steiger, E., and Enterline, H.T.: Squamous carcinoma of the breast. *Am J Clin Pathol* **55**:410, 1971.

2. Hasleton, P.S., Misch, K.A., Vasudev, K.S., and George, D.: Squamous carcinoma of the breast. *J Clin Pathol* **31**:116, 1978.

3. McDivitt, R.W., Stewart, F.W., and Berg, J.W.: *Tumors of the Breast.* Armed Forces Institute of Pathology, Washington, D.C., 1968.

3

Squamous Cell Carcinoma of the Stomach

PURE SQUAMOUS cell carcinoma of the stomach, or even a combination of adenocarcinoma and squamous cell carcinoma (adenosquamous cell carcinoma), is a rare disease. In considering squamous cell carcinoma of the stomach, lesions in the region of the cardia should be excluded because more often than not it is impossible to determine whether they arise within the distal esophagus or in the upper stomach.

Squamous cell carcinomas comprise only a small fraction of all gastric carcinomas, approximately 0.04–0.7%.[5] There is a definite male predominance, the ratio of male to female patients being in the range of 4:1. Of the 49 reported cases, the sex has been recorded in 46, with 37 men and 9 women. All patients were adults, the neoplasm occurring with greater frequency during the sixth decade of life.[3,5]

PATHOLOGY

The tumors are exophytic in character, protruding within the lumen of the stomach. They all have attained considerable size at the time of the resection.[4] The majority of the tumors (two-thirds of the cases) have developed in the region of the pylorus, and the remaining one-third were found in the body of the stomach[4] (Fig. 3-1).

Histologically, the features of squamous cell carcinoma are to be found. The pleomorphic squamous cells exhibit keratin pearl formation and intercellular bridges,

features typical for this particular histology[3-5] (Fig. 3-2). A number of theoretical proposals exist as to the pathogenesis of squamous cell carcinoma of the stomach. The most prevalent view seems to be that of squamous metaplasia of the glandular mucosa from which, eventually, squamous cell carcinoma arises.[5]

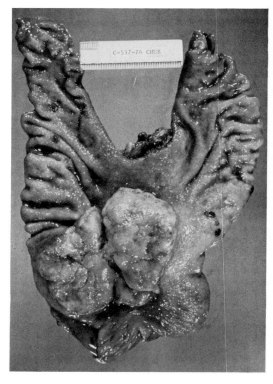

FIG. 3-1. Squamous cell carcinoma of the stomach. Surgical specimen showing a large fungating tumor located near the antrum. (Courtesy A. Rioux and S.R. Massé. *Can J Surg* **22**:238, 1979.)

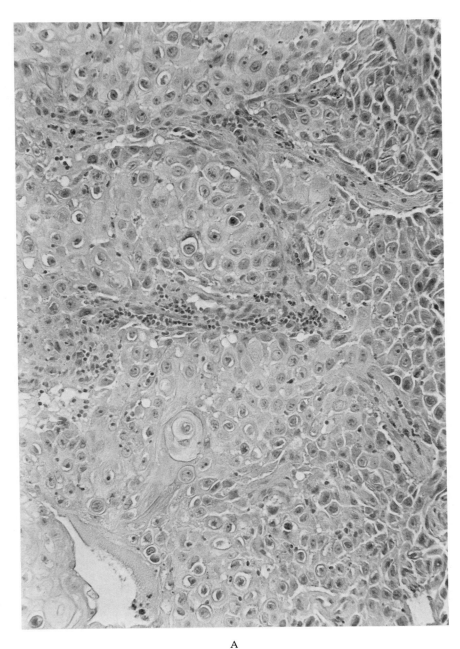

A

CLINICAL

The symptomatology is that of carcinoma of the stomach in general. Patients present with epigastric distress or pain, anorexia, indigestion, nausea, or vomiting. On clinical examination, quite often an epigastric mass is palpable. The diagnosis is established radiographically and the disease further evaluated by means of gastroscopy.[2,4,5]

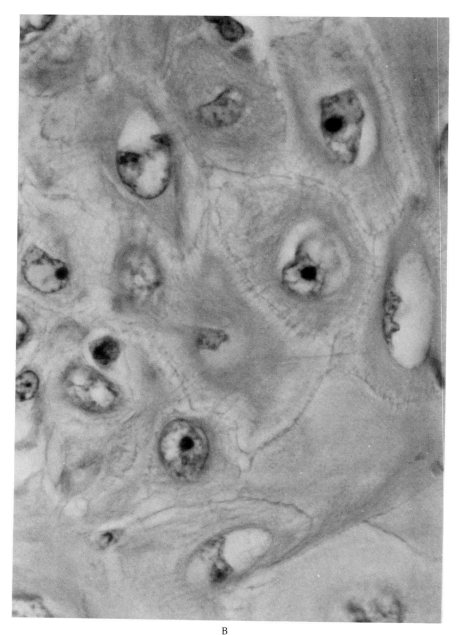

B

FIG. 3-2.   Squamous cell carcinoma of the stomach. (A): The tumor consists of keratinizing squamous carcinoma composed of sheets and masses of epithelial cells with pearl
formation. (B): High-power view showing intercellular bridges. (Courtesy A. Rioux and
S.R. Massé. *Can J Surg* **22**:238, 1979.)

The treatment has been surgical. For those patients who appear to be candidates for definitive resection, a total or subtotal gastrectomy has been performed.[1,2,4,5] It appears that a larger number of patients have gross tumor confined only to the stomach and therefore a larger number, in comparison to those with adenocarcinoma, have had definitive surgery.

Unfortunately, the disease behaves like an adenocarcinoma. As Boswell and Helwig[1] pointed out, only 5 of 18 squamous cell carcinomas reported in the literature had metastasized at the time of publication. In contrast, all but one of their own 12 cases, retrieved from the files of the Armed Forces Institute of Pathology, were dead with metastases or had evidence of metastases when adequate follow-up time was provided. All deaths occurred within seven months or less from the time of the diagnosis.[1]

REFERENCES

1. Boswell, J.T., and Helwig, E.B.: Squamous cell carcinoma and adenoacanthoma of the stomach. A clinicopathologic study. *Cancer* **18:**181, 1965.
2. Dreyer, B., and Louw, J.H.: Squamous-cell carcinoma of the stomach. *Br J Surg* **44:**425, 1956–1957.
3. Milstoc, M.: Squamous-cell carcinoma of stomach with liver metastasis. *NY State J Med* **69:**2913, 1969.
4. Rioux, A., and Masse, S.R.: Pure squamous cell carcinoma of the stomach. *Can J Surg* **22:**238, 1979.
5. Straus, R., Heschel, S., and Fortmann, D.J.: Primary adenosquamous carcinoma of the stomach. A case report and review. *Cancer* **24:**985, 1969.

4

Squamous Cell Carcinoma of the Colon

SQUAMOUS CELL carcinoma of the anal canal is an established clinicopathological entity, often involving, by direct extension, the lower rectum. Squamous cell carcinoma of the colon above the lower rectum, however, is distinctly rare. Schmidtmann[5] in 1919 described a squamous cell carcinoma involving the cecum in the region of the ileocecal valve. To the present time approximately 30 cases of primary squamous cell carcinoma of the colon have been reported. Most of the tumors are to be found in the rectum.[1,2] Other areas of involvement in decreasing frequency are the cecum, ascending colon, transverse colon, hepatic flexure, descending colon, and sigmoid colon.

There is no clear sex predominence and most patients are in their fifth or sixth decade of life at the time of the diagnosis. Burgess et al.[1] have reported on a 43-year-old male with squamous cell carcinoma of the cecum, and Hicks and Cowling[3] reported on a 90-year-old female with a tumor of the ascending colon.

Histologically, the neoplasms are squamous cell carcinomas, poorly or well differentiated. Penetration of the bowel wall by the tumor and involvement of the regional lymph nodes has been found in approximately one-third of the cases at the time of surgery. The tumor origin remains a subject of discussion. Some of the existing hypotheses include origin from embryonic nests, from squamous metaplasia of glandular epithelium, from neighboring epithelium, and from indeterminate basal cells during the replacement of the damaged glandular epithelium.[1-4]

It is generally agreed that effective therapy requires a wide surgical resection. The use of radiation therapy has been very limited in the few cases reported. There is evidence to suggest that the tumor is radioresponsive.[2] Review of the literature indicates that cures have resulted from definitive surgical therapy, namely, hemicolectomy or primary resection with end-to-end anastomosis. This surgical approach, however, is not feasible when intraabdominal metastases are to be found during laparotomy.[3] Most patients definitively treated were alive and free of disease for periods ranging from one to two years postoperatively. Due to the small number of cases and the lack of information, the survival rate cannot be expressed more specifically.[1,4]

REFERENCES

1. Burgess, P.A., Lupton, E.W., and Talbot, I.C.: Squamous-cell carcinoma of the proximal colon: Report of a case and review of the literature. *Dis Colon Rectum* **22**:241, 1979.
2. Comer, T.P., Beahrs, O.H., and Dockerty, M.B.: Primary squamous cell carcinoma and adenoacanthoma of the colon. *Cancer* **28**:1111, 1971.
3. Hicks, J.D., and Cowling, D.C.: Squamous-cell carcinoma of the ascending colon. *J Pathol* **70**:205, 1955.
4. Horne, B.D., and McCulloch, C.F.: Squamous-cell carcinoma of the cecum. A case report. *Cancer* **42**:1879, 1978.
5. Schmidtmann, M.: Zur Kenntis seltener Krebsformen. *Virchows Arch [Pathol Anat]* **226**:100, 1919.

5

Squamous Cell Carcinoma of the Prostate

KERATINIZING SQUAMOUS cell carcinoma of the prostate arises in the periurethral prostatic ducts. It is perhaps the rarest form of prostatic cancer. Kahler[4] in a histopathological review of 195 prostatic tumors found six (3%) to be of the squamous cell variety. Arnheim[1] found, in a postmortem examination of 176 prostatic carcinomas, four cases of squamous cell tumor. In more recent reports, however, the incidence of squamous cell prostatic carcinoma has been considerably lower than that just mentioned. Dixon and Moore[2] evaluated 500 cases of prostatic carcinoma, among which they found only one definite epidermoid tumor with keratin pearls present. Sieracki[5] in 1955 and Gray and Marshall[3] reported on four patients with histologically well-documented squamous carcinomas. The average age of the patients is 65 years.

PATHOLOGY

In diagnosing squamous cell prostatic carcinoma it is important to exclude a neoplasm of the urinary bladder which has invaded the prostate by extension. The patient described by Gray and Marshall[3] exhibited cells with intercellular bridges and abundant keratinization. In at least one patient described by Sieracki[5] definite keratinization was seen.

CLINICAL

The tumors produce obstruction of the prostatic urethra and therefore the com-monest presenting symptom is prostatism with trabeculation of the urinary bladder. Hematuria may be present.

On clinical examination, an enlarged prostate is to be found as the tumor grows. There is a tendency for iliac lymph node metastasis from which subsequently the disease spreads to the periaortic lymph nodes. All three patients described by Sieracki[5] were found to have disease in those regions at autopsy. It also tends to extend locally beyond the prostate into the surrounding structures, namely, the symphysis pubis, the perineum, the bladder, and the rectum.[3,5]

TREATMENT AND PROGNOSIS

The patient reported by Gray and Marshall[3] underwent radical prostatectomy, complete urethrectomy, and bilateral pelvic lymph node dissection. Three months later, however, he developed perineal recurrence, eventually dying of his disease in about one year from the onset of the symptoms.[3] Two of three patients reported by Sieracki[5] died without prior major therapy. The third patient was treated with total perineal prostatectomy followed by stilbesterol therapy and orthovoltage radiation to the pelvis. He did well for 11 months, at which point the pelvic disease recurred. He died eventually of his tumor 14 months after his initial surgery and 26 months from the onset of the symptoms.[5]

The number of reported cases is too small for any conclusions to be drawn. It is possible that this histological pattern will benefit from a combined surgical and radiotherapeutic approach.

REFERENCES

1. Arnheim, F.K.: Carcinoma of the prostate: A study of the postmortem findings in one hundred and seventy-six cases. *J Urol* **60**:599, 1948.

2. Dixon, F.J., and Moore, R.A.: *Tumors of the Male Sex Organs*. Armed Forces Institute of Pathology, Washington, D.C., 1958.

3. Gray, G.F., Jr., and Marshall, V.F.: Squamous carcinoma of the prostate. *J Urol* **113**:736, 1975.

4. Kahler, J.E.: Carcinoma of the prostate gland: A pathologic study. *J Urol* **41**:557, 1939.

5. Sieracki, J.C.: Epidermoid carcinoma of the human prostate. Report of three cases. *Lab Invest* **4**:232, 1955.

6

Carcinoma of the Pilonidal Sinus

PILONIDAL CYSTS and pilonidal sinuses represent a special form of the so-called "epidermal inclusion cysts." They are midline formations arising from the skin that overlies the sacrococcygeal region, formed by invagination of the surface epithelium. Sebum secretion and subsequent inflammation accompanied by ingrowth of hair shafts predispose to bacterial infection, usually by coliform bacilli and staphylococci. The pilonidal cyst may or may not communicate with the surface; the pilonidal sinus represents a similar formation that is associated with a sinus tract reaching the surface of the skin. After long presence with several inflammatory exacerbations, lateral sinus extensions develop within the adjacent subcutaneous tissues. It is on this background of particularly chronic suppurative disease that carcinomas occasionally arise.[2,5]

The incidence of carcinoma is small in spite of the fact that pilonidal sinuses and cysts represent a rather common disorder; only 0.1% of patients with this diagnosis have been found to develop malignancy. It appears that an essential factor for this event is the long-standing duration of chronic inflammatory process. All patients with carcinomas of the pilonidal sinus had a long history, which averaged 24 to 25 years.[2] That chronic inflammation is the major etiological factor is further supported by the fact that this tumor has not been encountered among the several thousands of military personnel who undergo operation for pilonidal disease.[1,4]

It is assumed that the young age and the prompt medical attention in this particular group of patients eliminate the chronic inflammatory stimulant.

There is a definite male predominance, reflecting the more common occurrence of pilonidal sinuses in males.[5] Thus, male patients were involved in 84% of the reported cases. The average age at the time of the diagnosis was 50 years.[4]

PATHOLOGY

The gross appearance of the lesion is suggestive of the diagnosis. In most cases the diagnosis was established upon the clinical suspicion of malignant neoplasm developing. Actually at times repeated biopsies were necessary in order to confirm the clinical impression.[1,4] The lesion is a fungating, ulcerated mass associated with infection, usually producing a foul-smelling discharge. It is to be found at the base of the sacrum overlying the coccyx and at times it almost extends to the anus (Fig. 6-1). The size of these tumors is considerable, their average diameter being in the range of 5–10 cm.[1,2,4] Histologically, of the 26 hitherto reported cases, 21 were squamous cell carcinomas, two were basal cell, one was an adenocarcinoma, and two were mixed squamous and basal cell carcinomas.[1,2] There is a gradual transition from the normal squamous cell epithelium of the skin to the areas of cellular atypia and tumor invasion[3] (Fig. 6-2).

15

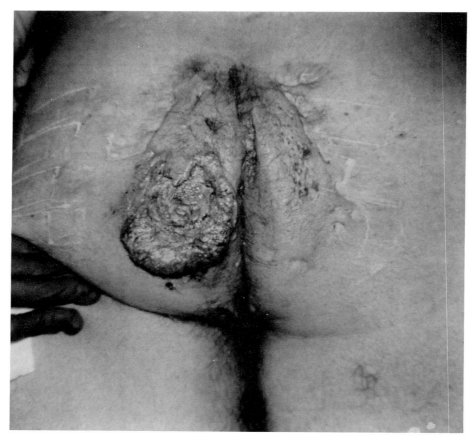

FIG. 6-1. Pilonidal sinus carcinoma in a 48-year-old male. The patient had a long-standing history of infected pilonidal cysts. He presented with a large, fungating, friable, foul-smelling mass that occupied the area from the base of the sacrum to practically the anus. (Courtesy H.J. Lerner and G. Deitrick. *J Surg Oncol* **11**:177, 1979.)

CLINICAL

Most patients present with a history of chronic drainage and discharge in the sacrococcygeal region. This as a rule has been resistant to medical therapy and has been associated with repeated flare-ups of acute inflammation. The development of a mass lesion associated with bleeding and foul discharge should raise the suspicion of malignant transformation.[3] Rectal examination and sigmoidoscopy are necessary in order to rule out primary anal or rectal carcinoma. In pilonidal sinus carcinomas the anus and the rectum are free of disease.[1,2,4]

The skin of the coccygeal region drains to the inguinal lymph nodes. Their incidence of involvement has been low, however. Enlargement due to inflammatory reaction may be present; however, only in two patients of the 26 reported was metastatic disease seen in the inguinal lymph nodes.[4,6]

TREATMENT AND RESULTS

Surgery has been the main therapy. The procedure entails primary excision of the lesion associated with wide local resection. This is accompanied by split-thickness skin grafting in order to close

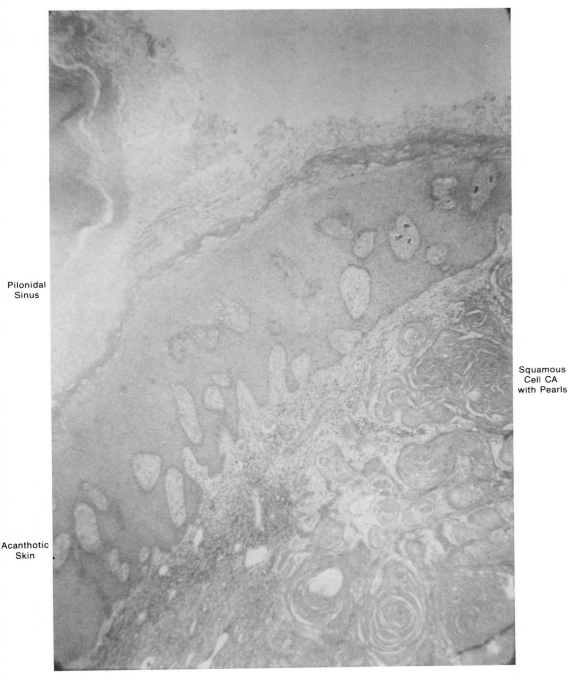

Pilonidal
Sinus

Squamous
Cell CA
with Pearls

Acanthotic
Skin

FIG. 6-2. Pilonidal sinus squamous cell carcinoma. Well-differentiated squamous cells with pearl formation are seen in the lower right part of the illustration, and the pilonidal sinus can be seen in the upper left part. Same patient as in Figure 6-1. (Courtesy H.J. Lerner and G. Deitrick. *J Surg Oncol* **11:**177, 1979.)

the defect.[2] There is clinical evidence to suggest that the tumors are radioresponsive; therefore radiation therapy should be considered in case of recurrence or in case of residual disease.[4] Due to the low incidence of involvement, lymph node dissection is not recommended; however, the status of the nodes should be carefully evaluated, clinically.

Among the 26 reported patients, seven developed recurrence. This usually led to failure of cure, with the exception of one patient who survived four years following recurrence.[2,4]

Puckett and Silver[4] in their literature review were able to identify 18 patients whose follow-up appeared to be adequate. Of these 13 (72%) were considered to have been cured of their disease by means of local resection.[4]

Emphasis should be placed on the complete pathological examination of the resected specimen, particularly in determining whether or not tumor is present at the margins of the submitted tissue. Local recurrence when it occurs is difficult to control and eventually leads to distant metastases and death.[1,3,4]

REFERENCES

1. Gaston, E.A., and Wilde, W.L.: Epidermoid carcinoma arising in a pilonidal sinus. *Dis Colon Rectum* **8**:343, 1965.
2. Lerner, H.J., and Deitrick, G.: Squamous-cell carcinoma of the pilonidal sinus: Report of a case and review of the literature. *J Surg Oncol* **11**:177, 1979.
3. Milch, E., Berman, L., and McGregor, J.K.: Carcinoma complicating a pilonidal sinus: Review of the literature and report of a case. *Dis Colon Rectum* **6**:225, 1963.
4. Puckett, C.L., and Silver, D.: Carcinoma developing in pilonidal sinus: Report of two cases and review of the literature. *Am Surg* **39**:151, 1973.
5. Robbins, S.L.: *Pathologic Basis of Disease*. W.B. Saunders, Philadelphia, 1974.
6. Terry, J.L., Gainsford, J.C., and Hanna, D.C.: Pilonidal sinus carcinoma. *Am J Surg* **102**:465, 1961.

7

Burn Scar Carcinoma

SCAR TISSUES of long-standing duration have a known propensity for malignant transformation. The most common scar tissue carcinoma is related to skin burns. Other such entities include carcinomas developing in chronic leg ulcers, in focuses of chronic osteomyelitis with sinus tract formations, and in chronic traumatic wounds. Finally, as described elsewhere in this volume, the carinomas seen in pilonidal sinus disease can be included in this group.[1,2]

Burn scar carcinomas have been known since antiquity. Marjolin in 1828 described the clinical entity in detail, hence the term "Marjolin ulcers" has been applied to denote malignant degeneration of burn scar. Judging from the literature, these tumors were much more common in the beginning of this century and earlier than they are at the present time. The use of electricity and central heating has decreased markedly the risk of thermal injury among the young. In certain parts of India and in Japan where people carry portable heaters in direct contact with their skin, a high incidence of thermal injuries and carcinomas continues to exist.[4,5]

Treves and Pack[5] reviewed the files of patients with skin cancer at the Memorial Hospital from 1917 until 1929. Among 1374 patients diagnosed, 28 had burn scar carcinomas, an incidence of 2%.

The neoplasms are primarily observed in adults, since a number of years are needed for their formation. In the series by Novick et al.[4] the average age at the time of the diagnosis was 58 years, with a range from 18 to 84 years.[4] The same average age, 58 years, was found in the series by Treves and Pack.[5] In the former series[4] 61% of the patients were male, whereas in the latter[5] the patients were equally divided among males and females. Similarly in the series by Giblin et al.[3] there was no difference in incidence as far as sex was concerned, the average age at the time of the diagnosis being 44 years.

PATHOLOGY

The majority of the patients have squamous cell carcinoma. A literature review indicates that 75 to 90% of burn scar carcinomas are squamous cell in character, the remaining being adenoacanthomas, basal cell carcinomas, and in rare instances sarcomas.[1,3–5] Usually the carcinomatous degeneration is confined to the periphery of the scar; however, eventually the center of the scar tissue becomes involved. The tumors extend deeply, ulcerate, and are associated with superimposed infections, discharge, and foul smell.

Treves and Pack[5] attributed the pathogenesis of burn scar carcinoma to multiple injuries affecting the thin epithelium that covers the scar tissue. Successive injuries result in successive attempts to regenerate and eventually this continuous stimulation at the margins of the scar leads to malignant transformation.[5] An alternative theory offered by the same authors suggests the release of toxins by the burn scar tissue.

CLINICAL

A long period, in the range of 20–40 years, usually elapses from the time of the thermal injury to the development of burn scar carcinoma. It has been shown that the younger the age at the time of the injury the longer the interval will be. Conversely, patients sustaining burns during their adult years are prone to develop carcinomas in shorter intervals.

The Marjolin ulcers are most often found in the upper and the lower extremities. In the series by Novick et al.[4] 56.5% of the cases were seen in the upper and lower extremities, the remaining occurring in the scalp, face, and the trunk. Practically identical percentages are presented by Arons et al.[1] As Treves and Pack[5] observe, burn scar carcinomas occur in areas where primary skin cancer is rather infrequent.

The initial appearance is that of an indurated papule that proceeds to diffuse tumor formation and eventually it ulcerates. The patients note increased pruritus or hyperesthesia prior to the development of the tumor. Usually there is a considerable lag between the onset of the disease and the time of the diagnosis. Often the ulcers have been quite prominent and quite large at presentation.[5] While advancing, the tumors are capable of invading underlying structures, burrowing through into muscles, tendons, and bones and metastasizing to regional lymph nodes. They also destroy walls of adjacent vessels and hemorrhages are seen in later stages.

The incidence of regional lymph node metastases is quite high. Thus, in the series by Arons et al.[1] lymph node metastases were observed in 36% of the cases; Treves and Pack[5] found 20% incidence of lymph node involvement; and Novick et al.[4] encountered 16 of 46 patients with nodal metastases. This development is a very significant and grave prognostic sign.

TREATMENT AND RESULTS

Apparently the best treatment is prevention. It has been well established that tumors of this type do not develop following skin grafting. Once a burn scar carcinoma is present, the preferred therapy has been surgical. It is recommended that the ulcerated area should be excised and a graft be performed thereafter. Obviously, this is not a feasible approach in advanced neoplasms. Consideration for prophylactic node dissection should be given in view of the fact that there is a high incidence of regional metastases.[1] Amputation may be necessary in order to avoid hemorrhage in cancers that invade deeply or in those that extend into bone and joints.[5]

There has been a general reluctance to utilize radiotherapy in the management of this neoplasm. It appears that for small or localized tumors, however, this therapy could be successful, as indicated by Treves and Pack.[5]

We have treated palliatively three patients with burn scar carcinomas by means of radiation therapy. In all three multiple previous surgical attempts were made to control the disease, which kept progressing and expanding toward the periphery and at depth. Although all three patients experienced relief in terms of pain and tumor regression, this response lasted only a few weeks. Tumor progression was soon obvious.

Burn scar carcinoma is a serious and often lethal disease whose natural history is different from that of a carcinoma of the skin. Recurrences occur often, especially when the approach is limited.

PROGNOSIS AND SURVIVAL

In the series by Treves and Pack[5] 54% of the patients were clinically free of cancer, surviving for more than three years at the time of publication. In the series by Arons et al.[1] metastases occurred in eight of 22 cases, with five patients dying of their disease. In the series by Giblin *et al.*[3] there were 14 patients of 21 evaluated surviving without evidence of disease for an average of 6.3 years following surgery. Finally in the series by Novick *et al.*[4] the five-year survival rate was 57% for lesions involving the face and the neck and 31% for lesions involving the lower extremities.

REFERENCES

1. Arons, M.S., Lynch, J.B., Lewis, S.R., and Blocker, T.G., Jr.: Scar tissue carcinoma. Part I. A clinical study with special reference to burn scar carcinoma. *Ann Surg* **161:**170, 1965.

2. Bowers, R.F., and Young, J.M.: Carcinoma arising in scars. Osteomyelitis and fistulae. *Arch Surg* **80:**564, 1960.

3. Giblin, T., Pickbell, K., Pitts, W., and Armstrong, D.: Malignant degeneration in burn scars: Marjolin's ulcer. *Ann Surg* **162:**291, 1965.

4. Novick, M., Gard, D.A., Hardy, S.B., and Spira, M.: Burn scar carcinoma: A review and analysis of 46 cases. *J Trauma* **17:**809, 1977.

5. Treves, N., and Pack, G.T.: The development of cancer in burn scars. An analysis and report of thirty-four cases. *Surg Gynecol Obstet* **51:**749, 1930.

8

Subungual Carcinoma

CARCINOMAS OF THE nail bed region are rare tumors. Actually, the commonest malignant subungual lesion encountered is malignant melanoma. Although it comprises only 2–3% of all cutaneous melanomas, it is still more common than are carcinomas.[6] To the present time, approximately 60 cases of subungual carcinomas have been described in the literature. The patients' ages have ranged from 24 to 82 years, the average age at the time of the diagnosis being 59 years. There is a preference for males, the ratio of men to women being 2:1.[2]

PATHOLOGY

The gross appearance is that of an exophytic ulcerated mass. It causes destruction of the overlying nail and in the majority of the cases infection and pus production are present as well.[7,9,10] The majority of the cases histologically have been squamous cell carcinomas. Six cases of basal cell carcinoma of the nail bed were encountered in the literature review by Hoffman.[7] Bowen's disease, or intraepidermal squamous cell carcinoma, of the nail bed has been diagnosed with increased frequency during the last 10–15 years. The clinical picture and the management is similar to that of carcinoma.[4,5]

CLINICAL

The appearance of these neoplasms is similar to that of an inflammatory process. In the majority of the patients pain and swelling are present. Ulceration and bleeding eventually develop, associated with purulent discharge from superimposed infection. The mistaken clinical diagnosis of chronic inflammatory disease is all too common. The rarity of this particular malignancy excludes it from the common differential diagnoses. Treatment for inflammatory disease delays proper therapy for a considerable period of time. In most patients the symptoms were present for more than a year prior to the diagnosis.[2,7,9,10] With the passage of time and as the disease progresses, involvement of the underlying osseous phalanx occurs. This development has been seen in approximately 18–20% of the cases.[2] Fortunately, lymph node involvement or distant metastases have not occurred, except for one patient who died with generalized disease.[3]

Approximately 80% of subungual carcinomas are seen in the fingers and the remaining 20% in the toes. The thumb is the commonest site.

Attiyeh et al.[2] in reviewing the experience at Memorial Sloan-Kettering Cancer Center found trauma and previous irradiation as definite predisposing factors. Among 12 cases, three had chronic paronychia in the involved digits and five had a previous history of professional exposure to radiation.[2]

TREATMENT AND RESULTS

Amputation of the distal phalanx of the involved finger is an effective way of treatment, resulting in cure of the patient, as the literature reveals. Due to the fact that regional lymph node metastases do not occur, axillary or inguinal node dissection is not recommended. With the exception of the patient already mentioned, all patients with subungual carcinomas have been cured following surgery. Therefore the five-year-survival rate, corrected for intercurrent deaths, approaches 100%.[2,3,5,7,9,10]

The role of radiation therapy in the management of these tumors is debatable. Thus, Inlow[8] reported on two patients with squamous cell carcinoma of the nail bed treated by means of definitive radiotherapy. The patients survived six and eight years following treatment, retaining good function of the involved digits. In the experience of others, however, such treatment has resulted in local recurrence. Weichert[11] reported on a patient whose tumor recurred following 6000 rad irradiation. Ashbell[1] along the same lines reported on two cases of squamous carcinoma of the nail bed recurring following

irradiation. Eventually these patients were cured by amputation.

REFERENCES

1. Ashbell, T.S.: Cancer of the nail bed. *JAMA* **241**:1893, 1979.
2. Attiyeh, F.F., Shah, J., Booher, R.J., and Knapper, W.H.: Subungual squamous cell carcinoma. *JAMA* **241**:262, 1979.
3. Campbell, C.J., and Keokarn, T.: Squamous-cell carcinoma of the nail bed in epidermal dysplasia. *J Bone Joint Surg* **48**:92, 1966.
4. Coskey, R.J., Mehregan, A., and Fosnaugh, R.: Bowen's disease of the nail bed. *Arch Dermatol* **106**:79, 1972.
5. Dieteman, D.F.: Bowen disease of the nail bed. *Arch Dermatol* **108**:577, 1973.
6. Dutra, F.R.: Cancer of the nail bed. *JAMA* **241**:239, 1979.
7. Hoffman, S.: Basal cell carcinoma of the nail bed. *Arch Dermatol* **108**:828, 1973.
8. Inlow, P.M.: Cancer of the nail bed. *JAMA* **241**:239, 1979.
9. Long, P.I., and Espiniella, J.L.: Squamous cell carcinoma of the nail bed. *JAMA* **239**:2154, 1978.
10. Shapiro, L., and Baraf, C.S.: Subungual epidermoid carcinoma and keratoacanthoma. *Cancer* **25**:141, 1970.
11. Weichert, K.A.: Cancer of the nail bed. *JAMA* **241**:239, 1979.

9

Sweat Gland Carcinoma

SWEAT GLAND CARCINOMAS are uncommon tumors of the skin, originating from the eccrine and apocrine glands. Tulenko and Conway[13] state that sweat gland tumors represent only 0.05% of all surgical pathological specimens and of these only 12% are carcinomas.

They mainly appear during the fifth and sixth decades of life but sometimes are seen at younger ages. Futrell et al.[6] reported on two cases, one occurring in the plantar surface of the foot and the other in the toe of two adolescent females aged 14 and 12 years, respectively. Hirsh et al.,[8] reporting on the experience at the University of Pennsylvania from 1938 through 1969, found seven patients with sweat gland carcinoma whose ages ranged from 16 to 69 years. Miller[10] in 1967 reviewed 34 cases from the literature and added five of his own. Of the total 39 patients, there were 21 males and 18 females whose ages ranged from 24 to 84 years, the average being 53 years. Review of the experience at Memorial Hospital included 83 patients, 44 of whom were female and 39 were male. Most patients were in their sixth and seventh decade of life; however, a youngster 7 years old was included in the same series.[3]

PATHOLOGY

There is a wide spectrum of histological patterns by which sweat gland carcinomas appear. They generally consist of glandular structures with mucin-producing cells ranging in appearance from low-grade well-differentiated to high-grade undifferentiated and anaplastic small cell tumors.[3] The glandular formations are lined with one, two, or more cellular layers and in most cases some portion of the tumor forms a papillary projection into the lumen, which is identified as a lumen of the sweat gland. It is within these lumens that mucin is found, as an intraluminal secretory material.[12] When the secretion of mucin is excessive, the histological pattern of mucinous (adenocystic) carcinoma of the sweat gland develops.[9]

It is important to separate well-differentiated carcinoma from adenoma because the former, in spite of the good histological picture, may recur or metastasize in due time.

CLINICAL

The tumor can occur in any part of the skin. The most common sites are the hands, the arms, and the skin of the head and neck. In Miller's[10] review these areas accounted for about 75% of the cases. The same author encountered cases involving the vulva, the groin, the leg, and the foot. In the review by El-Domeiri et al.,[3] 28 of 83 patients (33.6%) presented with lesions in the head and neck area. The remaining tumors were evenly distributed between the torso and the extremities. Among them, skin lesions were seen in the region of the perineum and the anal canal, the vulva, and a number of cases in the axillae, fingers, and toes.

Sweat gland tumors occurring in the eyelids can be differentiated histologically from sebaceous gland carcinomas because they do not contain stainable fat. The neoplasms in this region arise from the Moll's glands of the eyelid.[1,5]

Sweat gland tumors developing in the region of the axilla or in the skin of the female breast present a problem from a differential standpoint. They have to be distinguished from carcinoma of the breast and this indeed can be a difficult task.[11]

Due to the rarity of the disease, the preoperative diagnosis of sweat gland carcinoma is scarcely, if ever, made. Clinically, they appear as small, single, slowly growing, usually painless nodules whose color ranges from white to red or violaceous. The nodules may be multiple. When neglected and long-standing, ulceration takes place.[3,8,11,14] Their size at the time of diagnosis is 1 or 2 cm, but in exceptional cases tumors up to 4 or 5 cm have been recorded.[3,8,9]

Regional lymph node metastases may be clinically evident at the time of the diagnosis.[8,9]

Typically, the tumors have a long quiescent period of several years and then suddenly, at a given point, they accelerate their growth. This period, according to Miller,[10] averages eight years. In the experience of all authors sweat gland carcinoma has a long history of presence in the skin prior to its diagnosis. Metastatic disease therefore has a chance to develop during these long intervals. The route of spread is by means of the lymphatic system. Jacobson et al.[7] in summarizing 33 cases of metastatic sweat gland carcinomas found regional lymph node disease in all of them. Sixteen of these patients (38%) developed in addition hematogenous metastases to distant sites, the most common being the skeletal system.[7] Of 23 metastatic cases reviewed by Teloh et al.,[12] regional lymph node metastasis was the

first sign of extension in 18 patients. Actually, in 12 of them there was no other metastatic spread. In the remaining 11 (48%) distant sites included several organs, such as the lungs, pleura, liver, adrenals, bones, thoracic and abdominal lymph nodes, and, of course, the regional lymph nodes.

El-Domeiri et al.[4] reported on eight patients who developed sweat gland carcinoma in a previously irradiated skin. The interval between irradiation and the detection of the tumor ranged from 6 to 40 years.

TREATMENT AND RESULTS

The tumor has a definite tendency for local recurrence if incompletely excised and there is a clear preference for lymphatic dissemination. These two parameters of the natural history define the mode of therapy. A wide surgical resection should be performed and additionally regional lymphadenectomy is recommended.[8,14] This approach gives the patient the best chance to avoid local recurrence and to eradicate metastatic disease in the regional lymph nodes.

The tumor is not radiosensitive, at least according to the existing literature reports. Chung and Heffernan[2] reported on a recurrent tumor in the left submandibular region, which was postoperatively irradiated at 4000 rad level in 20 elapsed days. During the following two years, the neoplasm continued to grow locally, eventually metastasizing. Stout and Cooley[11] presented among their patients a 59-year-old man with recurrent axillary lymph nodes that were implanted with radium needles, receiving 7740 mg hours. There was persistent local disease and eventually metastases led to death. Hirsh et al.[8] state that radiotherapy in their experience had no effect.

PROGNOSIS AND SURVIVAL

Miller[10] found during his literature review that 28 of 39 patients eventually developed metastatic disease. Of these, 11 were known to have died because of their tumor at intervals ranging from 6 months to 30 years following the diagnosis. The author comments on the fact that reported cases may have some special or unusual feature and as such they may not be representative of all sweat gland carcinomas. El-Domeiri et al.[3] in their review series, found 34 patients alive at five years among 68 evaluable. This represents a survival rate of 50%. It is to be noted that of 34 patients alive, only 26 were free of disease; for this reason, the 10-year-survival rate was lower, namely, 37%.

The course of patients with metastatic carcinoma is not necessarily a short one. Hirsh et al.[8] reported on three patients who developed metastases and lived 10, 20, and 30 years following the diagnosis.

Patients with negative lymph nodes have a better prognosis. Their five-year-survival rate was 67%, as opposed to 29% for those with positive nodes. In addition to the lymph node status, the histological differentiation is another major prognostic factor. Well-differentiated tumors afforded a 70% five-year-survival, whereas the survival of patients with poorly differentiated sweat gland carcinomas was 37%. Tumors undifferentiated in character have the worst prognosis, with no patient surviving at five years.[3]

REFERENCES

1. Aurora, A.L., and Luxenberg, M.N.: Case report of adenocarcinoma of glands of Moll. *Am J Ophthalmol* **70:**984, 1970.
2. Chung, C.K., and Heffernan, A.H.: Clear cell hidradenoma with metastasis. Case report with a review of the literature. *Plast Reconstr Surg* **48:**177, 1971.
3. El-Domeiri, A.A., Brasfield, R.D., Huvos, A.G., and Strong, E.W.: Sweat gland carcinoma: A clinico-pathologic study of 83 patients. *Ann Surg* **173:**270, 1971.
4. El-Domeiri, A.A., Huvos, A.G., and Beattie, E.J.: Sweat gland carcinoma arising in irradiated skin. *AJR* **114:**606, 1972.
5. Futrell, J.W., Krueger, G.R., Chretien, P.B., and Ketcham, A.S.: Multiple primary sweat gland carcinomas. *Cancer* **28:**686, 1971.
6. Futrell, J.W., Krueger, G.R., Morton, D.L., and Ketcham, A.S.: Carcinoma of sweat gland in adolescents. *Am J Surg* **123:**594, 1972.
7. Jacobson, Y.G., Rees, T.D., Grant, R., and Fitchett, V.H.: Metastasizing sweat gland carcinoma: Notes on the surgical therapy. *Arch Surg* **78:**574, 1959.
8. Hirsh, L.F., Enterline, H.T., Rosato, E.F., and Rosato, F.E.: Sweat gland carcinoma. *Ann Surg* **174:**283, 1971.
9. Mendoza, S., and Helwig, E.B.: Mucinous (adenocystic) carcinoma of the skin. *Arch Dermatol* **103:**68, 1971.
10. Miller, W.L.: Sweat-gland carcinoma. A clinicopatholigic problem. *Am J Clin Pathol* **47:**767, 1967.
11. Stout, A.P., and Cooley, S.G.E.: Carcinoma of sweat glands. *Cancer* **4:**521, 1951.
12. Teloh, H.A., Balkin, R.B., and Grier, J.P.: Metastasizing sweat-gland carcinoma. Report of a case. *Arch Dermatol* **76:**80, 1957.
13. Tulenko, J.F., and Conway, H.: An analysis of sweat gland tumors. *Surg Gynec Obstet* **121:**343, 1965.
14. Wertkin, M.G., and Bauer, J.J.: Sweat gland carcinoma. Current concepts of surgical management. *Arch Surg* **111:**884, 1976.

10

Sebaceous Gland Carcinoma

THE HIGHEST CONCENTRATION of sebaceous glands is in the skin of the head and neck. The greatest number of ectopic sebaceous glands is in the oral mucous membranes and within the parotids.[3]

Sebaceous gland adenocarcinomas are to be considered serious and potentially life-threatening tumors.[13]

They are distinctly uncommon. Allen[2] reported their relative incidence to the other skin malignancies to be 1 per 2000, (0.05%). Warren and Warvi[14] found 28 cases among 4000 cutaneous carcinomas (0.7%).

In the region of the eyelids, however, sebaceous gland carcinomas are present with considerable regularity. Here they constitute 2% of all eyelid tumors and their presence requires awareness in terms of differential diagnosis. They arise from the meibomian glands and because of their relative frequency they outnumber all other sebaceous gland carcinomas anywhere else in the body.[5,14]

Miller and White[9] in a literature review found the average age of patients with this tumor to be 60 years, with a male to female ratio of 3:2. In the series by Warren and Warvi[14] the average age was found to be 65 years; however, no sex predisposition was obvious. Tumors of meibomian gland origin develop late in life also. According to most authors, the average patient's age for these neoplasms is 60 years. Rarely, they have been seen in earlier ages and again no definite sex predominence has been shown.

PATHOLOGY

Sebaceous cell adenocarcinomas arise from the epithelium of the sebaceous glands in the dermis of the skin. In order for them to be called sebaceous, they must exhibit, at least in part of the tumor, the features of a normal gland. Because of the presence of lipid secretory products, the cells are light-staining and they have a vacuolated cytoplasm. It is because of this lipid collection that the neoplasms have a yellow color.[14,15] These essential characteristic features vary from tumor to tumor according to the differentiation. In poorly differentiated lesions numerous mitotic figures are present and the lipoid globules may be very scarce.[14]

Urban and Winkelmann[13] reviewed the experienced at the Mayo Clinic and suggested three categories of sebaceous malignancy on the basis of the histology. The first group is composed of basal cell carcinomas with sebaceous cell differentiation, the second has squamous cell carcinomas with sebaceous gland differentiation, and the third contains pure sebaceous gland carcinomas.[13] Histologically, a pure sebaceous cell adenocarcinoma is far less common than the other two varieties, namely, basal cell or squamous cell carcinoma with sebaceous cell differentiation.[3,13]

In the parotid salivary glands, sebaceous gland ectopias can be found in approximately 25% of all individuals. It is possible that these elements create the dominant histological features seen in certain mixed tumors or in mucoepidermoid carcinomas of the parotid.[10] Akhtar *et al.*[1] are of the opinion that sebaceous tumors of the salivary glands derive their origin from ductal epithelial cells that have an inherent multipotential differentiation.[1]

CLINICAL

With the exception of meibomian gland carcinoma, the scalp and the face are the next most common sites of origin. Batsakis *et al.*[3] in a literature review found that these two areas accounted for 75% of all tumors. The trunk accounted for 15% and the remaining occurred in the extremities.

Meibomian gland tumors have a preference for the upper eyelid, which is involved twice as frequently as the lower, possibly because it contains more glands. Both eyelids may be involved simultaneously.[6]

The clinical appearance is that of a hard yellow nodule which grows slowly. Their size at the time of the diagnosis ranges from 0.5 to 5–7.0 cm. In most advanced cases ulceration takes place. Their yellow color has been considered an important differential diagnostic criterion.[13] Apparently there is a long period between the onset of the tumor and the diagnosis. In most cases this is more than one year's duration and actually in several patients many years have elapsed prior to diagnosis and therapy.[14]

In the meibomian glands the presentation may be one of recurrent inflammation of the eyelids in the middle of which the nodular neoplasm is present. Less often the nodule in the eyelid may be quite benign in appearance without any reaction around it.[3,6] Here, too, the length of symptoms is considerable in the range of one to three years.[8,11,12] These prolonged intervals are the main reason for the subsequent clinical problems. Orbital invasion takes place in 17% of the patients and lymph node metastases occur in 28%.[4]

Ginsberg[8] found a high local recurrence rate in the range of 32%. In his series there was ipsilateral lymph node involvement in 17% of the cases and orbital invasion with subsequent death occurred in 6%.

The tumors of the skin grow slowly and ulcerate late. The main problems are local recurrence and metastases. Both these problems are related to the duration of the disease and the inadequacy of the resection.

TREATMENT AND RESULTS

The tumor is treated by surgical resection. In the skin the resection should include an adequate margin of healthy tissue in order to avoid local recurrence. Lymph node dissection is not indicated as a primary form of therapy unless the lesion is large or unless it has ulcerated. A close follow-up, however, is recommended and examination and palpation of the regional lymph nodes should always be performed at regular intervals.

Radiation therapy has been applied to advanced inoperable or recurrent tumors and some temporary response has been elicited. Warren and Warvi[14] reported on a 66-year-old woman whose recurrent tumor in the region of the upper lid and nasal septum was treated with very modest amounts of radiation (1000 rad). Control was obtained for 2.5 years, after which the tumor resumed its growth.

Systemic chemotherapy in the form of cyclophosphamide, methotrexate, vincristine, and 5-fluorouracil has not been effective; however, no recent reports are available.[10]

Tumors of the meibomian gland require resection in their early stage. Adequate margins should be taken and checked by means of a frozen section examination intraoperatively.[6] Prophylactic lymphadenectomy is not a part of management but may be necessary later on. The need for follow-up is great. As Boniuk and Zimmermann[4] reported, 15 of 88 patients required orbital exenteration following the original surgery because they developed local recurrence. Lymph node metastases will require unilateral radical neck dissection.[4,6]

Sebaceous cell carcinoma of the parotid gland should have as a minimum therapy total parotidectomy, according to Batsakis *et al.*[3] Local excision or partial parotidectomy have been successful in the management of small lesions; however, it is after this type of procedure that local recurrence develops.[7,10]

PROGNOSIS AND SURVIVAL

Sebaceous cell carcinoma of the skin diagnosed early and adequately treated is a curable lesion carrying a good prognosis. If metastasis to the regional lymph nodes or local recurrence develops, the treatment should be vigorous because cure is still possible.[14] Miller and White[9] found 15 recurrences among their 75 evaluable cases, an incidence of 20%. Of those patients with recurrent disease, 10 died of their tumor. Shulman *et al.*[10] in a review of eight cases of parotid gland sebaceous carcinomas encountered three patients with local recurrence, two of whom subsequently proceeded with regional and distant metastases.

The five-year survival rate for patients with meibomian gland carcinomas as reported by Boniuk and Zimmermann[4] was 70%. Ginsberg[8] in a review of 142 cases of meibomian gland carcinomas found the mortality rate to be approximately 6%.

REFERENCES

1. Akhtar, M., Gosalbez, T.G., and Brody, H.: Primary sebaceous carcinoma of the parotid gland. *Arch Pathol* **96**:161, 1973.
2. Allen, A.C.: *The Skin.* Grune & Stratton, New York, 1967.
3. Batsakis, J.G., Littler, E.R., and Leahy, M.S.: Sebaceous cell lesions of the head and neck. *Arch Otolaryngol* **95**:151, 1972.
4. Boniuk, M., and Zimmermann, L.E.: Sebaceous carcinoma of the eyelid, eyebrows, caruncle, and orbit. *Trans Am Acad Ophthalmol Otolaryngol* **72**:619, 1968.
5. Brauninger, G.E., Hood, C.I., and Worthen, D.M.: Sebaceous carcinoma of lid margin masquerading as cutaneous horn. *Arch Ophthalmol* **90**:380, 1973.
6. Cavanagh, H.D., Green, W.R., and Goldberg, H.K.: Multicentric sebaceous adenocarcinoma of the Meibomian gland. *Am J Ophthalmol* **77**:326, 1974.
7. Constant, E., and Leahy, M.S.: Sebaceous cell carcinoma. *Plast Reconstr Surg* **41**:433, 1968.
8. Ginsberg, J.: Present status of meibomian gland carcinoma *Arch Ophthalmol* **73**:271, 1965.
9. Miller, R.E., and White, J.J.: Sebaceous gland carcinoma. *Am J Surg* **114**:958, 1967.
10. Shulman, J., Waisman, J., and Morledge, D.: Sebaceous carcinoma of the parotid gland. *Arch Otolaryngol* **98**:417, 1973.
11. Straatsma, B.R.: Meibomian gland tumors. *Arch Ophthalmol* **56**:71, 1956.
12. Sweebe, E.C., and Cogan, D.G.: Adenocarcinoma of the meibomian gland. A pseudochalazion entity. *Arch Ophthalmol* **61**:282, 1959.
13. Urban, F.H., and Winkelmann, R.K.: Sebaceous malignancy. *Arch Dermatol* **84**:113, 1961.
14. Warren, S., and Warvi, W.N.: Tumors of sebaceous glands. *Am J Pathol* **19**:441, 1943.
15. Wills, P.I., and Fechner, R.E.: Pathologic quiz, case 2. *Arch Otolaryngol* **101**:76, 1975.

11

Parathyroid Carcinoma

PARATHYROID CARCINOMA is a rare but well-established tumor. It represents an intriguing diagnostic problem because of the endocrine function it exhibits. The majority of the reported cases have hyperparathyroidism as their cardinal feature and several authors have considered this to be an essential element in making the diagnosis. It must be said, however, that a few cases of nonfunctioning parathyroid carcinoma have been published in the literature.[6,7,15]

The tumor is an infrequent cause of primary hyperparathyroidism. It accounts for about 3–4% of all such cases. Schantz and Castleman[12] found 20 parathyroid carcinomas among 487 patients with hyperparathyroidism (4%). Farr et al.,[5] reviewing the experience at Memorial Sloan-Kettering Cancer Center, encountered three functioning and one nonfunctioning parathyroid carcinomas among 100 patients with parathyroid tumors. The remaining tumors were 87 functioning and 7 nonfunctioning adenomas.

The average age at the time of the diagnosis has been about 44–45 years.[7,12] In contrast to parathyroid adenomas, the majority of which are to be found in females, parathyroid carcinomas have shown no statistically significant preference for either sex.[7,11,12]

PATHOLOGY

The gross tumor is ovoid or lobulated in shape, the average diameter being 3.0 cm.[12] Unlike the adenomas, they tend to adhere and infiltrate adjacent structures.[7] Pollack et al.[11] in a literature review found an equal distribution between the right and the left side of the neck, 60% and 40%, respectively. All of them occurred in the lower parathyroid glands.[11] Early parathyroid carcinomas may present as mediastinal masses. This is due to the fact that parathyroid glands may be found anywhere from the larynx down to the pericardium.[8,10,17]

Histologically, mitotic figures, thick fibrous bands, and capsular blood vessel and lymphatic vessel invasion are features of malignancy.[12] The absence of mitotic figures is not an absolute criterion, since tumors without mitoses have metastasized.[15] The following criteria have been considered as suggestive of parathyroid carcinoma: 1) adherence to surrounding structures, 2) clinically palpable tumor, 3) gland with thick capsule, 4) invasion through the capsule by the tumor, 5) invasion of venous blood vessels, and 6) the presence of mitoses.

There is a consensus that the histological pattern has to be viewed in conjunction with the physical and operative findings in order to arrive at the diagnosis of parathyroid carcinoma.

CLINICAL

Hyperparathyroidism dominates the clinical presentation and the symptomatology. Bone disease, manifested by severe pain in the bones and joints associated with pathological fractures, occurs in 60–70% of the cases. Urolithiasis is found of 30% of the patients and parenchymal renal disease as a result of hyperparathyroidism is seen in 21%.[2,7,12]

The serum calcium levels are elevated above 14 mg/100 ml in the majority of the cases. Only 22% of the patients had values below 13 mg/100 ml. In association with the hypercalcemia, hypophosphatemia develops. The serum parathyroid hormone levels, as measured by radioimmunoassay techniques, are elevated.[5] There is increased bone resorption, increased absorption of calcium from the gastrointestinal tract, increased tubular reabsorption of calcium, and reduced renal tubular reabsorption of phosphate.

Radiographically, typical pathological changes of osteitis fibrosa cystica are seen associated with generalized osteoporosis and pathological fractures. Frequently, the osseous changes produce the so-called "brown tumors," which represent solid masses arising from the bones, containing marrow osteoblasts and osteoclasts.

In addition to the skeletal symptoms, cardiac irregularities, psychotic episodes, depression and weakness, nausea, thirst, weight loss, vomiting, and abdominal cramps occur. All these symptoms are due to the severe hypercalcemia. Pancreatitis develops in 15% of the cases.[7]

The hypercalcemia in carcinomas is more severe than that observed in adenomas. This fact combined with the presence of a neck mass that is palpable in 50% of the cases should alert to the possibility of parathyroid carcinoma. The mean average values of serum calcium for carcinomas were 15.9%, versus 12% for those seen in adenomas.[11] Paralysis of the left vocal cord associated with functioning or nonfunctioning parathyroid carcinomas has been reported.[7]

Renal disease occurs in 32% of the cases. Urolithiasis and nephrocalcinosis may lead to renal colic. Renal damage results from nephrocalcinosis and this leads to uremia and hypertension.

Metastatic disease develops in approximately 30% of the cases.[12] In a review by Holmes et al.[7] metastases were found in 52% of the patients. The commonest sites were the regional lymph nodes, which were involved in 32%, followed by the lungs (26%).

Approximately 70% of the patients developed recurrence following resection, according to Pollack et al.[11] In an even earlier review by Stephenson,[15] all 19 cases examined had developed recurrence. It is possible that these cases were more prone to local recurrence, reflecting limitations of the surgical techniques.[15]

The primary cause of death is not the local recurrence or the metastatic deposits, but mainly the toxic effects of the hyperparathyroid state, such as chronic cachexia and wasting, cardiac arrhythmias, and uremia. Pancreatitis has accounted for a small number of deaths as well.[2,7]

Hyperparathyroidism appearing several months or years following surgery for parathyroid tumor is very suggestive of recurrent parathyroid carcinoma.[3,4,6,16]

For tumors mediastinal in location, the association of the radiographic findings with hypercalcemia leads to a differential diagnosis, which should include, in addition to parathyroid carcinomas or adenomas, bronchogenic carcinoma with parathyroid activity, bronchogenic carcinoma with extensive bone metastasis, and sarcoidosis.[8]

Selective venous catheterization in the region of the recurrence or the metastatic disease may reveal elevated serum parathyroid hormonal levels and thus establish successfully the presence of the neoplasm.[9]

TREATMENT AND RESULTS

Surgery is the recommended therapy for primary parathyroid carcinomas. Many authors have emphasized the importance of recovering en bloc the tumor with all existing adherences to the surrounding structures in order to prevent local recurrence.[2,7,12,15] The performance of radical lymph node dissection is a point of conjecture. Holmes et al.[7] advocate removal of the ipsilateral thyroid lobe, the isthmus of the thyroid gland, skeletonization of the trachea, and excision of any skeletal muscle intimately associated with the tumor. Because they found an overall 32% incidence of regional lymph node involvement, they recommend unilateral cervical neck dissection. On the other hand, the experience at Massachusetts General Hospital revealed only 13% regional node involvement. For this reason, the authors believe that node dissection is not necessary during the initial procedure.[12]

Recurrent disease should always be excised, if feasible, with a curative attempt. Metastases should be considered along the same lines because surgical excision is the most effective means of diminishing the toxic metabolic effects produced by the tumor. This procedure should be viewed as palliative, in an attempt to reduce the hypercalcemia.[7]

Radiation therapy has been given to a number of patients following recurrence. There is no evidence in the literature that any of the irradiated tumors was affected significantly; however, in almost all of the cases the adequancy of the radiation dosage is questionable.[2,7,11] Sigurdsson et al.[13] reported on a 53-year-old male whose severe hypercalcemia due to parathyroid carcinoma responded to the administration of stilbestrol diphosphate. The serum calcium level was reduced from 8.5 to 5.8 mEq/liter after daily intravenous injections of 1000 mg stilbestrol diphosphate for four days. This was followed by oral therapy, 200 mg three times per day. The incapacitating generalized bone pains diminished markedly. The authors believe that the effect was the result of direct inhibition of bone resorption.[13]

Calcitonin has been administered in the recommended dosage intramuscularly or intravenously. The results have been transient and their effects temporary.[6,13] Au[1] in a case report showed prolongation of the calcitonin effect with concomitant administration of prednisone. Eventually this combination ceased to be effective, in a matter of a few months.[1] Mithramycin has been used against hypercalcemic conditions. Singer et al.[14] reported on its application in a patient with metastatic parathyroid carcinoma. The drug was administered intravenously at a dosage of 55 μg/kg of body weight. There was a fall in the plasma calcium from 15 to 10 mg%. In seven days the plasma calcium level returned to the original values, however, and the injection was repeated. There was no influence on the plasma parathyroid hormone levels. The hypocalcemic action was thought to be the result of direct inhibition of bone resorption.[8] The effects of mithramycin, as reported to the present, have been temporary in character.[13]

PROGNOSIS AND SURVIVAL

Generally, the prognosis is guarded because parathyroid carcinoma is apt to develop local recurrence and distant metastases. Only one-third of patients with recurrent disease can be cured with additional surgery. In all cured, the recurrence had occurred late—two years or more—after the initial procedure in the series of Schantz and Castleman.[12] Obviously therefore recurrence within the first year carries a poor prognosis.

Holmes et al.[7] in their retrospective study obtained follow-up information on 43 of 46 patients. The cumulative survival at 5- and 10-year levels was 50 and 13%, respectively. For those patients who are known to have died from their disease, the survival time has been four to five years.[2,11]

REFERENCES

1. Au, W.Y.W.: Calcitonin treatment of hypercalcemia due to parathyroid carcinoma. Arch Intern Med 135:1594, 1975.

2. Barnes, B.A., and Cope, O.: Carcinoma of the parathyroid glands. Report of 10 cases with endocrine function. *JAMA* **178:**556, 1961.
3. Davies, D.R., Dent, C.E., and Ives, D.R.: Successful removal of single metastasis in recurrent parathyroid carcinoma. *Br Med J* **1:**397, 1973.
4. Ellis, H.A., Floyd, M., and Herbert, F.K.: Recurrent hyperparathyroidism due to parathyroid carcinoma. *J Clin Pathol* **24:**596, 1971.
5. Farr, H.W., Fahey, T.J., Nash, A.G., and Farr, C.M.: Primary hyperparathyroidism and cancer. *Am J Surg* **126:**539, 1973.
6. Hill, C.S., Jr., Ouais, S.G., and Leiser, A.E.: Long-term administration of calcitonin for hypercalcemia secondary to recurrent parathyroid carcinoma. *Cancer* **29:**1016, 1972.
7. Holmes, E.C., Morton, D.L., and Ketcham, A.S.: Parathyroid carcinoma: A collective review. *Ann Surg* **169:**631, 1969.
8. Lee, Y.T., and Hutcheson, J.K.: Mediastinal parathyroid carcinoma detected on routine chest films. *Chest* **65:**354, 1974.
9. Murray, T.M., Patt, N.L., and Muzaffar, S.A.: Parathyroid carcinoma: Location of pelvic metastases by parathyroid hormone assay. *Can Med Assoc J* **110:**809, 1974.
10. Nathaniels, E.K., Nathaniels, A.M., and Wang, C.: Mediastinal parathyroid tumors: A clinical and pathological study of 84 cases. *Ann Surg* **171:**165, 1970.
11. Pollack, S., Goldin, R.R., and Cohen, M.: Parathyroid carcinoma. A report of two cases and review of the literature. *Arch Intern Med* **108:**583, 1961.
12. Schantz, A., and Castleman, B.: Parathyroid carcinoma. A study of 70 cases. *Cancer* **31:**600, 1973.
13. Sigurdsson, G., Woodhouse, N.J.Y., Taylor, S., and Joplin, G.F.: Stilboestrol diphosphate in hypercalcaemia due to parathyroid carcinoma. *Br Med J* **1:**27, 1973.
14. Singer, F.R., Neer, R.M., Murray, T.M., Keutmann, H.T., Deftos, L.J., and Potts, J.T.: Mithramycin treatment of intractable hypercalcemia due to parathyroid carcinoma. *N Engl J Med* **283:**634, 1970.
15. Stephenson, H.U., Jr.: Malignant tumors of the parathyroid glands. A review of the literature with report of a case. *Arch Surg* **60:**247, 1950.
16. Tange, J.D.: Carcinoma of the parathyroid. *Br J Surg* **46:**254, 1958.
17. Weissman, I., Worden, J.P., and Christie, J.M.: Mediastinal parathyroid carcinoma with metastases. Report of a case and review of the literature. *Radiology* **68:**352, 1957.

12

Carcinoma of the Urachus

CAMPBELL BEGG[2] in 1931 presented a detailed publication pertaining to the clinical and pathological features of the colloid adenocarcinomas that arise from the dome of the bladder and from the epithelium of the urachus. Several case reports of these tumors had been presented up to that point in the literature. It was thought that they originated in local "embryonic rests." Indeed, embryologically, the rectum, the bladder, and the urachus all derive their origin from the primitive hindgut, or cloaca, which is lined by a layer of cuboidal epithelial cells. This structure is eventually divided by a septum into the rectum posteriorly, and the bladder and the urachus anteriorly. On the rectal side, the epithelium changes from cuboidal to columnar, whereas the epithelium of the bladder is transformed into transitional. In the urachus it remains cuboidal but retains the capacity to become columnar, as in the bowel.

Ordinarily, following birth, the urachus becomes obliterated, at which point the name changes to ligamentum umbilicale medianum. A patent urachus results from failure of obliteration and this can be total, extending from the bladder to the umbilicus, or partial, involving a segment of its length.

Carcinomas of the urachus arise from both the vesical and supravesical portions of this structure. Approximately 80% of these tumors are seen in males, and most patients are in their fifth and sixth decades.[7]

Franksson[3] in a review of 434 cases of urinary bladder carcinoma found 11 of urachal origin. This represents an incidence of 2.5%.

PATHOLOGY

Urachal carcinomas appear grossly as papillomas or as ulcerating lesions at the apex of the urinary bladder.[5] This appearance, of course, is noted when the tumor arises from the intramucosal and intramural portions or from a urachus that is completely patent, communicating with the dome of the bladder. Urachal tumors originating in the supravesical part present as masses in the anterior abdominal wall.[4]

Histologically, the majority of the neoplasms are mucin-producing adenocarcinomas. Other histological entities encountered include simple adenocarcinomas, sarcomas, benign adenomas, and fibromas.[2] The mucinous adenocarcinomas are multiloculated and they contain jellylike fluid. Microscopically, they are formed of cysts and acini, which are lined by columnar epithelium producing mucus. These cells carry the usual malignant characteristics and in several respects they resemble the histological appearance of rectal carcinomas. The epithelium creates papillary folds and within the cystic spaces mucinous material is present. Inside the cystic cavities calcium deposits are also often to be found.[1]

Mostofi et al.[6] in 1955 proposed a set of

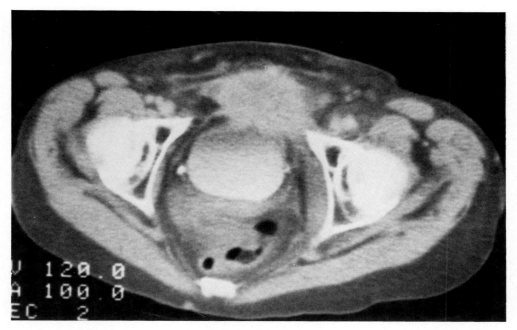

FIG. 12-1.   Carcinoma of the urachus in a 52-year-old female. A computerized tomography (CT) scan demonstrates a mass located anteriorly to the urinary bladder. The mass infiltrates the anterior abdominal wall. At surgery the urachus was involved in its entire length, from the umbilicus to the bladder. Histologically, this was a mucin-producing adenocarcinoma. (Courtesy W. P. Cockshott. *Radiology* **137:**731, 1980.)

criteria for the diagnosis of urachal carcinomas, particularly those associated with the urinary bladder. Thus, the neoplasms should arise from the dome of the bladder, be intramural in location, and exhibit several ramifications within the bladder wall. It is also necessary that malignant tumor elsewhere has been ruled out.

CLINICAL

Urachal carcinomas invading the urinary bladder present with hematuria, frequency, or dysuria, all symptoms similar to those of carcinoma of the bladder. In addition the passage of mucous and of necrotic material may be noticed.[1,5,7] On cystoscopic examination, a lesion at the dome of the bladder is to be found. This area is characteristic in terms of origin and the possibility of urachal carcinoma should come to mind.

A palpable mass located in the anterior abdominal wall, in an area extending from the symphysis pubis to the umbilicus and not necessarily midline in location, is the commonest presentation of urachal tumors arising from the supravesical portion (Fig. 12-1). Hayes and Segal[5] emphasized the importance of bimanual examination and stressed its value in detecting these masses for carcinomas connected with the bladder, when located behind the symphysis pubis.

Radiographically, plain films of the abdomen may reveal stippled calcifications within the tumor (Fig. 12-2). An intravenous pyelogram need not necessarily be abnormal. Defects of the dome of the bladder have been described when the tumor is exophytic in character. Bilateral ureteral displacement is another radiographic finding.[4]

Ultrasonography is quite appropriate in delineating these masses, because the

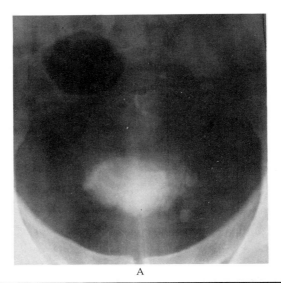

A

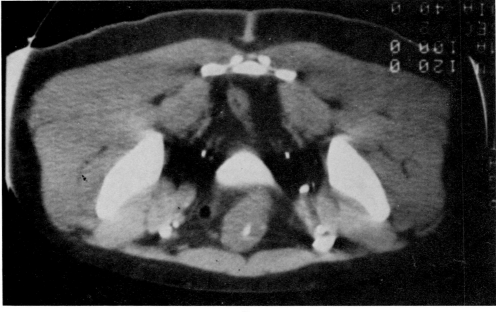

B

FIG. 12-2.   Carcinoma of the urachus in a 28-year-old male. (*A*): There is a curvilinear calcific density above the urinary bladder. A smaller calcification is seen to the left and slightly higher to the first one. Both are midline in location. (*B*): CT scan shows an ovoid midline mass, located anteriorly to the urinary bladder. The mass contains the above-mentioned calcifications. The patient presented with painless hematuria associated with mucoid urethral discharge. At surgery a urachal mucinous adenocarcinoma was found, involving the lower urachus and the dome of the bladder. (Courtesy W. P. Cockshott. *Radiology* **137**:731, 1980.)

growths are extraperitoneal and for this reason there is no interference from the bowel gas.[4]

When metastases occur, they involve primarily the lungs, the peritoneum, the omentum, and the liver.[7]

TREATMENT AND RESULTS

Limited operations, such as fulguration and transurethral resection, are inadequate therapeutic measures. It is considered incorrect to manage urachal carcinomas in a fashion similar to that of cancer of the bladder. Largely due to this tendency, 50% of the treatment failures are local recurrences.

It is important that the diagnosis be made preoperatively and the procedure be planned as such. Campbell Begg[2] described a surgical method that takes into account the anatomical and embryological circumstances of the region. He advocates removal of a block of tissue beginning just below the umbilicus and containing the transversalis fascia as well as the peritoneum down to the bladder. This has a shape approximating a triangle and in the same block of tissue a large cuff from the vault of the urinary bladder should be included. There should be no attempt made to preserve the peritoneum.[2] Since then several authors knowledgable with the subject have concurred and have strongly advocated this approach.[5,7]

We have participated in the management of a 26-year-old male having a urachal adenocarcinoma associated with the dome of the bladder. The presenting symptom was hematuria. Unfortunately, and perhaps typically, the original form of therapy was transurethral resection. Local recurrence was diagnosed six months later. This was further handled by means of a partial cystectomy. A second recurrence occurred in four months, at which point the patient was considered for radiotherapy. He was treated on a 6 MeV linear accelerator to the pelvis, receiving a total of 6000 rad in 30 treatments over 43 elapsed days. In addition he received radiation to a strip of the anterior abdominal wall, by means of electron beam, from superior border of the pelvic field to the umbilicus, for a total tumor dose of 5000 rad. Liver metastasis developed six months thereafter, and small bowel obstruction followed. Upon exploration, he was found to have massive peritoneal and omental metastases. In addition he had locally recurrent disease in the urinary bladder with bilateral ureteral obstruction that necessitated urinary diversion. The patient died from his disease two years following the original diagnosis.

There are no data available regarding the effects of systemic chemotherapy on this tumor. Certainly the histological similarity with bowel cancers should be kept in mind.

PROGNOSIS AND SURVIVAL

In most cases local recurrence and distant metastases have developed within two to three years from the time of the diagnosis. Although several patients have been lost to follow-up, it appears that a number may survive for many years with persistent disease, eventually dying from it. It also can be shown that few patients have been completely cured.[5]

It is believed that the cure rate and the survival could improve by adopting the treatment policy outlined previously. The recognition of this tumor preoperatively is therefore most important.[7]

REFERENCES

1. Bandler, C.C., and Roen, P.R.: Mucinous adenocarcinoma arising in urachal cyst and involving the bladder. *J Urol* **64**:504, 1950.
2. Campbell Begg, R.: The colloid adenocarcinomata of the bladder vault arising from the epithelium of the urachal canal: With a critical survey of the tumours of the urachus. *Br J Surg* **18**:422, 1931.
3. Franksson, C.: Tumors of the urinary bladder. *Acta Chir Scand [Suppl]* **151**:1, 1950.
4. Han, S.Y., and Witten, D.M.: Carcinoma of the urachus. *AJR* **127**:351, 1976.
5. Hayes, J.J., and Segal, A.D.: Mucinous carcinoma of the urachus invading the bladder. *J Urol* **53**:659, 1945.
6. Mostofi, F.K., Thomson, R.V., and Dean, A.L., Jr.: Mucinous adenocarcinoma of the urinary bladder. *Cancer* **8**:741, 1955.
7. Whitehead, E.D., and Tessler, A.N.: Carcinoma of the urachus. *Br J Urol* **43**:468, 1971.

13

Carcinomas of the Bartholin's Gland

BARTHOLIN'S GLANDS, or the greater vestibular glands, are part of the female genital system. They are located in the posterior section of the introitus, posterior to the vestibular bulb and beneath the bulbocavernosus muscle on either side. Cullen[5] in 1905 described their anatomy in detail. Each gland measures approximately 2 by 13 mm in size and leads to a main excretory duct, the external os of which is to be found medially to the medial border of the labium minorum, just external to the hymen, and near the middle of the vaginal orifice. The duct is lined with squamous epithelium composed of many cell layers in its distal part which proximally changes into transitional. The gland itself, according to Cullen's description, has an appearance similar to a bunch of grapes as the individual lobules communicate to the main duct with secondary terminals. The entire structure is well encapsulated.[5]

This is a mucus-secreting organ whose function is parallel to that of Cowper's gland in the male. The mucus is secreted during the genital stimulation. The lymphatic drainage of Bartholin's glands is similar to that of the vulva and the lower vagina. The regional lymph node groups are the superficial and deep inguinals, as well as the pelvic lymph nodes. There appears to be cross lymphatic communication, since contralateral metastases have been observed.[2,9]

Bartholin's gland carcinomas are obviously uncommon tumors, representing a small percentage of all vulvar neoplasms.

Barclay et al.[2] reported eight cases of Bartholin's gland carcinoma among 117 patients with carcinoma of the vulva. This is an incidence of 7.25%. Dodson et al.[6] found the incidence to be 5.3%. Wahlström et al.[10] in reviewing 337 cases of vulvar carcinomas identified six that fulfilled the criteria of primary carcinoma of Bartholin's gland, an incidence of 1.8%.

The age spectrum has been wide, ranging from the late teens up to the ninth decade of life. Numerically, the average age at the time of the diagnosis quoted by most authors is 50 years.[4,6,9]

PATHOLOGY

Grossly, during the early stages the malignancy presents as a mass, small, hard, and lying deep in the posterior portion of the labial fat. It is mobile at this stage and apparently it remains so for a considerable length of time. Eventually it extends beyond the capsule of the gland and invades the surrounding fat and muscles. At a later stage, it causes destruction of the pubic bone.[3,9]

Histologically, 90% of the tumors are adenocarcinomas or squamous cell carcinomas, both of which are seen with equal frequency.[2] The remaining 10% consist of such neoplasms as melanomas, sarcomas, and tumors with unclear histological pattern. Transitional cell carcinoma has been diagnosed only in one instance.[10] Among the adenocarcinomas, a subgroup has been identified, that of adenoid cystic carcinoma.[1,7] Histologically, adenoid cystic carcinoma has the characteristic appearance of large masses of neoplastic cells containing cystic spaces filled with amorphous basophilic material and surrounded by dense connective tissue stroma.

Squamous cell carcinoma and adenocarcinoma of the Bartholin's gland eventually metastasize to the regional lymph nodes. In the series by Barclay et al.[2] three of seven patients who underwent lymphadenectomy had positive lymph nodes. The involved nodes included deep femoral, inguinal, obturator, and hypogastric chains.[2] Three of six patients reported by Wahlström et al.[10] had metastatic lymphadenopathy. Two of five patients had metastasis to the nodes in the series reported by Trelford and Deos.[9] In the series by Chamlian and Taylor,[4] of 13 patients whose lymph node status was known, there were five with positive and eight with negative nodes. It appears that adenoid cystic carcinoma does not favor this route of spread. Nine patients treated by radical vulvectomy and some form of lymphadenectomy and reported by Addison and Parker[1] and the single patient reported by Eichner[7] showed no lymph node metastases.

Differential diagnosis between Bartholin's gland carcinoma and vulvar carcinoma is made on both clinical and anatomical grounds. Homan's criteria established in 1897 and quoted by recent authors or a variation of them provide a guideline to that effect. These include correct anatomical position of the tumor deep in the labium, an intact overlying skin, the presence of some element of glandular epithelium with an apparent transition from the normal elements to those that are neoplastic, and the absence of another primary tumor elsewhere.[2,4]

CLINICAL

In the early development the tumor presents as a painless mass in the posterior part of the major labium. As it enlarges, pain ensues. These two symptoms, namely, the feeling of a mass and that of pain are the commonest presenting signs. Dyspareunia is also quoted. Later on pruritus, bleeding, and discharge occur as ulceration of the skin develops. In the original stages the mass is movable; later, however, it becomes fixed to the skin and the underlying symphysis pubis.[2,3,6,8] The interval between the first symptoms and the diagnosis appears to be long. Masterson and Goss[8] found it to be, in their world literature survey, 8.3 months. Chamlian and Taylor[4] reviewed retrospectively 24 patients from the files of the Armed Forces Institute of Pathology. In no less than 12 patients (50%) the original diagnosis by the examining physician was that of an inflammatory or benign disease. These patients were treated accordingly, receiving antibiotics, sitz baths and undergoing incision and drainage. Marked delays in diagnosis resulted.[4] The experience of these authors is not unique, and others have written similarly.[6,8,9] The delay in diagnosis is unfortunate because this organ is superficial in location and early treatment will lead to good results. For this reason, it is advocated that whenever bartholinitis is considered, a biopsy should be taken if the symptoms persist, after an appropriate anti-inflammatory regimen.

TREATMENT AND RESULTS

Surgical procedures varying in scope and depth have been employed in the management of these patients. Excision of the tumor is the simplest form of therapy and, although on theoretical grounds such an approach is criticizable, in practice, however, a number of patients have been reported cured following such a procedure.[4,8] In order to encompass all the potential tumor-bearing structures, a radical vulvectomy associated with bilateral lymphadenectomy will give the maximal potential of sterilization. Barclay et al.[2] advocate such an approach and they encompass in the lymph node dissection the inguinal, femoral, external iliac, common iliac, hypogastric, obturator, and lower periaortic and vena caval nodes. In addition to their extensive vulvectomy, included is partial resection of the levator muscle and a wide vaginal excision on the involved side.[2] The authors reported on seven such patients; however, in spite of this radical therapy they were able to identify only two survivors at five years. Trelford and Deos[9] utilizing a more conservative approach that included radical vulvectomy and inguinal node dissection reported five cases successfully treated whose follow-up ranged from six months to four years.[9] Radical vulvectomy accompanied by bilateral inguinal lymphadenectomy and postoperative radiotherapy was used in five patients reported by Wahlström et al.[10] Of these, two patients were alive and well at seven years, one was alive with pulmonary metastases at four years, and the remaining two were dead from distant metastases at six months and five years. Radiation therapy, with the exception of this report[10] and an earlier report by Bowing and Fricke[3] dealing with local radium techniques in the management of Bartholin's gland tumor, has not been considered to be, and perhaps rightly so, a primary form of therapy.

In spite of the superficial position of the tumor, more often than not this is a fatal disease. The reason for this poor outcome appears to be the great delay between the onset and the diagnosis. Both the patients, due to their neglect, and the physicians, due to the fact that they consider the lesion benign in many instances, are responsible for this. Chamlian and Taylor[4] in their review of 24 patients with Bartholin's gland tumors found eight patients who were five-year or longer survivors. Five patients had radical vulvectomies, in four of which it was accompanied by bilateral lymphadenectomy. The remaining three patients had local excisions, in

one of which it was associated with a radium needle implant. Failure of local excision occurred in one patient, necessitating radical vulvectomy and bilateral lymphadenectomy.[4]

From these data, we conclude that radical vulvectomy and bilateral lymphadenectomy is the most promising form of therapy. This approach is recommended particularly when dealing with younger patients. The extent of the lymph node dissection is debatable. Certainly because a risk exists in terms of metastasis to the pelvic nodes, lymph nodes should be included in the surgical resection, particularly in a patient who is clinically able to tolerate the procedure well.

Adenoid cystic carcinoma of the Bartholin's gland appears to have a better prognosis and a different natural history. In their literature review Addison and Parker[1] found the average age of patients with this variety to be 44 years. This is younger than that of the rest of the group. The behavior of adenoid cystic carcinoma in this location is that of a less aggressive tumor, which is characterized by local recurrence and by long intervals of dormant existence. In general, lymph node metastases are absent and for this reason radical vulvectomy without lymphadenectomy appears to be the most appropriate approach.[1]

PROGNOSIS AND SURVIVAL

The prognosis should be good due to the fact that the tumor is in a superficial location, can be diagnosed early, is of a relatively low aggressiveness, and can be resected *in toto*. However, delay in the diagnosis has resulted in poor cure rates and low five-year survival, particularly as reported in earlier series.[3,8] We have compiled the three- and five-year-survival rates on the basis of the more recent series.[4,6,9,10] Some improvement is to be noted. Thus, whereas Masterson and Goss[8] in their literature review published in 1955 found the survival to be less than 10%, the results of more recently treated patients indicate increased rates of control, the three- and five-year survival rates being, respectively, 68 and 55%.

REFERENCES

1. Addison, A., and Parker, R.T.: Adenoid cystic carcinoma of Bartholin's gland. A review of the literature and report of a patient. *Gynecol Oncol* **5**:196, 1977.
2. Barclay, D.L., Collins, C.G., and Macey, H.B., Jr.: Cancer of the Bartholin gland. A review and report of 8 cases. *Obstet Gynecol* **24**:329, 1964.
3. Bowing, H.H., Fricke, R.E., and Kennedy, T.J.: Radium therapy for carcinoma of Bartholin's glands. *AJR* **61**:517, 1949.
4. Chamlian, D.L., and Taylor, H.B.: Primary carcinoma of Bartholin's gland. A report of 24 patients. *Obstet Gynecol* **39**:489, 1972.
5. Cullen, T.A.: Cysts of Bartholin's glands, with brief remarks on the anatomy of the normal gland structure. *JAMA* **44**:204, 1905.
6. Dobson, M.G., O'Leary, J.A., and Averette, H.E.: Primary carcinoma of Bartholin's gland. *Obstet Gynecol* **35**:578, 1970.
7. Eichner, E.: Adenoid cystic carcinoma of the Bartholin gland. Review of the literature and report of a case. *Obstet Gynecol* **21**:608, 1963.
8. Masterson, J.G., and Goss, A.S.: Carcinoma of Bartholin gland. Review of the literature and report of a new case in an elderly patient treated by radical operation. *Am J Obstet Gynecol* **69**:1323, 1955.
9. Trelford, J.D., and Deos, P.H.: Bartholin's gland carcinomas: Five cases. *Gynecol Oncol* **4**:212, 1976.
10. Wahlström, T., Vesterinen, E., and Saksela, E.: Primary carcinoma of Bartholin's glands: A morphological and clinical study of six cases including a transitional cell carcinoma. *Gynecol Oncol* **6**:354, 1978.

14

Carcinoma of the Cowper's Gland

FEWER THAN 15 cases of adenocarcinoma arising in the Cowper's gland have been reported. It is possible their actual incidence is somewhat higher than this figure indicates. The location of the organ is such that a carcinoma in the Cowper's gland could be considered to be of urethral, prostatic, or even rectal origin.[4]

Cowper's glands are two small round, flat organs located in the urogenital floor at the level of the apex of the prostate, between the deep surface of the bulb and the superficial surface of the membranous urethra. They measure 1.0–1.5 cm in size, leaving between them a space of 4–5 mm. Their excretory ducts measure 3.0–4.0 cm in length and follow a forward and medial course, entering obliquely into the urethra.[3] The glands are mucous secreting, tubular alveolar structures, lined by low columnar cells.

PATHOLOGY

The consistency of the tumors is hard and their shape oval or irregular at times.[1-3] They are mucin-producing adenocarcinomas, arranged in glandular neoplastic formations with tubular configurations. A dense fibrous stroma and granulomatous reactions are, as a rule, present.[2]

CLINICAL

The initial complaints are urinary. The patients experienced frequency, dysuria and nocturia. As the tumor enlarges, perineal pain develops, which becomes more obvious when the patient is in a sitting position, radiating toward the thighs. Eventually, the tumor can be felt as a perineal mass. Approximately 50% of the patients will experience some pain or discomfort during defecation as a result of the growth.[1,2]

On physical examination, the mass is readily palpable. Obviously, this requires a certain size; however, in most reported cases a mass of 2–5 cm was felt in the anterior part of the perineum. This is hard in consistency and tender on pressure. Intravenous urography may show some degree of stasis and retrograde urethrography will identify the irregularity and narrowing of the lumen of the posterior urethra.[2]

Regional lymph nodes are the internal iliac groups. For this reason no inguinal adenopathy is probable. Carcinoma of the Cowper's gland is a disease that in the majority of the cases has shown a propensity for local growth and eventual extension rather than for distant metastases.[2]

It is important to establish the diagnosis of malignancy and to differentiate the disease from an inflammatory process occurring in the posterior urethra. In addition it is important to identify this as a tumor of the Cowper's gland rather than carcinoma of the prostate or the rectum. This is not a hormone-dependent tumor and therefore orchiectomy is contraindicated.

TREATMENT AND RESULTS

As a rule, during the investigational period, several transurethral approaches are attempted. These procedures are traumatic, causing hemorrhage and inflammatory reaction, further accentuating the patient's symptoms and therefore hindering the diagnosis.

The majority of the patients have been treated by means of a local surgical resection of the tumor. A transperineal procedure similar to the one described by Gutierrez[3] has been used by most authors. A transverse incision in the perineum is made between the scrotum and the rectum and following tissue dissection the tumor is identified and resected. Through this approach, the relationship of the neoplasm to the anterior wall of the rectum and to the apex of the prostate is appreciated. Unfortunately, local resection does not yield good results. All patients treated in this fashion have died of their disease due to local recurrence. It is for this reason that Arduino and Nuesse[1] advocate a radical approach. They treated their patient—a 17-year-old with Cowper's gland carcinoma—en bloc dissection removing in continuity the penis, the entire urethra, all of the urogenital diaphragm, the prostate, and the seminal vesicles. The operation was a combined perineal and retropubic one. At the same time bilateral pelvic lymph-adenectomy was performed. The patient was followed for at least 30 months and no signs of recurrence were present.

Due to the fact that distant metastases are uncommon and because local recurrence is the rule, the need for local control is obvious.

REFERENCES

1. Arduino, L.J., and Nuesse, W.E.: Carcinoma of Cowper's gland: Case report. *J Urol* **102**:224, 1969.
2. Bourque, J.L., Charghi, A., Gauthier, G.E., Drouin, G., and Charbonneau, J.: Primary carcinoma of Cowper's gland. *J Urol* **103**:758, 1970.
3. Gutierrez, R.: Primary carcinoma of Cowper's gland. *Surg Gynecol Obstet* **65**:238, 1937.
4. Le Duc, E.: Carcinoma of Cowper's gland, report of the eleventh case. *Calif Med* **96**:44, 1962.

15

Adenocarcinoma of the Rete Testis

ADENOCARCINOMA OF THE rete testis is one of the rarest neoplasms. Approximately 20 case reports of this entity are to be found in the literature, many of them with inadequate follow-up data. Gisser *et al.*[1] in the latest review of the subject have accepted only 14 cases as being unquestionably true rete carcinomas.

The average age of the patients in the earlier review by Schoen and Rush[2] was 42 years. The average age of patients accepted by Gisser *et al.*[1] as adenocarcinoma of the rete testis in their review was 56 years. Obviously, this is a tumor of the adult male and has not been encountered in a man younger than 30 years.

PATHOLOGY

A finding that characterizes many confirmed cases of adenocarcinoma of the rete testis is the location of the tumor. It involves primarily the mediastinum of the testis and the region of the epididymis, leaving the bulk of the testicular parenchyma free. The visceral and the parietal layers of the tunica vaginalis may also be involved, and secondary hydrocele is frequently present.[2-4]

The histological criteria, which can be a guide to the diagnosis, include involvement of the mediastinum of the testis rather than the main parenchyma of the organ, evidence of transition between the non-neoplastic rete epithelium and the neoplasm through zones of cytologically atypical epithelium, and the absence of a teratomatous testicular neoplasm.[1]

Histologically, the pattern is one of adenocarcinoma, forming papillary and ductlike tubular structures. The areas of transition between the tumor growth and the adjacent normal rete structures are quite helpful in establishing the diagnosis. The tumor epithelium blends gradually into the flat epithelium of the rete tubules.[1,2]

CLINICAL

The commonest clinical symptom is scrotal enlargement. This is due to the presence of the tumor but quite often it is exaggerated by a secondarily induced hydrocele. The symptom duration in most patients has been in the order of three to six months. The disease does tend to metastasize, favoring primarily the local inguinal, iliac, and periaortic lymph nodes as well as the mediastinal lymph nodes.[1-4]

TREATMENT AND RESULTS

Orchiectomy has been the basic form of therapy for the majority of the patients and remains the recommended treatment. In some patients bilateral orchiectomy has been performed due to the local extension.

In the absence of distant metastases, and in view of the fact that the inguinal, pelvic, and periaortic lymph nodes are at risk, consideration for postoperative radiotherapy may be given. There is evidence to suggest that radiation in the early stages may be effective in stemming local recurrence.[1,2] On the other hand, when massive disease is present the effectiveness of radiotherapy is questionable.[4] A literature review with regard to the effects of systemic chemotherapy discloses failure of methotrexate, 5-fluorouracil, cyclophosphamide, vincristine, and actinomycin D in controlling the disease. However, in this particular tumor, as in other rare malignant neoplasms, the true effectiveness of modern systemic combination chemotherapy is unknown.[1]

The survival data of the 14 patients summarized by Gisser et al.[1] are as follows: There were five patients dying of their disease from one month to 1.5 years from the time of the diagnosis. Three patients were lost to follow-up; however, all had distant metastases and all were pre-

sumed to be dead of their disease. There were three patients dying from other causes, but at least two of these were known to have active disease. Only three were alive and well, surviving four, six, and eight months after their therapy. The over-all mortality rate was 65%.[1]

REFERENCES

1. Gisser, S.D., Nayak, S., Kaneko, M., and Tchertkoff, V.: Adenocarcinoma of the rete testis: A review of the literature and presentation of a case with associated asbestosis. *Hum Pathol* **8:**219, 1977.
2. Schoen, S.S., and Rush, B.F., Jr.: Adenocarcinoma of the rete testis. *J Urol* **82:**356, 1959.
3. Turner, R.W., and Williamson, J.: Adenocarcinoma of the rete testis: Report of a case. *J Urol* **109:**850, 1973.
4. Whitehead, E.D., Valensi, Q.J., and Brown, J.S.: Adenocarcinoma of the rete testis. *J Urol* **107:**992, 1972.

16

Tumors of the Seminal Vesicles

THE EMBRYONIC origin of the seminal vesicles is similar to that of the prostate gland. As with the prostate, they are hormonally dependent organs requiring testosterone for their full development.[5] Experiments in rats have shown seminal vesicle growth stimulation by testosterone administration and marked atrophy following orchiectomy.[3] The hormone dependency of the seminal vesicles should be kept in mind when treating epithelial neoplasms arising here.

Their malignant tumors, rare as they are, can be divided into those of epithelial and those of mesenchymal origin. Among the former, papillary adenocarcinoma is the commonest, whereas in the latter group various forms of soft tissue sarcomas are encountered.

Carcinoma of the seminal vesicles is a disease of the older male. Dalgaard and Giertsen[2] in their literature review found the average age of the patients to be 60.7 years, with a median age of 65 years at the time of the diagnosis. It is possible, however, for the tumor to appear in younger men.

PATHOLOGY

Seminal vesicle carcinomas may reach considerable size. According to Mostofi and Price[5] it is common for a mass of 10–15 cm to be found, producing obstruction of the prostatic urethra, of the internal urethral meatus, or of the lower portion of one or both ureters. Extension to the rectum is not too common. A primary literature review on the subject by Lazarus[4] in 1946 and the subsequent study by Dalgaard and Giertsen[2] in 1956 revealed that most of these tumors are papillary adenocarcinomas. Mixtures of adenocarcinoma and undifferentiated carcinoma can be found occasionally. The cells are clear columnal forming acinar and papillary structures.

CLINICAL

Many of the symptoms that the patients present with are similar to those of prostatic hypertrophy or prostatic carcinoma. Voiding difficulties, such as frequency in urination, dysuria, and incontinence, are often reported. In addition hematuria and hemospermia have occasionally been noted. Several patients have pain in the region of the perineum or pain radiating to the scrotum and the back. In contrast to prostatic hypertrophy or prostatic carcinoma the duration of the symptoms is relatively brief with tumors of the seminal vesicle.[2] In order to diagnose carcinoma of the seminal vesicle a primary prostatic carcinoma extending to the seminal vesicles must be ruled out. This is a more frequent clinical situation and when tumor is found involving both the prostate and the seminal vesicle it should be considered to be a prostatic primary, unless proved otherwise.

On clinical examination in the typical case, a mass is felt distinctly above the prostate separated from it through a shallow sulcus. However, in more advanced cases the differentiation is virtually impossible.[2] On cystoscopic examination, upward displacement of the bladder trigone associated with congestion and edema of the trigone and the posterior urethra can be found. The radiographic findings on the intravenous pyelogram are similar in character, namely, asymmetrical upward displacement of the bladder floor or even a filling defect present. Carcinoma of the rectum is another clinical entity that enters the differential diagnosis. On histological grounds following transrectal biopsy of the tumor, the differential diagnosis from primary colonic and primary prostatic carcinomas can be based on the papillary adenocarcinoma findings. This is a histological pattern distinctly different from that of prostatic or rectal carcinoma.[2]

TREATMENT AND RESULTS

In most cases the disease has been quite advanced locally at the time of the diagnosis. As a result, most patients have not been candidates for definitive therapy and they have been treated palliatively with cystostomy in order to alleviate their urinary symptoms. Three patients treated with radical surgery and followed for 5, 18, and 25 months were doing well.[2]

The disease pursues a rather rapid course with metastases occurring to the regional lymph nodes (66.6%), the lungs (33.3%), and the liver (41.6%).[4]

Local radiotherapy at definitive dose levels—6000 rad—should be considered if the neoplasm is deemed to be inoperable. There is clinical evidence to suggest that such a course of therapy will control the disease locally.[3] There is also ample clinical evidence that administration of estrogens in the form of stilbesterol will reverse a downhill course and will effectively provide comfort and prolong the patient's life. Kindblom and Pettersson[3] reported on a patient with multiple osteolytic metastases to the ribs, vertebrae, and pelvis

whose deteriorating general condition cleared rapidly on estrogens. At follow-up examination one year later, the patient had gained weight and was free of pain. In addition x-ray examinations showed sclerosis of the previous osteolytic areas and the bone scan showed marked regression of the previously observed abnormalities.[3]

Williamson[6] reported on a 50-year-old patient who presented with generalized peritonitis following rupture of a carcinomatous and infected seminal vesicle. The local tumor mass regressed on stilbesterol therapy and the patient was in continuous improvement six months following the initiation of his treatment.

On the basis of these reports and others published earlier, it is recommended that orchiectomy or estrogen administration be strongly considered in patients with locally advanced or metastatic seminal vesicle carcinoma. Patients managed without the benefit of hormonal therapy have had in general a poor prognosis. The majority were dead within one year from the time of the diagnosis.[5] Urinary obstruction associated with infection and uremia is the commonest mechanism of death.

Mesenchymal tumors of the seminal vesicles are less frequent than carcinomas. Buck and Shaw[1] reviewed the literature and encountered four such cases of sarcoma of the seminal vesicle. The authors added a case of their own. Histologically, fibrosarcomas, leiomyosarcomas, and pleomorphic sarcomas have been encountered.[1] Williamson[6] in 1978 reported on a 26-year-old man with a seminal vesicle sarcoma, most probably a fibrosarcoma. This particular tumor had an indolent course, recurring in a period of three years locally without signs of distant metastases. A case reported by Lazarus[4] of pleomorphic cell sarcoma was locally resected and postoperatively irradiated at 6000 rad. The patient was well two years later (Fig. 16-1). The patient reported by Buck and Shaw,[1] a 57-year-old man with a

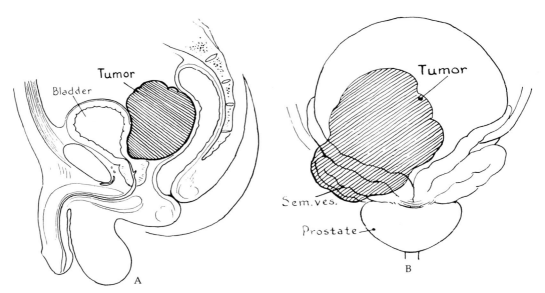

FIG. 16-1.   Sarcoma of the seminal vesicle. Schematic illustration in the sagittal view (A) and in the posterior view (B). (Courtesy J.A. Lazarus. *J Urol* **55**:190, 1946.)

low-grade fibrosarcoma of the seminal vesicles, was doing well without signs of local recurrence or distant disease six months following tumor resection.

REFERENCES

1. Buck, A.C., and Shaw, R.E.: Primary tumours of the retro-vesical region with special reference to mesenchymal tumours of the seminal vesicles. *Br J Urol* **44**:47, 1972.
2. Dalgaard, J.B., and Giertsen, J.C.: Primary car-cinoma of the seminal vesicle. Case and survey. *Acta Pathol Microbiol Scand* **39**:255, 1956.
3. Kindblom, L.G., and Pettersson, G.: Primary carcinoma of the seminal vesicle. Case report. *Acta Pathol Microbiol Scand* **84**:301, 1976.
4. Lazarus, J.A.: Primary malignant tumors of the retrovesical region with special reference to malignant tumors of the seminal vesicles; report of a case of retrovesical sarcoma. *J Urol* **55**:190, 1946.
5. Mostofi, F.K., and Price, E.B., Jr.: *Tumors of the Male Genital System*. Armed Forces Institute of Pathology, Washington, D.C., 1973.
6. Williamson, R.C.N.: Seminal vesicle tumours. *J R Soc Med* **71**:286, 1978.

17

Clear Cell Carcinoma of the Endometrium

CLEAR CELL carcinoma of the endometrium is an uncommon tumor, representing 4.7% of all endometrial cancers.[2] The presence of clear cell carcinoma in the uterus, an organ of müllerian origin, provides very strong support for the theory that clear cell tumors are indeed of müllerian and not of mesonephric origin.

The patients are older females, the majority being postmenopausal with an age distribution similar to that seen in adenocarcinoma of the endometrium. The mean age in the series by Kurman and Scully[1] was 68 years at the time of presentation.

PATHOLOGY

The gross appearance is that of a polypoid friable tumor, pink or grayish-white in color.

Microscopically, the tumor cells are arranged in various patterns, papillary, tubular, and cystic, or they form solid masses. These cells contain clear cytoplasm and they are flattened and hobnail in shape with regular nuclei. When tubules and papillae are formed, cystic spaces are lined by the clear cells. In most tumors an admixture of patterns and solid areas is to be found.[1,2] In some patients the clear cell carcinoma is associated with areas of typical endometrial adenocarcinoma.[2] Silverberg and DeGiorgi[2] have included in their series four patients with the so-called "secretory pattern." In a subsequent review Kurman and Scully[1] believed that this does not represent a special pattern but rather the result of progesterone stimulation upon a diffusely or focally well-differentiated adenocarcinoma.

CLINICAL

The presenting symptom in all patients is vaginal bleeding, the duration of which has varied from a few days to two to three years. The few premenopausal patients in whom the tumor has occurred presented with irregular bleeding with or without discharge.[1,2] Obesity, hypertension, and diabetes were encountered in 30–40% of the cases.

As with the clinical presentation, staging of clear cell carcinoma of the endometrium parallels that of adenocarcinoma of the endometrium. Thus, in the series by Kurman and Scully[1] of 21 patients, 15 (71%) were Stage I, five were Stage II, and one was Stage IV. In the series by Silverberg and DeGiorgi[2] of 10 women whose staging was available at the time of the review, five were Stage I, two were Stage II, and three were Stage III.

TREATMENT AND RESULTS

Various treatment programs have been used in management of the disease. This is understandable because the patients have been seen by various physicians over several years. Surgical treatment in most cases has been total abdominal hysterectomy and bilateral salpingo-oophorectomy. Radiation therapy in the form of preoperative radium or postoperative external beam therapy has also been frequently used. Many patients have been treated by combination of surgery and radiation therapy. Because myometrial invasion was present in 7 of 15 patients with Stage I in the series reported by Kunman and Scully,[1] the authors suggest that this is a more aggressive neoplasm than the usual endometrial carcinoma. Four of these patients with myometrial invasion died of their tumor. From the same series of five patients with Stage II disease, three died of metastatic carcinoma, one died of unknown cause, and only one was surviving 13.5 years after treatment.[1] In the series by Silverberg and DeGiorgi[2] one patient with Stage II disease treated by combined approach was surviving without evidence of tumor five years later.[2]

Metastatic sites include the retroperitoneal lymph nodes, the mediastinum, the lung, and the brain. The omentum and the peritoneum may also be involved. At this time, there are no reports available regarding the effectiveness of chemotherapeutic agents on this particular neoplasm.

PROGNOSIS AND SURVIVAL

It appears that there is a correlation between survival and staging as well as between survival and depth of myometrial invasion. Thus, of 20 patients with Stage I

disease, five died of their tumor and two of unknown causes, three of six patients with Stage II died of cancer and one of unrelated cause, and two of three patients with Stage III died shortly after the diagnosis was made. The third was surviving four years later without evidence of disease. A patient with Stage IV tumor was dead in nine months.[1,2] The depth of myometrial invasion is an important prognostic factor. Three of four patients with Stage I disease and deep invasion of the myometrium died of their tumor.[1]

The actuarial five-year-survival rate in the series by Silverberg and DeGiorgi[2] was calculated to be 20.6%. The actuarial survival in the series by Kurman and Scully[1] was found to be 55.3% at five years. These figures should be viewed with some reservation because both series are composed of a small number of cases and in both series several patients died from intercurrent disease. Perhaps the suggestion can be made that clear cell carcinoma of the endometrium appears to be somewhat more aggressive than the typical endometrial adenocarcinoma.

REFERENCES

1. Kurman, R.J., and Scully, R.E.: Clear cell carcinoma of the endometrium. An analysis of 21 cases. Cancer 37:872, 1976.
2. Silverberg, S.G., and DeGiorgi, L.S.: Clear cell carcinoma of the endometrium. Clinical, pathologic, and ultrastructural findings. Cancer 31:1127, 1973.

18

Clear Cell Adenocarcinoma of the Vagina and the Cervix

CARCINOMA OF THE vagina is relatively uncommon, accounting only for 1–2% of all female genital malignancies. The majority (85–90%) are squamous cell carcinomas.[4,13] Primary vaginal adenocarcinomas constitute 6% of all vaginal tumors.[17] Clear cell carcinomas belong to this group.

Allyn et al.[3] in 1971 reviewed the world literature pertaining to the so-called vaginal "mesonephromas." They concluded that two distinct groups could be identified: endodermal sinus tumors occurring in infancy and associated with poor prognosis, and clear cell carcinomas usually seen in adolescent and mature women and having a better outlook. The concepts of histogenesis have changed with the passage of time and at this point the term "clear cell carcinoma" is used. It is believed that these lesions are not mesonephric but essentially müllerian in origin. Their existence in both the cervix and the vagina is well established.[15] Their rarity is also known.

Clear cell or "mesonephric" carcinoma of the cervix is another rare but established tumor.[7] In a review of the subject by Hameed[7] 38 cases were identified in the literature from 1935 until 1968. The average patient's age was 33.4 years. It was the author's conclusion following the review that biologically clear cell carcinoma of the uterine cervix represented a less aggressive neoplasm with better prognosis, as compared with adenocar-cinoma of the cervix. For this reason, it represented a separate biological entity.

Interest in these rare tumors was greatly increased within the last 10 years following an article by Herbst and Scully.[8] It was their view that the tumors are müllerian in origin and because vaginal adenosis was simultaneously present in most cases, the carcinomas were considered malignant expression of this disorder. Several publications followed along the same lines. The development of most vaginal and cervical tumors as well as the presence of vaginal adenosis in younger females were eventually linked to maternal ingestion of diethylstilbesterol (DES) or related compounds during pregnancy. For this reason the Registry of Clear-Cell Adenoma of the Genital Tract in Young Females was established in order to centralize the data and provide a guide to management and prognosis.[1,2]

As of 1979, 346 cases of clear cell adenocarcinoma of the vagina and the cervix had been accessioned into the Registry. The mean age of the patients was 19.5 years. The youngest patient was 7 and the oldest was 29 years of age.[11]

PATHOLOGY

The gross appearance of the tumors is polypoid and their commonest location is the anterior wall of the upper one-third of the vagina. Occasionally they can be found in the posterior wall or the lower vaginal third.[10,17] Their size varies from a few millimeters to several centimeters. When involving the cervix, they are primarily exophytic in character.

According to the Registry reports, cytological examination is positive in terms of identifying, or at least directing suspicion toward the correct diagnosis in 76% of the cases.[10] The microscopic appearance is similar to clear cell carcinomas in other locations. Tubular and papillary formations are to be observed composed of clear cells exhibiting the hobnail shape pattern (Fig. 18-1). The majority of the tumors have a few mitotic figures present.[10]

Anatomical abnormalities non-neoplastic in character are to be found in high percentages of patients with clear cell adenocarcinoma. These include transverse ridges in the upper part of the vagina near the cervix and occasionally in the lower part of the vagina. Similarly, in the cervix,

ridges have been observed. Cervical erosions and vaginal adenosis are quite frequent.[10] Stafl et al.[18] found vaginal adenosis in 91% of the patients and extensive eversion of the columnar epithelium of the ectocervix in 9% of the patients among 63 young females whose mothers took DES in the first trimester of pregnancy. These patients were examined during a screening procedure and none of them had clear cell carcinoma present. Burke et al.[5] examined 250 patients having a history of exposure in utero to DES. There was a high incidence of gross abnormalities associated with the anatomy of the genital tract. Thus, cervical columnar epithelium was found in 150 women (60%) and a cervicovaginal hood was identified in 147 (58.8%). The external genitalia were normal in all patients. Adenosis, biopsy proved, was found to be present in the vaginal walls, the fornices, or the hood in 185 cases (74%). In spite of earlier reports, the au-

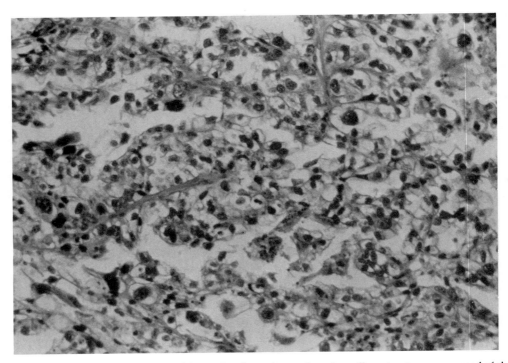

FIG. 18-1.   Clear cell adenocarcinoma of the vagina. Irregular cystic and papillary structures composed of clear cells with large variations in nuclear size and shape.

thors were unable to identify significant squamous precancerous changes related to DES exposure.[5] In a more recent report Kaufman et al.,[12] performing hysterosalpingograms in 60 young women exposed to DES in utero, identified anatomical changes in 40. These changes, consisting of hypoplastic uterus, a T-shaped uterus and a uterine cavity containing constricting bands, as well as polypoid defects and synechiae, were attributed to the intrauterine exposure to DES.

Forsberg,[6] after injecting neonatal female mice with estradiol 17β and with DES, observed the development of heterotopic columnar epithelium in the anterior part of the vagina, the vaginal fornices, and the uterine cervix. These experiments strengthened the view that the development of vaginal adenosis as well as the anatomical changes are related to DES exposure in utero in humans and that subsequently a number of patients proceed to develop clear cell carcinomas.[6] These conclusions are to be viewed with a certain degree of caution because not all patients with clear cell carcinoma have a history of exposure to DES in utero.

Sandberg[16] demonstrated the presence of occult submucosal glands in 9 of 22 postpubertal patients (41%) who were examined during autopsy. This finding suggested that the incidence of occult vaginal adenosis and the potential of development of gross lesions is far greater than generally believed. The study included 35 consecutive postmortem examinations of human females.[16]

CLINICAL

The case has been made that the relatively high incidence of clear cell carcinoma involving the vagina and the cervix in young females which has been observed in the last 10 or so years is due to exposure in utero to DES.[9,10,14,17] Most of these patients were born in the 1950s at a time when stilbesterol and similar com-

pounds were used for the so-called "high-risk pregnancies."[10] In the most recent report from the Registry, two-thirds of the 317 patients were exposed to DES or similar compounds while in utero, but in the remaining no history of maternal hormone therapy could be elicited.[11]

Silverberg and DeGiorgi[17] reported on four patients with clear cell carcinoma of the vagina of which only one had prenatal exposure to DES. The authors are of the opinion that maternal estrogen intake is a definite contributing factor, but not absolutely essential, in the development of these tumors.[17] Nordqvist et al.[14] reviewed and reported on 21 women with the diagnosis of clear cell adenocarcinoma of the cervix and/or vagina. In seven a positive history of maternal intake of estrogens was elicited. In the remaining 13 the possibility of exposure existed only for three who were born during the period when estrogen therapy was feasible and actually applied as a management for threatened abortions.[14]

Vaginal bleeding and discharge are the commonest presenting symptoms. A small proportion of patients have been diagnosed during a screening procedure while totally asymptomatic.[11]

Approximately two thirds of the vaginal clear cell adenocarcinomas are Stage I, the tumor being confined to the vagina.[10] As far as carcinoma of the cervix is concerned, 35% represent Stage I, 50% are Stage II, and the remaining are Stage III disease.[10] Work-up procedures should be similar to those of carcinoma of the cervix.

In the experience of the Registry, patients with Stage I have a 16% risk of developing pelvic lymph node metastases.[11]

TREATMENT AND RESULTS

A variety of treatment programs have been used. These have been based on the extent of the disease and on the opinion of the individual physician as to their optimal management. Thus, several small vaginal carcinomas have been locally excised. In patients with Stage I and Stage II, the procedure has been partial or total vaginectomy. Anterior or total exenteration with removal of the bladder and rectum have been performed in more advanced cases. Cervical clear cell adenocarcinomas have been treated by means of Wertheim's hysterectomy, which includes pelvic lymph node dissection, mostly with preservation of one or two ovaries. Radiation therapy has also been used both in the early cases and in more advanced ones. Chemotherapeutic programs have been tried in patients with reluctant disease or distant metastases.

Nordqvist et al.[14] are of the opinion that radical hysterectomy with pelvic lymph node dissection is appropriate treatment for cervical lesions, Stage I and Stage II. They also recommend that vaginectomy be performed in Stage II disease and that reconstruction of the vagina be done at the same session. The authors favor preservation of the ovaries. In their experience lymphatic invasion is of paramount importance in terms of prognosis. All four patients who were found to have metastases in their lymph nodes died of their disease irrespective of treatment. Radiation was given only to advanced cases.[14]

Herbst et al.,[11] analyzing the results in 346 cases of clear cell adenocarcinoma entered in the Registry, examined the effectiveness of treatment, particularly in patients with Stage I disease. Four modes of therapy were identified: local radiotherapy, standard internal and external beam radiotherapy, local resection, and radical hysterectomy with partial or complete vaginectomy and pelvic lymph node dissection. The lowest recurrence rate (8.1%) was to be found among patients who underwent radical surgery. Patients receiving external beam radiotherapy accompanied by radium implant had a higher recurrence rate (36.8%); however, most of them had large vaginal tumors. These recurrence rates were tabulated at the end of the five-year period.[11]

The majority of the recurrences (60%) occurred in the pelvis. Distant metastases developed primarily in the lungs (36%) and in the supraclavicular lymph nodes (20%).

At this point no single agent or combination chemotherapy is known to be effective in the management of recurrent or metastatic clear cell carcinoma. Occasional responses have been elicited from the use of single alkylating agents, 5-fluorouracil, Adriamycin, and actinomycin D.[11]

PROGNOSIS AND SURVIVAL

In the series by Nordqvist et al.,[14] which included patients treated at Memorial Sloan-Kettering Cancer Center from 1946 until 1974, the two-year-survival rate was 62.5%. From the same series among the 12 patients who were eligible for five-year follow-up, seven (58%) were alive without evidence of disease at that time.[14] As reported by Herbst et al.,[11] the actuarial five-year-survival rate based on the cases accessioned into the Registry was 78%. Overall recurrence rate for all cases was 23% at five years. Patients with Stage I disease, as expected, fare better. Their five-year-survival was 87% in carcinoma of the vagina and 91% in carcinoma of the cervix.[11]

REFERENCES

1. Adenocarcinoma Registry. Obstet Gynecol Surv 27:395, 1972.
2. Adenocarcinoma Registry. Obstet Gynecol 39:841, 1972.
3. Allyn, D.L., Silverberg, S.G., and Salzberg, A.M.: Endodermal sinus tumor of the vagina. Report of a case with 7-year survival and literature review of so-called "mesonephromas." Cancer 27:1231, 1971.
4. Anderson, W.A.D.: Pathology. C.V. Mosby, St. Louis, 1966.
5. Burke, L., Antonioli, D., and Rosen, S.: Vaginal and cervical squamous cell dysplasia in women

exposed to diethylstilbestrol in utero. *Am J Obstet Gynecol* **132**:537, 1978.

6. Forsberg, J.G.: Estrogen, vaginal cancer, and vaginal development. *Am J Obstet Gynecol* **113**: 83, 1972.

7. Hameed, K.: Clear cell "mesonephric" carcinoma of uterine cervix. *Obstet Gynecol* **32**:564, 1968.

8. Herbst, A.L., and Scully, R.E.: Adenocarcinoma of the vagina in adolescence. A report of 7 cases including 6 clear-cell carcinomas (so-called mesonephromas). *Cancer* **25**:745, 1970.

9. Herbst, A.L., Kurman, R.J., Scully, R.E., and Poskanzer, D.C.: Clear-cell adenocarcinoma of the genital tract in young females. Registry report. *N Engl J Med* **287**:1259, 1972.

10. Herbst, A.L., Robboy, S.J., Scully, R.E., and Poskanzer, D.C.: Clear-cell adenocarcinoma of the vagina and cervix in girls: Analysis of 170 Registry cases. *Am J Obstet Gynecol* **119**:713, 1974.

11. Herbst, A.L., Norusis, M.J., Rosenow, P.J., Welch, W.R., and Scully, R.E.: An analysis of 346 cases of clear cell adenocarcinoma of the vagina and cervix with emphasis on recurrence and survival. *Gynecol Oncol* **7**:111, 1979.

12. Kaufman, R.H., Binder, G.L., Gray, P.M., Jr., and Adam, E.: Upper genital tract changes associated with exposure in utero to diethylstilbestrol. *Am J Obstet Gynecol* **128**:51, 1977.

13. McGowan, L.: *Gynecologic Oncology.* Appleton-Century-Crofts, New York, 1978.

14. Nordqvist, S.R.B., Fidler, W.J., Jr., Woodruff, J.M., and Lewis, J.L., Jr.: Clear cell adenocarcinoma of the cervix and vagina. A clinicopathologic study of 21 cases with and without a history of maternal ingestion of estrogens. *Cancer* **37**:858, 1976.

15. Novak, E., Woodruff, J.D., and Novak, E.R.: Probable mesonephric origin of certain female genital tumors. *Am J Obstet Gynecol* **68**:1222, 1954.

16. Sandberg, E.C.: The incidence and distribution of occult vaginal adenosis. *Am J Obstet Gynecol* **101**:322, 1968.

17. Silverberg, S.G., and DeGiorgi, L.S.: Clear cell carcinoma of the vagina. A clinical, pathologic and electron microscopic study. *Cancer* **29**:1680, 1972.

18. Stafl, A., Mattingly, R.F., Foley, D.V., and Fetherston, W.C.: Clinical diagnosis of vaginal adenosis. *Obstet Gynecol* **43**:118, 1974.

19

Clear Cell Carcinoma of the Ovary

CLEAR CELL CARCINOMAS of the ovary owe their name to their histological similarity with clear cell carcinomas of the kidney. This is a descriptive term that does not indicate the histogenesis of these tumors. Actually their origin and their classification have been the subject of several works. Originally described by Schiller[5] in 1939, they were called mesenophromas. Teilum[7] in 1950 separated from them the so-called "yolk sac tumor" (endodermal sinus tumor or embryonal carcinoma of the ovary). The remainder of the group are now called clear cell carcinomas or mesonephroid carcinomas.[7]

Clear cell tumors of the ovary were thought to arise from mesonephric remnants in the region of the ovary. This position, however, has been changed in recent years because increasing evidence supports a müllerian rather than a mesonephric origin.[2,4,6]

In contrast to the endodermal sinus tumor with which it was earlier confused, clear cell carcinoma of the ovary occurs later in life and it has a good prognosis. Most patients are between 40 and 60 years of age at the time of diagnosis.[3,4]

They comprise approximately 4.5% of all ovarian carcinomas.[2]

PATHOLOGY

Their gross appearance is basically that of a solid mass. As they increase in size, cystic areas may develop within.[3]

They may grow excessively, reaching up to 30.0 cm in diameter. Usually they are about 15.0 cm.[2,4] In the series by Rogers et al.,[4] most of the tumors (94.7%) were unilateral, whereas in the series by Fine et al.[2] bilaterality was noted in 12 of 31 cases.

Microscopically, the appearance is in many respects similar to that of renal cell carcinoma. A glandular growth pattern develops in the form of tubular structures with central small spaces. Interspersed between these tubular formations, solid and papillary areas are to be found. There are two main cell types, those with clear cytoplasm, the clear cells, and those containing eosinophilic granules.[1–4]

The current view on their histogenesis is that they are of müllerian origin. According to Scully,[6] there are many reasons to substantiate this hypothesis. Clear cell carcinomas of the ovary often coexist with endometrioid carcinoma, a tumor of established müllerian origin. They also coexist often with pelvic and ovarian endometriosis and they have been reported to arise from the epithelium of endometriotic cysts. Clear cell carcinomas further are known to occur within the endometrial cavity arising from the endometrium and more recently have been related to vaginal adenosis of a müllerian type in young female patients who were exposed *in utero* to diethylstilbestrol.[6] On the other hand, there are definite differences between ovarian clear cell carcinomas and clear cell carcinomas of the kidney.[6] The latter are tumors of mesonephric origin.

For practical purposes, all clear cell ovarian tumors should be considered as carcinomas.[6]

CLINICAL

The presenting symptoms, as with most ovarian tumors, are nonspecific and they consist of vague abdominal discomfort and distention, gastrointestinal complaints, and only occasionally severe abdominal pain. Uncommon is the presence of irregular or abdominal vaginal bleeding. This in most instances is related to other genital tract pathology.[2–4]

In the series by Rogers et al.[4] a large percentage of patients (68%) had the tumor confined to one ovary. This is a high number of stage I ovarian carcinomas as compared to Stage I adenocarcinoma of the ovary. Stage II disease was seen in 19% of the patients: stage III, in 11.6%; and stage IV, in 1.2%, as reported by the same authors.[4] Ten of 40 patients (25%) reported by Norris and Robinowitz[3] had tumor spread beyond the ovary in the form of local pelvic metastasis at the time of laparotomy. Ascites was seen in 8.4% at the time of the surgery.[3] The presence of ascites seemingly does not represent a grave sign in the early period, since two of three patients with stage Ic disease were alive and well at five years. There were no survivors, however, in Stage II and III when ascites was present.[4]

TREATMENT AND RESULTS

The extent of the surgery, as in all ovarian carcinomas, and the type of procedure are dictated by the clinical staging. Total abdominal hysterectomy and bilateral salpingo-oophorectomy is the recommended treatment for stage I tumors and debulking procedures, in an effort to reduce the tumor volume, should be considered and practiced whenever feasible for higher stages. In the series by Rogers et al.[4] 21 of 33 patients (63.5%) were alive at the end of five years following total ab-

dominal hysterectomy and bilateral salpingo-oophorectomy. From the same series among a group of 10 patients with Stage Ia disease treated by unilateral adnexal resection, eight (80%) were alive and well at five years.[4] Although this is not a recommendable cancer procedure, it certainly demonstrates the better biological behavior of clear cell ovarian carcinoma.

The results obtained by Fine et al.[2] are somewhat less optimistic. The authors reviewed the therapy and the subsequent course in 31 cases of which 22 underwent bilateral salpingo-oophorectomy and hysterectomy, six had bilateral salpingo-oophorectomy, and three were considered inoperable. Metastases to the peritoneum, omentum, or the liver were seen in 14 cases at the time of the primary surgery. In the authors view postoperative radiotherapy and single agent chemotherapy failed to alter the course of the disease. Follow-up in 29 cases gave them a 20.6% five-year survival with six patients surviving at that period of time. Intraabdominal metastases with involvement of the peritoneum, the abdominal lymph nodes, and the liver was the primary cause of death; however, in six patients extraabdominal extension to the chest and the retroperitoneal space was observed.[2]

Due to the rarity of this particular histological type, no concrete statement can be made about the efficacy of adjuvant therapy. Systemic chemotherapy most probably will be as successful as it is in the management of patients with adenocarcinoma. Radiotherapy also could be considered in the treatment of local tumor bulk.

PROGNOSIS AND SURVIVAL

With the exception of the series reported by Fine et al.[2] in which the five-year-survival rate was found to be 16%, corrected for deaths due to intercurrent disease, most authors have found clear cell carcinoma of the ovary to be of better prognosis. Thus, Norris and Robinowitz,[3] on the basis of follow-up data obtained on 39 patients, calculated the actuarial survival to be 47% at five years and 42% at 10 years.

Unilateral clear cell carcinoma confined to one ovary yielded a cummulative survival of 80% at five years in the series reported by Czernobilsky *et al.*[1] Rogers *et al.*[4] had an over-all salvage rate for all stages of 43.5%. However, if the analysis was to be made according to the stage at the time of the diagnosis, patients with Stage I disease had 63.5% five-year survival; Stage II, 16.6%; and there was no survivor at five years among patients with Stage III and Stage IV tumors.

The main prognostic factor is the stage at the time of the diagnosis. Tumor size and the various histological patterns and admixtures that these tumors present with have no significant influence upon the prognosis.[3,4]

REFERENCES

1. Czernobilsky, B., Silverman, B.B., and Enterline, H.T.: Clear-cell carcinoma of the ovary. A clinicopathologic analysis of pure and mixed forms and comparison with endometrioid carcinoma. *Cancer* **25:**762, 1970.

2. Fine, G., Clarke, H.D., and Horn, R.C., Jr.: Mesonephroma of the ovary. A clinical, morphological, and histogenetic appraisal. *Cancer* **31:**398, 1973.

3. Norris, H.J., and Robinowitz, M.: Ovarian adenocarcinoma of mesonephric type. *Cancer* **28:** 1074, 1971.

4. Rogers, L.W., Julian, C.G., and Woodruff, J.D.: Mesonephroid carcinoma of the ovary: A study of 95 cases from the Emil Novak Ovarian Tumor Registry. *Gynecol Oncol* **1:**76, 1972.

5. Schiller, W.: Mesonephroma ovarii. *Am J Cancer* **35:**1, 1939.

6. Scully, R.E.: Ovarian tumors. A review. *Am J Pathol* **87:**686, 1977.

7. Teilum, G.: Mesonephroma ovarii (Schiller). An extra-embryonic mesoblastoma of germ cell origin in the ovary and testis. *Acta Pathol Microbiol Scand* **27:**249, 1950.

20

Endometrial Carcinoma of the Prostate

MELICOW AND PACHTER[2] were the first to describe in 1967 a prostatic carcinoma of the endometrial variety. The tumor histologically resembled adenocarcinoma of the uterus and it was the authors' suggestion that it arose in the region of the utricle. In the opinion of most investigators who subsequently have dealt with the subject, these tumors are a distinct entity to be separated from the other papillary tumors found in the area of the prostatic urethra and the prostatic ducts.[6] It is an uncommon neoplasm, at least uncommonly reported. Merchant et al.,[4] reviewing the literature in 1976, found nine published cases and added a tenth of their own.[4] The age of the patients has ranged from 61 to 79 years, the average being 68 at the time of the diagnosis.

PATHOLOGY

The histological appearance is strikingly similar to that of endometrial adenocarcinoma of the uterus. It is thought that the neoplasia develops in the region of the utricle. This structure is found at the apex verumontanum. The latter arises from the dorsal wall of the posterior urethra and protrudes into the lumen. The utricle develops from the müllerian ducts and it is thought by some to be homologous to the female vagina, although others maintain that it is homologous to the uterus, which seems to be the prevalent opinion. The tissues in that specific region are responsive to estrogen administration. Prominent squamous cell changes have been observed here, in patients with prostatic cancer receiving estrogens.[2]

Carney and Kelalis[1] have described the histopathological criteria. There is a papillary appearance with occasional ciliated columnar cell lining. The cytoplasm of the cells is darkly eosinophilic, there is subnuclear cytoplasmic vacuolization, and there are secretions negative to mucicarmine staining.[1] The overall appearance is that of irregular acinar spaces exhibiting a cribriform pattern with complex papillary infoldings very much reminiscent of endometrial adenocarcinoma.[6] The most convincing evidence that this tumor originates in the utricle is the microscopic findings of ciliated tumor cells. These are occasionally seen in endometrial carcinoma in the female but have never been described in prostatic tumors of either ductal or acinar origin.[1] In spite of the substantial evidence, actual proof of its origin is lacking, since the prostatic utricle is a minute structure usually destroyed completely at the time of the diagnosis. The question of ductal origin has been raised on the basis of electron microscopic studies by Zaloudek et al.[7]

CLINICAL

Because of the central location, there is early interference with the urethral lumen. As a result, hematuria and bladder outlet obstruction are usually the presenting symptoms. In contrast to the commonly seen acinar adenocarcinoma, where more often than not the neoplasm grows in one of the lobes, here the diagnosis is made during the early stages. All 10 patients had urinary obstruction, and gross hematuria was seen in seven.

It follows, that rectal examination is nonrevealing in the early stages and that transrectal needle biopsy may fail to provide the diagnosis. The latter is established by means of transurethral resection.[6]

Because of the proximity to the bladder, the trigone and the ureteral orifices may be involved, resulting in hydronephrosis.[3]

Metastases to the skeletal system do take place. Dense sclerotic deposits in the spine and the pelvis have been reported.[3,4]

TREATMENT AND RESULTS

Transurethral resection has been the primary mode of therapy in most patients.[3,4,7] Radiotherapy has been applied in three, locally to the prostate and for metastatic bone disease.[3,4] Local recurrences have developed following transurethral resection; therefore it is recommended that postoperative radiotherapy follows this procedure. The tumor has been radioresponsive. In general, orchiectomy or estrogen administration have been avoided on the premise that this tumor is identical biologically to female endometrial carcinoma. However, Young and Lagios[6] reported an objective regression of the prostatic tumor mass following orchiectomy.

PROGNOSIS

There is a relatively indolent course and no deaths have been reported among the 10 reviewed patients. Actually the majority were living free of disease.[4,5,7]

REFERENCES

1. Carney, J.A., and Kelalis, P.P.: Endometrial carcinoma of the prostatic utricle. *Am J Clin Pathol* **60**:565, 1973.
2. Melicow, M.M., and Pachter, M.R.: Endometrial carcinoma of prostatic utricle (uterus masculinus). *Cancer* **20**:1715, 1967.
3. Melicow, M.M., and Tannenbaum, M.: Endometrial carcinoma of uterus masculinus (prostatic utricle). Report of 6 cases. *J Urol* **106**:892, 1971.
4. Merchant, R.F., Jr., Graham, A.R., Bucher, W.C., Jr., and Parker, D.A.: Endometrial carcinoma of prostatic utricle with osseous metastases. *Urology* **8**:169, 1976.
5. Satter, E.J., and Blumenfeld, C.M.: Endometrial carcinoma of the prostatic utricle. *J Urol* **112**:505, 1974.
6. Young, B.W., and Lagios, M.D.: Endometrial (papillary) carcinoma of the prostatic utricle—response to orchiectomy. A case report. *Cancer* **32**:1293, 1973.
7. Zaloudek, C., Williams, J.W., and Kempson, R.L.: "Endometrial" adenocarcinoma of the prostate. A distinctive tumor of probable prostatic duct origin. *Cancer* **37**:2255, 1976.

21

Transitional Cell Carcinoma of the Prostate

THIS IS A well-established but uncommon prostatic malignancy. Rhamy et al.[7] in reviewing 800 cases of prostatic carcinoma found the incidence of transitional cell type to be 2.5%. The tumor is thought to arise from the transitional epithelium that covers the distal portion of the prostatic ducts. It was first described by Melicow and Hollowell[6] in 1952 and since that time several reports have appeared in the literature. Greene et al.[2,3] reviewing the material from the Mayo Clinic presented the clinicopathological findings of 39 patients with this diagnosis. Ende et al.[1] found seven patients with transitional cell carcinoma among 200 cases seen at the Veterans Administration Hospital in Nashville, Tennessee.

The average patients' age at the time of the diagnosis is 65 years.[1,2,4,7]

PATHOLOGY

The tumors arise centrally in the region where the prostatic ducts join the prostatic urethra.[4] Histologically they resemble transitional cell carcinoma of the urinary bladder, the majority of them being Grade III, poorly differentiated invasive neoplasms (Fig. 21-1). Masses of necrotic tumor are found plugging medium-sized ducts and inflammatory changes, including microabscesses, may be quite prominent. In the cases reviewed by Rhamy et al.[7] 20% had adenocarcinoma elements coexisting with transitional cell carcinoma. The necrotic features and the prominent tumor plugs within the ducts are emphasized by many authors.[2,4,5]

CLINICAL

The most important presenting symptom is obstruction of the urinary outflow, which, due to the anaplastic character of the tumor, is of rapid onset. More than 80% of the patients have prostatism as the main complaint.[2,4,7] Another symptom is pronounced hematuria that is associated with anemia.

One of the typical and perhaps characteristic symptoms of transitional cell carcinoma of the prostate is rectal obstruction. The extensive local growth within a period of a few months effectively occludes most of the rectal lumen.[4,6]

The serum acid phosphatase remains normal.

Intravenous urography reveals a grossly enlarged prostate in most patients and rectal examination confirms this finding. The gland is hard and encroachment upon the rectal lumen is readily appreciated in advanced cases. Transurethral resection effectively discloses the diagnosis, but transrectal or perineal biopsy has a lower yield.[8]

The progress of the disease is overwhelming, in terms of local growth. This is associated with severe lower pelvic and perineal pain. The tumor extends upward into the bladder and characteristically downward along the urethra in a manner similar to other transitional cell car-

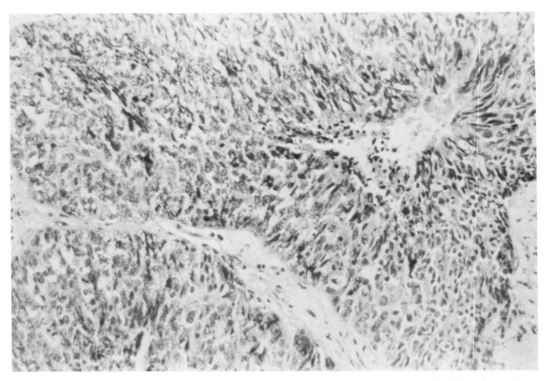

FIG. 21-1.   Transitional cell carcinoma of the prostate. Poorly differentiated transitional cell carcinoma in a 65-year-old patient.

cinomas of the urinary tract.[2,7,8] Extensive pelvic lymph node involvement is to be found in postmortem studies, and osteolytic or osteoblastic bone metastases as well as brain and lung metastases have been reported.[2]

TREATMENT AND RESULTS

This is not a hormone-dependent prostatic carcinoma. Estrogen administration and orchiectomy have failed to affect the progress of the disease and therefore are not indicated.[1,2]

Prostatectomy and radiation therapy have been used in the management of these patients. In the series by Rhamy *et al.*[7] supervoltage radiation therapy to the level of 7000 rad has been employed, but failing, according to the authors, to control the tumor in all patients. In the series by Greene *et al.*[3] four patients who under-

went radical prostatectomy survived an average of 43 months. The average survival of nine patients treated definitively by radiation therapy was 26 months, and finally patients managed with hormonal manipulation lived only 11 months from the time of the diagnosis. Johnson *et al.*[4] reported on six patients seen at M.D. Anderson Hospital with tumor localized to the prostate at the time of diagnosis. They were treated with radiotherapy, receiving 4000–6000 rad as a tumor dose, and two received in addition estrogen therapy. Four other patients from the same series were treated in excess of 6000 rad to the prostate. Apparently the level of the radiation dosage made no difference in terms of survival, which ranged from 12 to 36 months, the average being 20 months.[4] Rhamy *et al.*[7] advocate radical cystoprostatectomy with ileal loop urinary diversion as the treatment of choice, this on theoretical grounds rather than on reality.

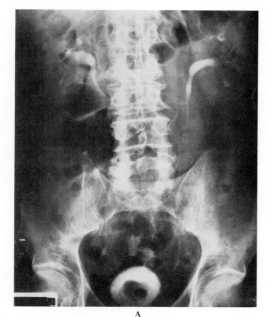

A

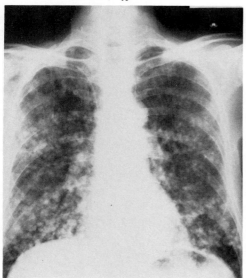

B

FIG. 21-2. Transitional cell carcinoma of the prostate in a 69-year-old male. Intravenous pyelogram shows large filling defect of the urinary bladder due to prostatic enlargement (A). Six months later chest radiograph shows extensive bilateral pulmonary metastases (B).

We have seen and treated recently a 69-year-old male with transitional cell carcinoma of the prostate. The patient was initially treated with orchiectomy, which did not affect the tumor growth. Four months later the prostate was grossly enlarged, partially obstructing the rectal lumen. The mass practically filled the pelvis and was fixed to both pelvic walls. There was no distant metastases obvious at the time. Radiation therapy to the pelvis by means of rotational technique at the rate of 400 rad every other day was delivered for a total of 4400 rad. This was in the form of a split therapy with an intermission of three weeks in the middle of the course. The total elapsed time was 54 days. There was good tumor response with marked shrinkage of the growth, the prostate returning to practically normal size. However, at the end of this therapy it was obvious that extension to the penile urethra had taken place and radiographically there were lung metastases. The patient died of his disease nine months after the diagnosis. (Fig. 21-2)

PROGNOSIS AND SURVIVAL

This is a lethal disease whose biological behavior shows no similarity to the commoner adenocarcinoma of the prostate. Untreated patients or those treated with hormonal manipulation are usually dead within four to eight months from the onset.[3] For those patients who had surgery or radiation therapy, the average survival was 20 to 24 months.[3,7] Eight of 10 patients reported by Rubenstein and Rubnitz[8] were dead within a year from the time of the diagnosis. The only survivors are to be found in the series by Greene et al.[3] There are two patients of a group of 39 whose disease was Stage A at the time of presentation. One was treated with prostatocystectomy, surviving 42 months later, and the second with radical prostatectomy surviving for 60 months. A third patient was dead at 48 months.

REFERENCES

1. Ende, N., Woods, L.P., and Shelley, H.S.: Carcinoma originating in ducts surrounding the prostatic urethra. *Am J Clin Pathol* **40**:183, 1963.

2. Greene, L.F., Mulcahy, J.J., Warren, M.M., and Dockerty, M.B.: Primary transitional cell carcinoma of the prostate. *J Urol* **110**:235, 1973.

3. Greene, L.F., O'Dea, M.J., and Dockerty, M.B.: Primary transitional cell carcinoma of the prostate. *J Urol* **116**:761, 1976.

4. Johnson, D.E., Hogan, J.M., and Ayala, A.G.: Transitional cell carcinoma of the prostate. A clinical morphological study. *Cancer* **29**:287, 1972.

5. Karpas, C.M., and Moumgis, B.: Primary transitional cell carcinoma of prostate gland: Possible pathogenesis and relationship to reserve cell hyperplasia of prostatic periurethral ducts. *J Urol* **101**:201, 1969

6. Melicow, M.M., and Hollowell, J.W.: Intraurothelial cancer: Carcinoma in situ, Bowen's disease of the urinary system. Discussion of thirty cases. *J Urol* **68**:763, 1952.

7. Rhamy, R.K., Buchanan, R.D., and Spalding, M.J.: Intraductal carcinoma of the prostate gland. *J Ruol* **109**:457, 1973.

8. Rubenstein, A.B., and Rubnitz, M.E.: Transitional cell carcinoma of the prostate. *Cancer* **24**:543, 1969.

22

Oat Cell Carcinoma of the Larynx and the Trachea

OAT CELL CARCINOMA, or anaplastic carcinoma, of the upper respiratory tract is an uncommon neoplasm. Although this histological variety represents approximately 11% of all primary lung tumors, only a few such cases have been reported involving the larynx and the trachea.

LARYNX

It was Olofsson and Van Nostrand[9] who described the first case of an oat cell carcinoma originating in the larynx. Since that communication, nine additional cases have been published. The average age at the time of the diagnosis is 63 years. Most of the patients are males and all heavy smokers.[1,4,5,7,9]

Pathology

Histologically, the tumors are composed of irregular clumps and cords of small cells, with round dark nuclei and numerous mitotic figures. Infiltration of the surrounding striated muscles is usually observed and lymph node metastases are the rule.[4,5,9]

Clinical

A common symptom is the appearance of a mass in the neck, representing metastatic lymphadenopathy. This is often accompanied by hoarseness of the voice and a feeling of sore throat. In a number of patients, due to the fast tumor expansion, the disease presents acutely with respiratory distress and dyspnea. The airway is being occluded by an exophytic mass.[2,3,7,8]

Direct laryngoscopy reveals a large growth, which in most cases occupies a large segment of the subglottic region with or without involvement of the vocal cords.[1,8–10] The epiglottis and the aryepiglottic folds have occasionally been the site of the primary.

Treatment and Results

The first step in the management of the patient with oat cell carcinoma of the larynx may be the performance of emergency tracheostomy. Due to the rapid tumor growth, obstruction can develop quickly, resulting in respiratory distress.[4,9]

In the earlier reports the main therapeutic impetus was on total laryngectomy. This was accompanied by lymph node dissection.[1,4,5,8,9] The realization that there is a high propensity not only for lymph node but also for hematogenous metastases associated with high mortality and the poor results of surgery alone has placed current emphasis on radiation therapy and chemotherapy.[2,3,8,10]

Total laryngectomy with lymph node dissection was performed in five of the earlier reported cases. Two received preoperative radiotherapy. Only one patient was alive and well 2.5 years after radiotherapy and surgery.[9]

Recent reports question the surgical approach, recommending instead chemotherapy and irradiation. An effective program has been cyclophosphamide, vincristine, methotrexate, and CCNU; another is cyclophosphamide, Adriamycin, and methotrexate; and yet another, vincristine, cyclophosphamide, and Adriamycin.[2,3,7,8,10]

Radiation therapy was given in the range of 4000 rad in four weeks. Three of four patients treated in this manner were surviving for periods in excess of one year, and the fourth died of metastatic disease.[2,3,8,10]

TRACHEA

Carcinomas of the trachea are rare. Rostom and Morgan[11] have estimated that about 2.6 new cases per one million population per year are seen. According to the same authors, the incidence of primary tracheal tumors is 0.35% of all malignant diseases.

Pathology

Squamous cell carcinoma comprises the majority, other histological variants being adenoid cystic carcinoma and adenocarcinoma. Oat cell carcinoma of the trachea is an uncommon disease indeed. In our literature review we encountered eight such cases.

Clinical

When available, the history of these patients records heavy smoking habits of long duration. The average age at the time of the diagnosis was 58 years.[6,11-13]

As with all of the tracheal neoplasms, increasing breathing difficulty over a period of a few months is the commonest presenting symptom. Hemoptysis and

cough can also be present, although they are encountered less commonly.

The shortness of breath is directly related to the mechanical occlusion of the lumen and in combination with the negative chest x-ray very often leads to the erroneous diagnosis of asthma and treated as such.[6,12] The shortness of breath finally becomes extreme and stridor develops.

The gross appearance of the lesion is that of an exophytic, cauliflower type mass protruding into the lumen. Histologically, an oat cell carcinoma of the trachea has appearances similar to an oat cell carcinoma of the lung.[6,12,13]

The diagnosis is based on bronchoscopic examination and biopsy.

Treatment and Results

Treatment of tracheal carcinomas presents formidable technical problems. Radical surgical resection followed by reconstruction procedures perhaps is the appropriate method for an adenoid cystic carcinoma or even a squamous cell carcinoma; however, in the case of an oat cell carcinomas radiotherapy should be given preference. Actually, patients adequately treated with radiotherapy for oat cell carcinoma of the trachea have died primarily of distant metastases.[11,12] The liver appears to be the usual metastatic site, as well as the regional lymph nodes. Jash reported on a 63-year-old female who was alive and well without clinical symptoms five months following the completion of definitive radiotherapy.[6] Systemic combination chemotherapy utilizing programs similar to those of oat cell carcinoma of the lung should be applied. No reports, however, are available on such treatments in the literature.

Prognosis and Survival

The over-all prognosis for oat cell carcinoma of the trachea has been extremely poor. With the exception of the previously mentioned case, all patients were dead of their tumor within a few months.[6,11,13]

References

1. Benish, B.M., Tawfik, B., and Breitenback, E.E.: Primary oat cell carcinoma of the larynx: An ultrastructural study. *Cancer* **36:**145, 1975.

2. Bitran, J.D., Toledo-Pereyra, L.H., and Matz, G.: Oat cell carcinoma of the larynx. Response to combined modality therapy. *Cancer* **42:**85, 1978.

3. Bone, R.C., and Deer, D.: Oat cell carcinoma of the larynx. *Laryngoscope* **88:**1190, 1978.

4. Ferlito, A.: Oat cell carcinoma of the larynx. *Ann Otol Rhinol Laryngol* **83:**254, 1974.

5. Gelot, R., Rhee, T.R., and Lapidot, A.: Primary oat-cell carcinoma of head and neck. *Ann Otol Rhinol Laryngol* **84:**238, 1975.

6. Jash, D.K.: Oat cell carcinoma of the trachea. *J Laryngol Otol* **87:**681, 1973.

7. Lorenz, S.A., III, and Arena, S.: Primary oat cell carcinoma of the larynx. *Pa Med* **82:**41, 1979.

8. Mullins, J.D., Newman, R.K., and Coltman, C.A., Jr.: Primary oat cell carcinoma of the larynx. A case report and review of the literature. *Cancer* **43:**711, 1979.

9. Olofsson, J., and Van Nostrand, A.W.P.: Anaplastic small cell carcinoma of larynx. Case report. *Ann Otol Rhinol Laryngol* **81:**284, 1972.

10. Reddy, G.N., Vrabec, D.P., and Bernath, A.M.: Primary oat cell carcinoma of the larynx. *Pa Med* **83:**22, 1980.

11. Rostom, A.Y., and Morgan, R.L.: Results of treating primary tumours of the trachea by irradiation. *Thorax* **33:**387, 1978.

12. Wengraf, C.: Oat cell carcinoma of the trachea. *J Laryngol Otol* **84:**267, 1970.

13. Zarowitz, H., and Hoffman, J.B.: Primary carcinoma of the trachea. *Arch Intern Med* **89:**454, 1952.

23

Melanoma of the Central Nervous System

MELANIN-CONTAINING CELLS are to be found in several areas of the central nervous system. Such are the leptomeninges, the labyrinth, the cerebrospinal and the sympathetic ganglia, the reticular formation of the medulla, the pons, the substantia nigra and the locus ceruleus.[6] Most authors feel that primary central nervous system melanomas are of meningeal origin.[1] Savitz and Anderson[6] published a detailed literature review. According to the authors, central nervous system melanomas can be classified into four groups:

1. Leptomeningeal melanomatosis. These tumors arise in areas of diffuse meningeal melanosis. They proceed to infiltrate the subarachnoid space, extending along the vessels. In addition they involve the roots of the cranial nerves. They simultaneously obstruct the foramina of Luschka and Magendie and they obliterate the arachnoid villi in the convexity of the brain. The result is a communicating hydrocephalus. Sixty-four such cases were encountered by the authors. Bojsen-Moller[1] published subsequently three similar cases. The patients are 40 to 50 years of age.
2. Neurocutaneous melanosis. The intracranial melanomatous tumor is associated with extensive hairy nevi, particularly of the back. This form has a peak incidence during the first decade of life, and it is rare after 30 years of age.[6]
3. Intracranial melanoma. Included

under this groups are isolated primary intracranial melanomas, 72 of which have been reported in the literature.[1,6] The patients are 30 to 40 years old. The growths have been located in the cerebral cortex, the medulla oblongata, the hypophysis, and the cerebellum.

4. Spinal cord melanoma. They can be distinguished into intramedullary, representing slightly more than 50% of the total, intradural, representing most of the remaining, and the very rare extradural tumors. Sixty-two such cases exist in the literature.[3,6]

With the single exception of a case described by King and Propst[5] in which during myelography black cerebrospinal fluid was obtained, the preoperative diagnosis of a malignant melanoma of the central nervous system has not been made.

The symptoms are similar to those of other tumors and related to the location of the lesion. During surgery it is common to obtain the clinical impression of an angiomatous mass.

Melanomas of the central nervous system, as the rest of the brain neoplasias, do not metastasize.[1] Conversely the central nervous system represents metastatic site for about 35% of patients suffering from cutaneous melanomas.[2] It goes without saying that no lesion should be accepted as a primary central nervous system melanoma if another focus is known.

The prognosis is poor and the treatment usually incomplete. According to Kiel *et al.*,[4] the survival of patients with malignant melanoma of the brain is in the order of six months. Three of the six patients reported by Bojsen-Moller[1] were long survivors, two dying two years after surgery, the third being alive at 18 months.

In tumors of the spinal cord the median survival has been 10 months from the onset of the symptoms.[4]

REFERENCES

1. Bojsen-Moller, M.: Primary cerebral melanomas. Report of six cases and a review of the literature. *Acta Pathol Microbiol Scand [A]* **85:**447, 1977.

2. Das Gupta, T.K., Brasfield, R.D., and Paglia, M.A.: Primary melanomas in unusual sites. *Surg Gynecol Obstet* **128:**841, 1969.

3. Hirano, A., and Carton, C.A.: Primary malignant melanoma of the spinal cord. *J Neurosurg* **17:**935, 1960.

4. Kiel, F.W., Starr, L.B., and Hansen, J.L.: Primary melanoma of the spinal cord. *J Neurosurg* **18:**616, 1961.

5. King, A.B., and Propst, H.D.: Melanomas of the central nervous system: Description of a primary spinal cord melanoma. *Guthrie Clin Bull* **21:**19, 1951.

6. Savitz, M.H., and Anderson, P.J.: Primary melanoma of the leptomeninges: A review. *Mt Sinai J Med NY* **41:**774, 1975.

24

Melanoma of the Oral Cavity
and the Oropharynx

THE INCIDENCE OF malignant melanomas in the head and neck region, arising from the mucous membranes, is given in the publication by Hormia and Vuori.[3] The authors searched the Finnish Cancer Registry for a 12-year period from 1953 to 1964, and they encountered 11 such tumors. Of these, five involved the nasal cavity, five were in the oral cavity, and one was occupying the larynx and the pharynx. During the same period of time 1047 cutaneous melanomas were registered. Thus, the ratio between mucosal melanomas of the head and neck and cutaneous melanomas in general is 1:105.

Along similar lines, Conley and Pack[2] found 50% of the mucosal melanomas in the oral cavity, 34.6% in the nasal cavity, and the remaining 15.4% in the pharynx and larynx.

There is a definite, almost in a ratio of 2:1, male preponderence.[5] The patients generally are old, the majority of them being in the sixth or the seventh decades of life.[2–5]

PATHOLOGY

The pathological staging of cutaneous melanomas cannot be applied in its entirety when dealing with mucosal melanomas. The classification is based primarily on the degree of tumor penetration and, in the skin, it utilizes such anatomical landmarks as the papillary dermis and the reticular dermis, in order to denote the tumor levels. These structures do not exist in the mucosal regions; however, as Shah et al.[5] demonstrated, the depth of penetration is an important prognosticating factor. It is their recommendation that the depth be measured with the help of an ocular micrometer and the penetration registered in millimeters.[5]

CLINICAL

In the oral cavity, the commonest location of melanomas is the palate (Fig. 24-1). Four of 5 cases in the Finnish series[3] and 11 of 26 cases in the series by Conley and Pack,[2] occurred here. They have also been reported in the gingiva and the buccal mucosa.[5] Less often they have been seen in the lips, floor of the mouth, the tongue, and the tonsils.[1–5]

Melanomas of the mucous membrane have some highly characteristic features in their early stages, according to Conley and Pack.[2] The deposition of pigment creates a brown-gray discoloration that appears deceptively benign. Often, melanoma of the mucous membrane is associated with melanosis. Within the area of melanosis, the tumor may be quite localized and only multiple peripheral biopsies will establish the diagnosis accurately.[2] As the lesions grow, they become slightly elevated bluish-black in color and they may or may

70

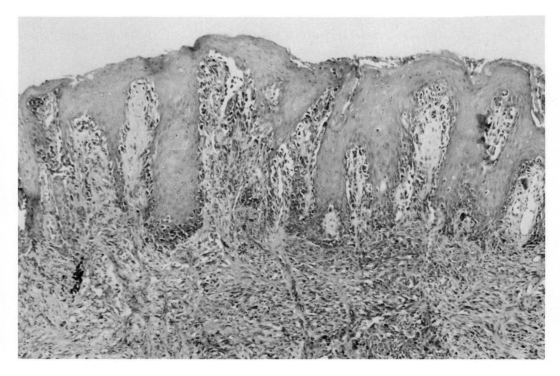

FIG. 24-1. Melanoma of the palate. Junctional activity and submucosal infiltration by malignant nevus cells are demonstrated.

not be accompanied by regional lymph nodes.[3]

The overall incidence of regional lymph node involvement is not too high. Among patients presenting with localized disease, 7.7% were found to have nodal involvement on initial examination and another 15.4% developed metastasis in the neck at a later time.[2]

In the series by Shah et al.,[5] 66% of the patients had localized disease (Stage I) at the time of diagnosis, 23% had regional nodes involved (Stage II), and the remaining 11% had disseminated melanoma (Stage III).

The incidence of local recurrence of melanomas in the oral cavity is in the range of 25%. This is lower than that observed in melanomas of the upper respiratory passages and is primarily due to the fact that surgery is easier accomplished. Local recurrence in the region of

the pharynx was 32% in the series by Conley and Pack.[2]

TREATMENT AND RESULTS

The majority of the tumors have as initial treatment local resection. Composite resection including removal of the tumor and the regional lymph nodes is considered the treatment of choice for melanomas of the inferior alveolus, the floor of the mouth and the lateral pharynx. Radical neck dissection, perhaps, does not add to the survival.[2]

Surgery alone, or surgery combined with radiotherapy, were used in the patients reported by Hormia and Vuori.[3] It is the authors' opinion that the best therapeutic method is radical resection. Catlin,[1] presenting the material from Memorial Hospital, had six five-year survivors of 16 patients who underwent radical neck dissections. There were an additional five patients without evidence of disease at five years whose treatment was wide excision. None of the four patients whose procedure was combined resection of the tumor and the regional lymphatics (the so-called "commando" procedure) survived.

All but two patients in the series by Shah et al.[5] had surgical excisions. In several, repeated procedures were performed in an attempt to control the disease at the primary site.

Given the overall poor results, and the peculiarities of clinical behavior of malignant melanoma, Conley and Pack[2] raise the question as to whether or not electrodesiccation may be used. It is their view that for early superficial tumors this method may offer the same probabilities of local control, while maintaining the anatomical integrity.

PROGNOSIS AND SURVIVAL

The depth of invasion of the primary lesion can provide limited prognostic guidance.[5] Surviving at five years were 3 of 10 patients (33%) with invasion to less than 0.5 mm, 4 of 22 patients (18%) with invasion of 0.6–1 mm, and only 1 of 10 (10%) with invasion deeper than 1 mm.

The five-year, disease-free survival rate was 15% in the series reported by Conley and Pack.[2]

Shah et al.[5] found 15 of 74 patients (20%) surviving at the end of the five-year period, but only seven were free of tumor. Thus, the disease-free survival in their series was 10%.

REFERENCES

1. Catlin, D.: Mucosal melanomas of the head and neck. *A J R* **99**:809, 1967.
2. Conley, J., and Pack, G.T.: Melanoma of the mucous membranes of the head and neck. *Arch. Otolaryngol* **99**:315, 1974.
3. Hormia, M, and Vuori, E.E.J.: Mucosal melanomas of the head and neck. *J Laryngol Otol* **83**:349, 1969.
4. Mesara, B.W., and Burton, W.D.: Primary malignant melanoma of the upper respiratory tract. Clinicopathologic study. *Cancer* **21**:217, 1967.
5. Shah, J.P., Huvos, A.G., and Strong, E.W.: Mucosal melanomas of the head and neck. *Am J Surg* **134**:531, 1977.

25

Melanoma of the Upper Respiratory Tract

MALIGNANT MELANOMAS of the upper respiratory tract have been subdivided into melanomas of the nose and the paranasal sinuses and melanomas of the larynx.

MELANOMAS OF THE NOSE AND THE PARANASAL SINUSES

Melanomas in this region, presumably, originate from preexisting melanocytes. Normally, however, such cells are not present in the mucous membrane of the nose and that of the sinuses.[8] A number of theories have been proposed in order to explain their histogenesis. Neural crest elements may be transformed into melanocytes and nevus cells; there may be metaplasia of squamous and glandular epithelium into pigment-producing cells; or there may be migration of melanoblasts to sites where they usually do not exist.[1,2,4,5,7,12,15]

Melanomas of the nose and sinuses comprise 0.5–1.7% of all melanomas.[6] The majority arise in the nasal cavity. Ravid and Esteves,[12] in their original review of 117 cases, found no melanoma involving the sinuses without concomitant involvement of the nasal cavity. Subsequently, primary melanomas of the paranasal sinuses were reported.[4,8]

There is a strong Caucasian predominance and very few black patients have been encountered. In terms of sex no difference in incidence is to be found. Most patients are between 50 and 70 years of age.[4,8,12]

Pathology

Grossly, most tumors are solid polypoid growths. Their consistency varies from firm to cystic to friable or necrotic. About two-thirds are dark, due to the melanin pigment, the remainder being pink or white.[5,8,12]

The pathological diagnosis can be easily made in the presence of melanin pigment.[4,12] When the tumor lacks pigment, such entities as anaplastic carcinoma, poorly differentiated squamous cell carcinoma, reticulum cell sarcoma, transitional cell carcinoma, rhabdomyosarcoma, malignant schwannoma, and angiomyosarcoma have been entertained. Special stains will help in arriving at the correct diagnosis.[8] Junctional changes can rarely be seen. The bulk of the disease has usually destroyed the original epithelium.

Clinical

The most prevalent symptom the patients present with is nasal obstruction, which usually is unilateral. Nasal obstruction alone, or associated with epistaxis, is seen in 85–90% of the patients.[4,12] Pain was present in 16% of the cases reported by Freedman et al.[4] Swelling of the face, nose, palate, and neck was encountered in 5–9%.[4] On the average, the symptoms' duration has been three to four months.

The nasal cavity, and particularly the nasal septum, is the commonest site. The inferior and the middle turbinates follow in order.[4,8]

On physical examination, a mass is found in the majority of the patients. The usual clinical impression is that this represents a nasal polyp, a common disorder. The size of the tumors varies from 1.0 cm to a large mass occupying the ipsilateral nasal cavity. Radiographically, the extent of the tumor can be well delineated and bony destruction can be detected. There is opacification of the involved sinus and posterior extension into the nasopharynx takes place.[3,4,9]

Ulceration of the tumors was present in 17 of 18 cases reported by Ancla et al.[1]

Metastases to the cervical lymph nodes, at the time of diagnosis, were present in 18% of the cases.[4]

Treatment and Results

Barton[2] in 1975 reported three cases of malignant melanoma involving the head and neck region, which were treated successfully by cryosurgery. One of these tumors arose from the nasal septum.[2]

Surgical resection, radiation therapy, and a combined approach have been the traditional forms of therapy. If surgery is to be used, wide resection is necessary. Malignant melanomas of the nose and paranasal sinuses in high percentages exhibit local tumor recurrence and extension to adjacent structures following surgery.[12] Freedman et al.[4] advocate surgery or a planned combination of surgery and radiation therapy as the best approach, adding that radiation therapy by itself has nothing to offer in the way of definitive treatment.[4] This statement, however, can be challenged by the reports of Ghamrawi and Glennie[6] and the report by Pande.[10] Both reports suggest good prospects of local control of malignant melanoma in the nasal cavity provided the dose-fractionation relationship follows the guidelines discussed in the introduction. This entails a high-dose, small-fractionation technique. All six patients included in these reports responded well

to radiotherapy, among them being three long-term survivors. Death from unrelated disease occurred in three patients.[6,10]

On the basis of these data, it is our recommendation that surgical resection be accompanied by definitive local radiotherapy, as already described.

Prognosis and Survival

The overall prognosis on the basis of the literature reports is poor. Ravid and Esteves[12] found the five-year survival rate to be 6%.

Local recurrences, eventually accompanied by dissemination of the disease, has been the fate of the majority. During the first year from the time of the original biopsy, 55% of the patients had either local recurrence or regional or distant metastases in the series described by Holdcraft and Gallagher.[8]

A more optimistic view is expressed by Freedman et al.,[4] reporting on their experience at the Mayo Clinic. The authors stress the real possibility of salvaging patients in spite of recurrent disease and they advocate repeated surgical procedures, radiotherapy, and chemotherapy, means by which they were able to help and extend the average survival of 18 such patients to 4.2 years. Patients with early lesions were treated primarily by means of surgery and the five-year-survival rate of this group was 61.3%. Patients with combined therapy had a 34.2% five-year survival.[4]

These are exceptionally good results. In the experience of most authors, as summarized by Gallagher,[5] the average survival is only 2.6 years after the onset of the symptoms. The author could find only 11% of 226 patients recorded in the world literature up to 1969 who had survived for five years.[5]

MELANOMAS OF THE LARYNX

Goldman et al.[7] encountered a case of extensive melanosis of the laryngeal mucosa while studying serial sections of cancerous and irradiated larynges. Following this encounter, the authors undertook a histological evaluation of laryngeal mucosas in an effort to identify melanocytes. They were able to recognize them as scattered foci in an appreciable number of specimens. These foci were mainly confined to the squamous mucosa of the vocal cords where they were seen within the epithelium and the adjacent superficial stroma.[7] It is implied that the laryngeal melanomas may arise from such melanocytic aggregates. The tumors represent a medical oddity, since only 23 cases could be found reported in the literature up to 1974.[2,7,9,11,13–15]

The tumor has been reported to occur without a special preference in all parts of the larynx, including the epiglottis, arytenoids, the ventricle and the false cords, the true cords, the pyriform fossa, as well as in some cases in several laryngeal regions simultaneously.

A vague discomfort or a peculiar feeling in the throat is the common presenting symptom without overwhelming pain. Upon inspection the tumor may be pigmented, or it may be gray-yellow in color. Often it has been thought of as being squamous cell carcinoma.[13–15] There may be a greater incidence among males and the average age at the time of diagnosis has been 56 years.[7]

Surgical resection, which in this case means laryngectomy, should be considered the treatment of choice. The question of radical neck dissection has not been settled, but probably such an approach should be considered to avoid future recurrences. Shanon et al.[14] reported on a patient who developed metastatic lymph nodes in the neck three years after his original therapy of supraglottic laryngectomy and postoperative radiotherapy. On the other hand, Barton,[2] noting the vagaries of the natural history of melanomas, is less enthusiastic about prophylactic neck dissection, advocating the use of cryosurgery for small tumors.

With a few exceptions, local recurrence and distant metastases have taken place. It is to be noted, however, that some long-term survivors, indeed, have been reported.[2,11,14]

REFERENCES

1. Ancla, M., de Brux, J., and Leroux-Robert, J.: Mélanomes primitifs des fosses nasales et de la bouche. Etude histologique de 19 cas. *Bull Cancer (Paris)* **57**:79, 1970.
2. Barton, R.T.: Mucosal melanomas of the head and neck. *Laryngoscope* **85**:93, 1975.
3. Conley, J., and Pack, G.T.: Melanoma of the mucous membranes of the head and neck. *Arch Otolaryngol* **99**:315, 1974.
4. Freedman, H.M., DeSanto, L.W., Devine, K.D., and Weiland, L.H.: Malignant melanoma of the nasal cavity and paranasal sinuses. *Arch Otolaryngol* **97**:322, 1973.
5. Gallagher, J.C.: Upper respiratory melanoma pathology and growth rate. *Ann Otol Rhinol Laryngol* **79**:551, 1970.
6. Ghamrawi, K.A.E., and Glennie, J.M.: The value of radiotherapy in the management of malignant melanoma of the nasal cavity. *J Laryngol Otol* **88**:71, 1974.
7. Goldman, J.L., Lawson, W., Zak, F.G., and Roffman, J.D.: The presence of melanocytes in the human larynx. *Laryngoscope* **82**:824, 1972.
8. Holdcraft, J., and Gallagher, J.C.: Malignant melanomas of the nasal and paranasal sinus mucosa. *Ann Otol Rhinol Laryngol* **78**:5, 1969.
9. Nsamba, C.: A case of malignant melanoma of the larynx. *J Laryngol Otol* **80**:1178, 1966.
10. Pande, Y.N.: Malignant melanoma of the postnasal space. *J Laryngol Otol* **84**:1065, 1970.
11. Pantazopoulos, P.E.: Primary malignant melanoma of the larynx. *Laryngoscope* **74**:95, 1964.
12. Ravid, J.M., and Esteves, J.A.: Malignant melanoma of the nose and paranasal sinuses and juvenile melanoma of the nose. *Arch Otolaryngol* **72**:431, 1960.
13. Sataloff, J., and Shorago, G.W.: The resident's page. *Arch Otolaryngol* **87**:114, 1968.
14. Shanon, E., Covo, J., and Loeventhal, M.: Melanoma of the epiglottis. A case treated by supraglottic laryngectomy. *Arch Otolaryngol* **91**:304, 1970.
15. Vuori, E.E.J., and Hormia, M.: Primary malignant melanoma of the larynx and pharynx. *J Laryngol Otol* **83**:281, 1969.

26

Melanoma of the Lung

PRIMARY MELANOMA of the lung is perhaps the most difficult of primary visceral melanomas to prove. Jensen and Egedorf[1] have proposed the following criteria in accepting the diagnosis: 1) no previous excision of skin tumors, 2) no previous excision of ocular tumors, 3) the lung tumor to be solitary in character, 4) the morphology to be compatible with a primary tumor, 5) no melanomas present in other viscera at the time of the diagnosis, and 6) at autopsy no melanomas to be detected in the skin or the eyes.

Taboada *et al.*[2] reported two cases of what they considered primary lung melanomas and reviewed the literature up to 1972. A total of 12 cases were found.

The commonest presenting symptom is that of hemoptysis and less common has been the presence of chest pain. Three patients were asymptomatic, the tumor being found on x-ray examination.

The average patient's age was 50 years, the youngest, 20 years, and the oldest, 60 years. There was practically an equal number of male and female patients.

Nine patients underwent surgery in the form of lobectomy of pneumonectomy and the remaining were treated symptomatically. There were only three patients surviving at three years without signs of active disease. Two additional patients were surviving for shorter periods without disease present. The remaining died of their tumor, surviving on the average 11 months from the time of the diagnosis.

REFERENCES

1. Jensen, O.W., and Egedorf, J.: Primary melanoma of the lung. *Scand J Respir Dis* **48:**127, 1967.
2. Taboada, C.F., McMurray, J.D., Jordan, R.A., and Seybold, W.D.: Primary melanoma of the lung. *Chest* **62:**629, 1972.

27

Melanoma of the Esophagus

THE ESOPHAGUS REPRESENTS a rare location for malignant melanoma to develop. Literature review reveals a number of reports, where, with relative confidence, primary malignant melanoma in this location has been diagnosed. The main question in all extracutaneous melanomas is whether they represent primary or metastatic lesions. Hendricks *et al.*[1] and earlier Moffat *et al.*[2] discussed the origin of esophageal melanoma. It was pointed out that the esophagus is a rare site of metastatic disease in patients with malignant melanoma of the skin and that this fact combined with an increasing accumulation of case reports of esophageal malignant melanomas without evidence of any other primary strengthens the argument that the tumors indeed began here.[1] Four cases have been described where the malignant esophageal melanoma coexisted with melanosis of other segments of the esophagus. Junctional changes in patients with malignant melanomas of the esophagus have also been observed.[3] Up to 1974, 33 cases had been reported.[1]

CLINICAL

The tumors are bulky and exophytic in character, producing obstruction of the lumen. The commonest presenting symptom is that of dysphagia and less often a discomfort in the back, pain in the chest, pressure, and at times a significant weight loss.[1-3]

Barium swallow reveals a large exophytic mass protruding into the lumen and actually causing local distention because of its expansion. This radiographic appearance is unlike the narrow irregular configuration or the apple-core picture of the common esophageal carcinomas.[1,2] Most of the tumors are located in the middle or the lower part.[3] On esophagoscopy, a polypoid tumor, dark or black in color, is to be seen projecting into the lumen, rather friable on touch, easily bleeding.

The clinical course is rather rapid. When feasible, the tumors have been treated by esophagogastrectomy, with esophagogastrostomy. In several patients metastatic disease to the liver or the regional lymph nodes was found at the time of the operation.

Regardless of the mode of therapy, there are no survivors. Metastatic disease develops rapidly, the lungs being the most often involved. Other metastatic locations are the liver, pancreas, brain, and, indeed, several other sites may be included in the list.[1-3]

The life-span of the patients is less than a year from the time of the diagnosis. We have tabulated the length of survival from the available reports and found it to be nine months, approximately.

REFERENCES

1. Hendricks, G.L., Jr., Barnes, W.T., and Suter, H.J.: Primary malignant melanoma of the esophagus. A case report. *Am Surg* **40**:468, 1974.

2. Moffat, R.C., Richard, L.B., and Gnass, J.E.: Primary malignant melanoma of the esophagus. A case report. *Can J Surg* **15**:306, 1972.
3. Piccone, V.A., Klopstock, R., LeVeen, H.H., and Sika, J.: Primary malignant melanoma of the esophagus associated with melanosis of the entire esophagus. First case report. *J Thorac Cardiovasc Surg* **59**:864, 1970.

28

Melanoma of the Gallbladder

METASTATIC GALLBLADDER melanoma is found in approximately 15% of the patients dying from this disease process.[2] Primary malignant melanoma of the gallbladder appears to be an extremely rare entity indeed. A literature review reveals only nine cases that perhaps qualify for this diagnosis, the last three being described by Peison and Rabin in 1976.[4] Six of the patients were males and 3 females, the average age being 50 years.

The histogenesis of the tumor is only speculative. Metaplasia of the mucosa to squamous epithelium and subsequent junctional changes within this squamous metaplasia may represent one mechanism, according to Walsh.[6] These melanocytes are within the squamous metaplasia rather than within the normal biliary epithelium. Others believe that melanocytes migrate during the 100 mm size embryonic stage from the neural crest not only to the skin but also to internal sites and from them eventually melanoma may arise.[4]

The tumors are polypoid in appearance, protruding into the gallbladder lumen. This in contradistinction to metastatic disease, which most often is serosal in character. Their size is in the range of 2–6 cm, approximately.[3–6]

The clinical presentation is that of gallbladder disease, namely, abdominal pain in the right upper quadrant, severe at times, radiating to the back and the shoulder.[1,4–6] Balthazar and Javors[1] presented the radiographic manifestation of the disease, which is primarily a large solitary defect within the gallbladder.

Cholecystectomy has been performed in six patients, the remaining three being diagnosed at the postmortem examination. Of the six patients operated upon, long-term follow-up was available only in two.[4,6] One patient was alive and well 14 years postoperatively and the second developed metastatic lymphadenopathy after a six-year, disease-free period.[4]

REFERENCES

1. Balthazar, E.J., and Javors, B.: Malignant melanoma of the gallbladder. Am J Gastroenterol 64:332, 1975.
2. DasGupta, Tk., and Brasfield, R.D.: Metastatic melanoma of the gastrointestinal tract. Arch Surg 88:969, 1964.
3. Jones, C.H.: Malignant melanoma of the gallbladder. J Pathol Bacteriol 81:423, 1961.
4. Peison, B., and Rabin, L.: Malignant melanoma of the gallbladder. Report of three cases and review of the literature. Cancer 37:2448, 1976.
5. Raffensperger, E.C., Brason, F.W., and Triano, G.: Primary melanoma of the gallbladder. Am J Dig Dis 8:356, 1963.
6. Walsh, T.S., Jr.: Primary melanoma of the gallbladder with cervical metastasis and fourteen and a half year survival. First histologically proven case. Cancer 9:548, 1956.

29

Melanoma of the Ovary

IT IS GENERALLY accepted that melanomas in this location arise from dermoid cysts. Normally, the ovary does not contain melanocytes. In order to diagnose primary ovarian melanoma, certain criteria are to be observed. Marcial-Rojas and Ramirez de Arelano[3] set as necessary prerequisites the absence of multiple metastases or other primary sources as well as the need for the initial symptoms to be pelvis-related.

Leo et al.,[2] in a subsequent literature review, added as an additional requirement the presence of intraepidermal junctional activity with a transformation of the epidermal cells into melanoblasts within the dermoid. In their opinion only six cases, including their own, could be found in the world's literature conforming to these criteria. Morrow and DiSaia[4] in their comprehensive review included six additional cases that the authors considered as primary ovarian melanomas. Jernstrom and MacMuffly[1] point out that failure to identify teratomatous elements should not necessarily exclude ovarian origin, since the growth of the tumor may obliterate such elements.

The average patient's age has been 50 years. The presenting symptoms are similar to those of ovarian tumors. There is abdominal enlargement, associated with the presence of a mass and on occasion with gastrointestinal symptoms. At surgery, sizable masses, the average diameter exceeding 10 cm, have been found. These at times appeared as typical dermoids, and at times pelvic extensions with peritoneal implants have been encountered.[2,4]

The treatment consisted of tumor resection in the majority of the cases. A few patients underwent bilateral salpingo-oophorectomy and hysterectomy.

The disease possesses the clinical behavior of both primary ovarian tumors and of melanomas. Metastases are to be found in the peritoneal cavity as well as distally in other organs.

The longest survivor to be reported is described by Jernstrom and MacMuffly.[1] She was alive and well 2.5 years following bilateral salpingo-oophorectomy, omentectomy, and post-operative radiotherapy for a 10 cm right ovarian tumor with omental implants. Of the remainder of the patients, there were four surviving without evidence of disease at the time of the publications with very short follow-up periods, in terms of a few months. Three patients were lost to follow-up, and four were dead of their melanoma. The average survival time of the latter was less than one year.

REFERENCES

1. Jernstrom, P., and MacMuffly, H.: Malignant melanoma of the ovary. Am J Clin Pathol 32:557, 1959.
2. Leo, S., Rorat, E., and Parekh, M.: Primary malignant melanoma in a dermoid cyst of the ovary. Obstet Gynecol 41:205, 1973.
3. Marcial-Rojas, R.A., and Ramirez de Arelano, G.S.: Malignant melanoma arising in a dermoid cyst of the ovary. Cancer 9:523, 1956.
4. Morrow, C.P., and DiSaia, P.J.: Malignant melanoma of the female genitalia: A clinical analysis. Obstet Gynecol Surv 31:233, 1976.

30

Melanoma of the Cervix

AS WITH all mucous membrane melanomas, it is important to establish that the tumor is a primary in this location and to exclude the possibility of metastasis. The presence of junctional activity in the area adjacent to the lesion has been of primary importance in this determination.[1]

To this date, 10 such patients have been reported in the literature.[1,2] In practically all the tumor involved simultaneously the cervix and the adjacent vaginal fornices. Vaginal bleeding and discharge have been the main symptoms; however, in some patients such as the one described by Jones et al.,[1] the tumor had been asymptomatic.

Surgery and radiotherapy to various extent has been used in their management. It appears that a radical surgical procedure, which includes abdominal hysterectomy, bilateral salpingo-oophorectomy, pelvic lymphadenectomy, and vaginectomy, might be the appropriate therapy to consider for a patient who clinically has no signs of metastases. Such an approach afforded an 11-year, disease-free survival in a patient. At that point, local recurrence developed and death followed six months later.[1] Puri et al.[2] applied radiation

therapy in managing their 70-year-old patient. By means of a linear accelerator, 5000 rad were given to the pelvis and 1800 mg hours were delivered via radium placement. The disease did not respond and the patient continued to deteriorate, dying 10 months from the time of the diagnosis.[2]

The length of survival of patients, with the exception of the one described by Jones et al.,[1] has been in the range of 13 months. Another long-term survivor is to be found in the literature, the patient described by Taylor and Tuttle,[3] who had been treated by vaginal hysterectomy, developing local recurrences four years later. She eventually died with local and disseminated disease 13 years from the time of diagnosis.

REFERENCES

1. Jones, H.W., III, Doregemueller, W.M., and Makowski, E.L.: A primary melanocarcinoma of the cervix. Am J Obstet Gynecol 111:959, 1971.
2. Puri, S., Yoonessi, M., and Romney, S.L.: Malignant melanoma of the cervix uteri. Obstet Gynecol 47:459, 1976.
3. Taylor, C.E., and Tuttle, H.K.: Melanocarcinoma of the cervix uteri and vaginal vault. Arch Pathol 38:60, 1944.

31

Melanoma of the Vagina

THE INCIDENCE OF primary vaginal melanoma is much smaller than that of vulvar origin. In the series by Das Gupta and D'Urso[2] from Memorial Hospital three cases of vaginal corresponded to 23 vulvar melanomas seen in the period from 1934 through 1959. The lesion is indeed rare comparing it with other primary malignant tumors occurring in the vagina (less than 3%) and with cutaneous melanomas (less than 0.1%).[10,11,13]

The origin of vaginal melanoma has attracted considerable discussion, primarily because the generally accepted view has been that melanocytes do not occur in the vagina. Norris and Taylor[9] have proposed as a possible mechanism the metaplasia of the mucous membranes.[9] Nigogosyan et al.[8] investigated the presence of melanocytes in the normal vaginal mucosa and were able to find them present in 3 of 100 specimens.

CLINICAL

Most patients are in the 50–60 age bracket. The disease, however, has been seen with less frequency in both younger and older ages. It is to be noted that all reported patients have been Caucasian.[3–5]

Vaginal bleeding associated with discharge has been the commonest presenting symptom. This is usually light in character and not in the form of hemorrhage. Another initial symptom is the presence of a mass discovered by the patient in approximately 20% of the cases. The tumors may be located anywhere in the vagina; however, the lower part and particularly the anterior wall are the favored sites.

In the series by Norris and Taylor[9] the duration of the symptoms prior to the diagnosis was approximately 3 months. In the series by Jentys et al.[5] the duration averaged 3.5 months.

On clinical examination, a polypoid mass protruding into the vaginal lumen is seen, the color of which may vary from black to light red–brown or yellow. Ulceration and necrosis are common. The tumor size varies from 1 to 7 cm.[4,12]

Metastases to the inguinal lymph nodes, if not present at the time of the diagnosis, are quite common later during the course of the disease. Common also is the tendency for local recurrence and hematogenous dissemination.

TREATMENT AND RESULTS

Unfortunately, vaginal melanoma is an entity difficult to treat and carries an ominous prognosis. Due to the rarity of the tumor and the differences of its extent at the time of the diagnosis, the treatment programs have been quite variable. Local excision, a procedure performed in earlier years or in patients with poor medical status, results in a mean survival time of nine months.[1,6] Taking into account the mode of spread, radical surgery seems to be the advisable procedure. Pack and Oropeza[10] recommend a radical hysterectomy, vaginectomy, and inguinal and pelvic lymphadenectomy as minimum required surgery. Das Gupta and D'Urso[2] recommend anterior exenteration. Although these programs may increase the survival time in terms of several months, they do not seem capable of bringing about cures.[4,12]

Deutsch *et al.*[4] reported on five cases of primary vaginal melanoma in which radiotherapy played a role in the management. The authors reviewed the treatment of 74 additional cases from the literature. As in other locations, the tumor may be influenced temporarily by local radiotherapy. Along these lines, this modality may be quite useful for palliative purposes in decreasing the pain and slowing the bleeding. As a rule, regrowth was observed in a matter of months. This has been the experience of others as well.[4,7,13]

REFERENCES

1. Collantes, T.M., Pratt, J.H., and Dockety, M.B.: Primary malignant melanoma of the vagina. *Obstet Gynecol* **29:**508, 1967.
2. Das Gupta, T., and D'Urso, J.: Melanoma of the female genitalia. *Surg Gynecol Obstet* **119:**1074, 1964.
3. Daw, E.: Primary melanoma of the vagina. *Am J Obstet Gynecol* **112:**307, 1972.
4. Deutsch, M., Fried, A.B., Parsons, J.A., and Sartiano, G.: Primary malignant melanoma of the vagina. *Oncology* **30:**509, 1974.
5. Jentys, W., Sikorowa, L., and Mokrzanowski, A.: Primary melanoma of the vagina. Clinico-pathologic study of 7 cases. *Oncology* **31:**83, 1975.
6. Laufe, L.E., and Bernstein, E.D.: Primary malignant melanoma of the vagina. *Obstet Gynecol* **37:**148, 1971.
7. Morrow, C.P., and DiSaia, P.J.: Malignant melanoma of the female genitalia. A clinical analysis. *Obstet Gynecol Surv* **31:**233, 1976.
8. Nigogosyan, G., De La Pava, S., and Pickren, J.W.: Melanoblasts in vaginal mucosa. *Cancer* **17:**912, 1964.
9. Norris, H.J., and Taylor, H.B.: Melanoma of the vagina. *Am J Clin Pathol* **46:**420, 1966.
10. Pack, G.T., and Oropeza, R.A.: A comparative study of melanomas and epidermoid carcinomas of the vulva: A reveiw of 44 melanomas and 58 epidermoid carcinomas (1930–1965). *Rev Surg* **24:**305, 1967.
11. Perez, C.A., Arneson, A.N., Galactos, A., and Samanth, H.K.: Malignant tumors of the vagina. *Cancer* **31:**36, 1973.
12. Ragni, M.V., and Tobon, H.: Primary malignant melanoma of the vagina and vulva. *Obstet Gynecol* **43:**658, 1974.
13. Rutledge, F.: Cancer of the vagina. *Am J Obstet Gynecol* **97:**635, 1967.

32

Melanoma of the Vulva

MALIGNANT MELANOMA OF the vulva represents the commonest of all melanomatous tumors seen in the female genital tract. The disease accounts for approximately 10% of all malignant vulvar tumors and, conversely, 3–4% of all melanomas in females are to be found here.[1,3] The age range has been rather wide. In the series by Chung et al.[2] the youngest patient in the group was 17 years and the oldest 84. Their mean age was 54.5 years, which was identical to that reported by Yackel et al.[6] and by Morrow and Rutledge.[3] As with melanomas in other locations, there is an overwhelming preponderance of Caucasian patients. The ratio of black to Caucasian is in the range of 1:30–1:40.[2,6]

PATHOLOGY AND HISTOLOGY

Morrow and DiSaia[4] in their detailed analysis of melanomas involving the female genitalia point out that approximately 80% of all vulvar melanomas arise in the mucous membranes, namely, the introitus, the clitoris, and the labia minora. The remaining 20% are to be found in the labia majora, the mons veneris, and in the perineum.[4]

Chung et al.[2] reviewed their experience at Memorial Hospital and retrospectively determined the type of tumor growth as defined by Clark et al.[1] It was shown that the majority of patients (82%) presented with tumors showing epithelial changes consistent with either superficial spreading melanoma or with melanoma of squamous mucosae. This latter variety has been seen in melanomas arising in various mucous membranes and in certain areas of modified skin. The remaining were nodular melanomas (18%). The same authors[2] proceeded to stage the tumors according to the levels of invasion, a classification also proposed and described by Clark et al.[1] Due to the differences between the vulvar skin and the squamous mucous membranes of the labia as compared to the skin in other locations, the classification was somewhat modified. It was found that of 33 examined lesions none was confined to level I, there were eight at level II, five at level III, 12 at level IV, three that extended at least to level IV, and five at level V.[2] The authors were able to demonstrate the prognostic significance of both the clinical and the histological classification as described.

CLINICAL

Pruritus and bleeding are the commonest presenting symptoms and next in frequency is the presence of an actual tumor mass.[2,4,6] Many patients were aware that these symptoms were associated with an enlargement of a previously existing mole.[5] Metastatic inguinal lymphadenopathy has occasionally been among the presenting signs. This is particularly true in earlier series, which presumably included more advanced cases.[2,3] The symptoms in most patients have been noticed a number of months prior to seeking medical evaluation.[3]

The average tumor size is between 2 and 3 cm and the incidence of inguinal lymph node involvement is in the range of 50% at the time of the diagnosis.[2,5]

The Federation of Gynecology and Obstetrics in 1971 introduced a clinical staging system for carcinoma of the vulva. It is based on T–N–M tumor evaluation and it includes four clinical stages. The system in the experience of Morrow and Rutledge[5] is quite useful when applied to melanoma of the vulva because it offers a good indication of the patient's prognosis.

TREATMENT AND RESULTS

Review of the literature indicates that a number of patients have been cured of their disease process by local wide excision or simple vulvectomy. However, in view of the present-day knowledge of the high incidence of inguinal and pelvic lymph node metastases and because the overall five-year-survival rate has been in most series in the range of 30%, most authors dealing with the subject advocate radical surgery. As a minimum, this should include en bloc dissection of the inguinal, femoral, and deep pelvic lymph nodes as well as radical vulvectomy. Vaginectomy and anterior, posterior, or total exenteration should also be considered if indicated by the size and the location of the tumor.[4,5] This recommendation, however, cannot be applied to all patients with vulvar melanoma. Morrow and Rutledge[4] found that clinically detectable groin metastases carry a grim prognosis and all patients with disease in the inguinal region died of their tumor in spite of radical surgery. In the series by Chung et al.[2] two of 12 patients with clinically and histologically positive lymph nodes who underwent node dissection survived five years. It appears therefore that a radical approach might be more appropriate at an earlier rather than at a later stage. Furthermore,

Chung et al.[2] have nicely illustrated that the ultimate outcome is more related to the level of invasion rather than to the form of therapy. In their series there were no deaths from melanoma among eight patients with level II disease irrespective of therapy. This contrasted to a 60% mortality rate at five years for patients with level III and level IV tumors, whereas the mortality at five years was 80% for lesions with level V.[1]

Radiotherapy and systemic chemotherapy, as well as immunotherapy, may be considered in inoperable situations. The former may offer palliation in the form of local implants with radioactive material, whereas the latter are adjuvant modalities for both local and systemic disease.

PROGNOSIS AND SURVIVAL

As with melanomas occurring in other locations, the level of invasion is the single most reliable prognostic indicator. The mortality rate relative to the clinical tumor growth type was highest for nodular melanomas (80%), followed by melanoma of squamous mucosae (55%), and finally was the least in patients with superficial spreading melanoma (43%).[1] Regional lymph node metastasis affects the survival as expected. Patients with clinically or histologically positive inguinal lymph nodes had a five-year-survival rate of 14.3% as compared to 56.1% for those with negative lymph nodes.[3]

The overall five-year survival has been in the range of 36%. It is to be mentioned that beyond that point local recurrence or distant metastases can still occur.

REFERENCES

1. Clark, W.H., Jr., From L. Bernardino, E.A. and Mihm, M.C. The histogenesis and biologic behavior of primary human malignant melanoma of the skin. *Cancer Res* **29:**705, 1969.
2. Chung, A.F., Woodruff, J.M., and Lewis, J.L., Jr.: Malignant melanoma of the vulva. A report of 44 cases. *Obstet Gynecol* **45:**638, 1975.

3. Das Gupta, T., and D'Urso, J.: Melanoma of female genitalia. *Surg Gynecol Obstet* **119:**1074, 1964.

4. Morrow, C.P., and DiSaia, P.J.: Malignant melanoma of the female genitalia: A clinical analysis. *Obstet Gynecol Surv* **31:**233, 1976.

5. Morrow, C.P., and Rutledge, F.N.: Melanoma of the vulva. *Obstet Gynecol* **39:**745, 1972.

6. Yackel, D.B., Symmonds, R.E., and Kempers, R.D.: Melanoma of the vulva. *Obstet Gynecol* **35:**625, 1970.

33

Melanoma of the Urethra

Male Uurthra

IN THE PRESENT review melanomas arising from the skin and the glans penis have been excluded.

Up to 1974, 12 patients with intrisic urethral melanomas had been described. Bracken and Diokno[2] reviewed the world literature at that time and added a case of their own. Of the 12 patients, the disease in six was confined to the urethra at the time of the diagnosis.

The recommended therapy is total phallectomy accompanied by inguinal and iliac lymphadenectomy. Apparently, regional lymphadenectomy performed after the occurrence of metastasis failed to control the disease in two cases.

Eight of the 12 patients were known to have died of their malignancy. There were two patients living, one dying at nine months without evidence of tumor, and one was lost to follow-up.

Female Urethra

The most recent report on the subject is the paper by Block and Hotchkiss.[1] The authors published on a patient of their own and proceeded with a literature review of 15 additional cases. Morrow and DiSaia[3] in their review of malignant melanoma involving female genitalia were able to identify at least 42 instances of urethral primary recorded in the world's literature.

They are seen distinctly in the older age group. The average patient's age is 64 years and the overwhelming majority are Caucasian. There is a rapid onset of symptoms, their duration lasting from a few weeks to a few months prior to the diagnosis. This is possibly due to the sensitivity of the location and to the fact that urinary symptoms, such as urgency, hematuria, dysuria, incontinence, and nonspecific perineal pain, are prominent. Associated is often a serosanguineous vaginal discharge with foul odor.

Upon examination, the tumor is seen in the region of the urethral meatus; it may easily be confused with a caruncle, having an identical appearance. It is usually pigmented. The color varies from black to blue or brown.[1,3] Apparently, there is a great propensity for regional spread via the superficial lymphatics to the vulva and the vagina and by means of the deep lymphatics to the inguinal lymph nodes and hematogenously to distant sites. It is, indeed, this rapid extension that renders the treatment very difficult and the prognosis very grave.

As with melanomas in other locations, radical attack against the primary and the regional lymphatics is an appealing concept; however, the realities of the situation may force a less radical approach. It is the recommendation of Morrow and Di-Saia[3] that in patients with otherwise good health surgery should be performed, encompassing en bloc excision of the urinary bladder, urethra, vagina, uterus, and vulva, accompanied by pelvic and inguinal lymphadenectomy. Most authors, however, noting the uniformly poor prognosis and the advanced age of the patients, are less enthusiastic. A review of the literature shows that only 3 of the 42 reported cases survived five years and of these two eventually died of melanoma.[3]

REFERENCES

1. Block, N.L., and Hotchkiss, R.S.: Malignant melanoma of the female urethra: Report of a case with 5-year survival and review of the literature. *J Urol* **105:**251, 1971.
2. Bracken, R.B., and Diokno, A.C.: Melanoma of the penis and the urethra: 2 case reports and review of the literature. *J Urol* **111:**198, 1974.
3. Morrow, C.P., and DiSaia, P.J.: Malignant melanoma of the female genitalia: A clinical analysis. *Obstet Gynecol Surv* **31:**233, 1976.

34

Melanoma of the Anal Canal

THE ANORECTAL REGION is a relatively uncommon area for malignant melanoma to
develop. In spite of that a substantial
number of case reports exist in the literature. The tumor has attracted the attention
of such authors as Laennec and Virchow
in the past. To date, approximately 200
cases have been described. In our view
this tumor is not that rare, especially in
major treatment centers. By most accounts
anal melanoma represents approximately
1% of all anorectal tumors and, conversely, 1.6% of all malignant melanomas
are to be found in this region.[1,9] According
to some, the relationship between malignant melanoma and anal carcinoma is
much higher, the former comprising 20%
or more of the growths in this location.[10,11]
These authors have excluded rectal lesions
when tabulating the incidence.

There is no sex predilection and the age
at onset is similar to that seen in patients
with malignant melanoma in other locations. The youngest patient recorded was
22 years old and the oldest, 95. The average is 55 years.

PATHOLOGY

There has been considerable debate as
to their origin, especially with regard to
the existence of melanoma within the rectum. Mason and Helwig[3] reviewed the
material of the Armed Forces Institute of
Pathology and discussed in their paper the

various theories of potential histogenesis.
It was their conclusion that melanoma is
associated almost always with the presence of pigmented cells. These cells are
absent above the anal pectinate line;
therefore melanotic tumors of the rectum
must be considered as metastatic in
character or as direct extensions of
melanomas arising in the anus.[3] The majority of melanomas occur in the
mucocutaneous junction or at the anal
verge.[6] This was the case in 65 of 68 cases
reviewed by Braastad et al.[1]

The gross appearance can be deceptive
and many of them have been initially
diagnosed as thrombosed hemorrhoids.
Their shape is that of a polypoid mass and
they are usually solitary tumors. However,
in 14% of the cases the lesions are multiple.[1,3,6,11]

In most cases the estimated diameter is
between 2 and 5 cm. The color may vary
from frankly black to violaceous but partial or complete depigmentation can be
seen.[1,3,6,7]

Histologically, the pigmentation of the
primary lesion may be markedly demonstrable, or demonstrable only by special
staining techniques. Approximately 50%
of the cases have strong pigmentation.[3]
The tumors are very cellular, containing a
large number of mitoses. Often they are so
anaplastic that, according to Morson and
Volkstädt,[4] the initial diagnosis in more
than 50% of the cases may be other than
malignant melanoma.[3,4,8]

Tumor extension can take place upward

along the submucosal layer into the rectum, manifesting eventually as a polyp within the rectal wall, laterally into the perianal tissues, as well as via the venous system and through the lymphatic system into the pelvic and inguinal lymph nodes.[4]

CLINICAL

Rectal bleeding is the usual presenting symptom. This may be accompanied by the presence of a mass, some disturbances in the bowel habits, and pain. In the more advanced cases and as the tumor enlarges prolapse through the anus of a penduculated mass can be seen.[8,11] The changes in the bowel habits could be either in the form of constipation or diarrhea.[2] The average duration of the symptoms prior to the diagnosis has been seven to nine months.[1,9]

On physical examination, the tumor is readily palpable in most instances; however, as mentioned, the clinical diagnosis often is incorrect. Most commonly, it has been called a thrombosed hemorrhoid or a nonspecific polypoid mass. The diagnosis is easier when strong pigmentation is present. Inguinal lymph node metastasis may exist at the time of the diagnosis.

TREATMENT AND RESULTS

The management of melanomas of the anorectum evolved from relatively simple local excision, to radical surgery, and then again, especially in recent years, to a more limited type of resection. It has become increasingly obvious that the prognosis is related to the pathological stage at the time of the diagnosis rather than to the extent of the surgery.[8,9] Braastad et al.[1] reviewed 86 cases of malignant melanoma in this region and they added eight more cases of their own. Of these, 61 underwent definitive surgery. In 34 instances the operation was a limited local removal and in the remaining 27 an abdominoperineal resection was carried out

combined in four cases with inguinal node dissection. The long-term results did not vary regardless of the type of surgical treatment performed. In eight patients radiotherapy was added, but it did not influence the survival either.[1]

Pack and Martins[6] advocated rather strongly radical surgery in the form of an abdominoperineal resection combined with pelvic lymph node dissection, bilateral inguinal and femoral node dissection, and removal of a wide strip of skin, subcutaneous tissue, and fascia intervening between the groin and the perineum. Unfortunately, their results do not support this form of management. The seven patients treated in this manner died from their disease, the average survival being 11 months.[6] Husa and Höckerstedt[2] reported in 1974 on 14 patients, of which five underwent abdominoperineal resection and seven, local excision. There was no tumor removal in the remaining two patients. The average survival time of the patients was 2.8 years and the survival curves looked identical for both the local excision and the abdominoperineal resection groups.[2]

The role of radiation therapy has been debated. In view of our own experience and that of others with high-dose radiotherapy in the management of malignant melanoma, it seems that radiotherapy in the form of local implantation may be considered if clinically indicated. The perineal region is known to be sensitive in tolerating high-dosage external beam programs.

PROGNOSIS AND SURVIVAL

The average life expectancy is in the range of 10–15 months. Patients with large, inoperable lesions live less than those on whom the disease is seemingly localized.[3,5,8] Actually, the extent of the disease at the time of the diagnosis appears to be the best prognostic indicator. This is well shown in the study by Husa and Höckerstedt.[2] The survival of patients with regional nodal involvement was 15% at 1.5 years. The survival of patients with localized tumors was 100% during the same interval of time. From this point on, however, the curve became identical to that of the advanced disease group.[2] In the series by Mason and Helwig[3] the average survival time was 15 months from the onset of the symptoms.

REFERENCES

1. Braastad, F.W., Dockerty, M.B., and Dixon, C.F.: Melano-epithelioma of the anus and rectum. Report of cases and review of literature. *Surgery* **25**:82, 1949.
2. Husa, A., and Höckerstedt, K.: Anorectal malignant melanoma. A report of fourteen cases. *Acta Chir Scand* **140**:68, 1974.
3. Mason, J.K., and Helwig, E.B.: Ano-rectal melanoma. *Cancer* **19**:39, 1966.
4. Morson, B.G., and Volkstädt, H.: Malignant melanoma of the anal canal. *J Clin Pathol* **16**:126, 1963.
5. Nyqvist, A., and Tillander, H.: Malignant melanoma of the anal canal. Report of two cases. *Acta Chir Scand* **135**:730, 1969.
6. Pack, G.T., and Martins, F.G.: Treatment of ano-rectal malignant melanoma. *Dis Colon Rectum* **3**:15, 1960.
7. Raven, R.W.: Anorectal malignant melanoma. *Proc R Soc Med* **41**:469, 1948.
8. Remigio, P.A., Der, B.K., and Forsberg, R.T.: Anorectal melanoma: Report of two cases. *Dis Colon Rectum* **19**:350, 1976.
9. Sergeev, S.L., Smirnova-Stetsenko, E.S., Golbert, S.V., Khrushchov, M.M., Simakina, E.P., and Oserskij, A.N.: Melanoma of the rectum. *Am J Proctol* **24**:411, 1973.
10. Sinclair, D.M., Hannah, G., McLaughlin, I.S., Patrick, R.S., Slavin, G., and Neville, A.M.: Malignant melanoma of the anal canal. *Br J Surg* **57**:808, 1970.
11. Singh, W., and Madaan, T.R.: Malignant melanoma of the anal canal. *Am J Proctol* **27**:49, 1976.

35

Mesothelioma of the Pericardium

THE MAJORITY OF malignant tumors of the pericardium are metastatic in character. Primary pericardial tumors are quite rare and of them mesothelioma is the one that has been described rather well in terms of clinical manifestations and histology. The incidence of pericardial mesothelioma is one case per year per 40 million population, according to epidemiological studies by McDonald et al.[6] Up to now, approximately 100 such cases have been reported in the literature.

In the present review, which includes older and more recent reports, we found the average age of the patients to be approximately 40 years. There is a higher incidence among males, the ratio of male to female being 3:1. The clinical histories thus far have not linked this specific site to asbestosis, as in the case of pleural and abdominal mesotheliomas.[1,3,9]

PATHOLOGY

In most cases the tumor is extensive. The pericardium is thick and tumor masses are present within the pericardial cavity. In this manner the myocardium is eventually invaded by the tumor. The superior and inferior vena cava are often encased by the masses, and, as a result, passive congestion of the face and of the upper and the lower extremities and hepatomegaly are encountered. A direct invasion of the cardiac muscle may produce conduction abnormalities and ero-

sion into a coronary artery may present as a myocardial infarct.

Pericardial mesotheliomas primarily expand by direct extension into the adjacent pleural spaces and less often they involve regional mediastinal lymph nodes. Metastases outside the thorax are quite rare.[4,9,7]

Histologically, pericardial mesotheliomas, have been classified as epithelial, fibrous, and mixed, as have those arising in the pleura. Stout and Murray[9] in 1942 on the basis of tissue culture studies showed that the fibrous spindle cell type of the neoplasm and the epithelial variety have common origin from mesothelial cells. It is therefore accepted now that they both represent a different histological appearance of the same tumor. Actually, in the majority of the cases the appearance is that of the fibrous variety or the mixed.[1] No prognostic significance related to the histology has been identified. The epithelial form consists of glandlike spaces and of large clefts that are lined by malignant tumor cells. The fibrous segments are composed of spindle or round cells whose arrangement may be orderly or they may be present without a distinct pattern.[1,3]

CLINICAL

The clinical manifestations are directly related to the constrictive action of the pericardial mesothelioma upon the heart and to the local extension of the tumor.

Thus, chest pain or discomfort associated with dyspnea and easy fatigability are the common prodromal signs. In addition elevated temperature, high pulse rate, and peripheral edema may accompany the clinical presentation.[4,10,11] Cough is sometimes productive, at other times not; venous hypertension, pericardial friction rub, and pulsus paradoxus have also been reported.[7]

Radiographically, chest examination on admission has shown in the majority of the cases an enlarged cardiac silhouette. This has led to the initial diagnosis of pericarditis or of heart failure. At this time, a nuclear scan determination will reveal a relatively small cardiac pool compared to the overall size of the heart, as seen on the films. Obviously, the thickness in question is due to the pericardial neoplasia and to the small pericardial effusions the neoplasm produces.[10] The electrocardiogram has not been very helpful. Signs of pericarditis are consistently reported. Radiographic vascular studies have shown irregularities of the chambers and compression upon major veins, the venae cavae, and the pulmonary artery.[4,10]

The patients as a rule have been diagnostic problems for their attending physicians. Their obvious heart failure is not responsive to cardiotonosis and it improves only moderately on diuretics. There has been often a good initial response when high doses of steroids were administered.[7,8] Steroids in conjunction with aspirin have brought about control of the temperature as well. Diagnostic pericardiocentesis has been attempted, since the diagnosis of pericarditis is commonly made. The cytological results have been variously reported; however, this may reflect the individual experience rather than the actual yield. It should be mentioned that the pericardial fluid in these cases is small in amount.

The disease has a rather rampant course. Following a short improvement brought about primarily because of the bed rest at the time of the initial diagnosis in most patients, readmission was required following their discharge within a short time and death came soon thereafter. It has been said that 60% of the patients are dead within the first six months.[5]

In earlier years, correct diagnosis was made during autopsy.[1] More recently, with advent of the cardiovascular surgical procedures, exploratory thoracotomy has been undertaken in practically all patients reported. Attempts at resecting the neoplasm have been made in a number of cases; however, the direct involvement by the tumor of the major vessels renders complete resection virtually impossible.[4,7,10] Radiation therapy at definitive dose levels has been used in the management of these patients. Sytman and MacAlpin[10] reported postoperative treatment of a fibrous mesothelioma, partially resected, by means of a cobalt-60 unit to a total tumor dose of 5128 rad. There was a marked reduction of the tumor size as observed radiographically, which was very short-lived. The patient died a few months later with local tumor present in the pericardium and, associated with it, metastatic deposits to the lungs and diaphragm.[10] Furman et al.[4] irradiated postoperatively at a tumor dose of 5100 rad a patient with partial resection of a biphasic mesothelioma. In nine months shortness of breath reappeared and nodular metastases to both lungs were evident.[4]

PROGNOSIS AND SURVIVAL

For practical purposes, this remains a lethal disease. Whether or not early diagnosis will lead to eventual salvage of some of these patients remains to be seen.[4] The diagnosis requires an extremely high index of suspicion. Pader and Kirschner[7] suggest that the following signs may be helpful: 1) recurrent pericardial effusion, hemorrhagic in character, in the absence of an inflammatory disease; 2) irregular

and enlarged cardiac silhouette radiographically; 3) refractory heart failure, and
4) unexplained chest pain. It is possible
that a well-circumscribed tumor can be
removed *in toto*; however, this represents
an uncommon situation.[2] The effects of
the currently available chemotherapeutic
agents on mesotheliomas are under study.

REFERENCES

1. Dawe, C.J., Wood, D.A., and Mitchell, S.: Diffuse fibrous mesothelioma of the pericardium. Report of a case and review of the literature. *Cancer* **6:**794, 1953.
2. Dooley, B.N., Beckmann, C., and Hood, R.H., Jr.: Primary mesothelioma of the pericardium. Successful surgical removal. *J Thorac Cardiovas Surg* **55:**719, 1968.
3. Fine, G.: Primary tumors of the pericardium and heart. *Cardiovasc Clin* **5:**208, 1973.
4. Furman, R., Bryant, L.R., Srivastava, T.N., Reeves, J., Weiss, D.L., and Castello, J.: Right ventricular mesothelioma with pulmonary obstruction. *Chest* **63:**642, 1973.
5. Mairot, A.: Contribution à l'étude des tumeurs primitives du pericarde. Thèse présenté a la faculté Mixte Medicine et de Pharmacie de Lyon. Mâcon, 1960.
6. McDonald, A.D., Harper, A., Attar, O.A., and McDonald, J.C.: Epidemiology of primary malignant mesothelial tumors in Canada. *Cancer* **26:**914, 1970.
7. Pader, E., and Kirschner, P.A.: Primary sarcoma of the pericardium. *Am J Cardiol* **14:**399, 1964.
8. Shin, M.S., Ho, K.J., and Liu, L.B.: Pericardial mesothelioma masquerading as rheumatic heart disease. *Arch Intern Med* **137:**257, 1977.
9. Stout, A.P. and Murray, M.R.: Localized pleural mesothelioma, investigation of its characteristics and histogenesis by the method of tissue culture. *Arch Path* **34:**951, 1942.
10. Sytman, A.L., and MacAlpin, R.N.: Primary pericardial mesothelioma: Report of two cases and review of the literature. *Am Heart J* **81:**760, 1971.
11. Vigneault, M., and Vanesse, R.: Sarcome primitif du coeur. Observation d'un cas de réticulosarcome du péricarde. *Can Med Assoc J* **100:**770, 1969.

36

Leiomyosarcoma of the Heart

THIS IS A RARE neoplasm among the primary cardiac tumors. Whorton[3] in a review of 100 cardiac primaries found only five leiomyosarcomas.

PATHOLOGY

The tumors attain a large size, involving primarily the ventricles. Histologically interlacing bundles of spindle and ovoid-shaped cells are found without cross striations.[1,2] The diagnosis of leiomyosarcoma requires exclusion of a primary site elsewhere in the body, with secondary involvement of the heart.

Due to the fact that all patients exhibit widespread metastases to several organs at the time of their death, it is indeed difficult to state with certainty whether or not primary leiomyosarcoma of the heart does actually exist.[1]

REFERENCES

1. Bearman, R.M.: Primary leiomyosarcoma of the heart. Report of a case and review of the literature. *Arch Pathol* **98**:62, 1974.
2. Kennedy, F.B.: Primary leiomyosarcoma of the heart. *Cancer* **20**:2008, 1967.
3. Whorton, C.M.: Primary malignant tumors of the heart. *Cancer* **2**:245, 1949.

37

Rhabdomyosarcoma of the Heart

THIRTY-FIVE CASES OF primary rhabdo-myosarcoma of the heart have been described. This uncommon cardiac neoplasm has been seen in patients of all ages, from young infants to octogenarians. Reviewing the literature, we found the median age to be 44 years. It appears that both sexes are equally affected.

PATHOLOGY AND HISTOLOGY

The tumor may arise in all the cardiac chambers, however the atria are more often involved than the ventricles.[1–5]

Microscopically there is polymorphism. Giant cells and mitoses are common. The tumor cells are rhabdomyoblasts and in order to establish the diagnosis, cross striations must be demonstrated within them. This can be easier done by electron microscopy.[1,4]

CLINICAL

The presenting symptoms are those of an intracardiac neoplasm, namely, pain in the chest, dyspnea, weakness, and dizziness. Radiographically, the heart is enlarged, with irregular borders. There are nonspecific electrocardiographic changes.

Practically all patients at the time of their death had disseminated metastatic disease. The commonest site of metastasis was the lungs, followed by the liver and the mediastinal lymph nodes. In several instances a widespread involvement of organs and tissues was encountered.[1–5]

TREATMENT AND RESULTS

Often the treatment has been only supportive and in most cases the diagnosis has been made during the postmortem examination. In more recent years, with the advent of modern radiology and cardiovascular surgery, isolated case reports have been published, detailing definitive therapy. Thus, Matloff *et al.*, reported on a 46-year-old female whose tumor arose in the left atrium. Following surgical resection, the first local recurrence developed five months later. At this time, the left atrial wall, including the atrial appendage with all gross tumor, were excised. Megavoltage radiotherapy to the heart followed, the patient receiving 4950 rad in 32 days. Simultaneously, she was placed on a maintenance dosage of Natulan, 100 mg/day. Death occurred 34 months after the original diagnosis, because of widespread extracardiac metastases to the brain, the liver, and the gastrointestinal tract.[3]

Gerdes *et al.*[2] presented a 68-year-old male with a presumptive diagnosis of atrial septum rhabdomyosarcoma, whose presenting sign was bilateral lung metastases. Following biopsy, radiotherapy was used for the lung tumors, which responded well to dosages of 5500 rad in five to six weeks. The patient died of congestive heart failure two years after the initial diagnosis. The cardiac tumor was found at autopsy.[2]

The just-described cases indicate that prolongation of life is possible by combining treatment modalities. Surgery remains the preferable choice, but it tends to be incomplete because of the extent and invasiveness of the tumors. It appears that ionizing radiation may cause regression of cardiac rhabdomyosarcomas and certainly it should be used in their management. Systemic combination chemotherapy is another consideration for this neoplasm.

REFERENCES

1. Bemis, E.L., Pemberton, A.H., and Lurie, A.: Rhabdomyosarcoma of the heart. *Cancer* **29:**924, 1972.

2. Gerdes, A.J., Parker, R.G., and Berry, H.C.: Pleomorphic rhabdomyosarcoma: Response to irradiation. *Radiol Clin (Basel)* **44:**97, 1975.

3. Matloff, J.M., Bass, H., and Dalen, J.E.: Rhabdomyosarcoma of the left atrium. Physiologic responses to surgical therapy. *J Thorac Cardiovasc Surg* **61:**451, 1971.

4. Porter, G.A., Berroth, M., and Bristow, J.D.: Primary rhabdomyosarcoma of the heart and complete atrioventricular block. A case report and review of the literature. *Am J Med* **31:**820, 1961.

5. Pund, E.E., Jr., Collier, T.M., Cunningham, J.E., Jr., and Hayes, J.R.: Primary cardiac rhabdomyosarcoma presenting as pulmonary stenosis. *Am J Cardiol* **12:**249, 1963.

38

Fibrosarcoma of the Heart

A NUMBER OF well-documented cases of fibrosarcoma of the heart exist in the literature. Apparently there is a wide age variation, from the very young to the very old.[1-5]

PATHOLOGY

The tumors can be found with equal frequency in all four cardiac chambers and in the pericardium.

Microscopically, they are composed of fibroblasts that are surrounded by variable quantities of collagen. The cells are round to oval and sometimes irregular in shape. Spindle-shaped forms can also be seen. There is considerable variation in the size, shape, and mitotic activity of the cells, as well as in the amount of the collagen material present.[2-4]

CLINICAL

The clinical signs are related primarily to the location of the tumor. When arising in the right ventricle, they produce pulmonary outflow obstruction. Arrhythmias are frequently present and when there is pericardial involvement pain, fever, and dyspnea exist. Actually, all patients have dyspnea as one of the presenting symptoms associated with weakness and fatigue. In general the clinical and electrocardiographic and radiographic signs are those of an intracardiac tumor.

TREATMENT AND RESULTS

The diagnosis was made in four patients by means of cardiac catheterization and selective angiocardiography preoperatively. These procedures permitted exploratory surgery and ventriculotomy to be performed in three cases.[2-4] During the operation, the bulk of the tumor was resected.[2-4] The patient described by Baldelli et al.[1] had a large-sized tumor of the right ventricle, which was judged to be inoperable. Following surgery, all four patients received postoperative radiotherapy. The patient described by Dong et al.[2] received a tumor dose of 5392 rad to the right ventricle in a six-week period. There was clinical and radiographical improvement. The previously stenotic pulmonary outflow tract returned practically to normal limits as repeat angiocardiography demonstrated.[2] He died one year postoperatively of brain metastases.[3] Sagerman et al.[5] delivered 6300 rad in 41 days to a 55-year-old female following the diagnosis of fibromyxosarcoma involving the anterior wall of the right ventricle, which was incompletely excised. The patient died free of cardiac symptoms one year later. Here, as in the previous patient, brain metastases was the cause of death.[4] Goldstein and Mahoney[3] reported on a 19-year-old female with a right ventricular fibrosarcoma. The tumor was grossly removed and following recovery the patient received postoperatively radiotherapy at the level of 7000 rad to the heart. She died of metastatic lung and liver disease in six months. The patient reported by Baldelli et al.[1] had a fibrosarcoma arising in the left ventricle. Following biopsy, the patient received 5400 rad in 38 days to the heart. The radiological pattern remained unchanged. The patient's condition deteriorated progressively and she died one year following the diagnosis.[1]

There are no reports on systemic chemotherapy for fibrosarcomas in this location.

REFERENCES

1. Baldelli, P., De Angeli, D., Dolara, A., Diligenti, L.M., Marchi, F., and Salvatore, L.: Primary fibrosarcoma of the heart. *Chest* **62:**234, 1972.
2. Dong, E., Jr., Hurley, E.J., and Shumway, N.E.: Primary cardiac sarcoma. *Am J Cardiol* **10:**871, 1962.
3. Goldstein, S., and Mahoney, E.B.: Right ventricular fibrosarcoma causing pulmonic stenosis. *Am J Cardiol* **17:**570, 1966.
4. McAllister, H.A., Jr., and Fenoglio, J.J., Jr.: *Tumors of the Cardiovascular System.* Armed Forces Institute of Pathology, Washington, D.C., 1978.
5. Sagerman, R.H., Hurley, E., and Bagshaw, M.A.: Successful sterilization of a primary cardiac sarcoma by supervoltage radiation therapy. *AJR* **92:**942, 1964.

39

Intracardiac Teratoma

THIS IS AN EXTREMELY rare tumor, five cases of which have been described in the English literature. Of these, three were malignant and two were benign teratomas. All patients, with one exception, were children.[2]

PATHOLOGY

The tumors have occurred primarily in the right cardiac chambers, originating from the interatrial and interventricular septum. Histologically, in the benign form derivatives of all three germ layers, including bone, cartilage, smooth muscle, and neural tissue, have been found. The malignant type is generally solid, composed of poorly differentiated epithelial cells forming glandlike structures intermingled with fibrocollagenous or myxomatous stroma.[2,3]

CLINICAL

The presenting symptoms in the case described by Arshadi and Watson[1] were dyspnea and tachycardia; however, the patients of Cabañas and Moore[2] and of Solomon[3] had as first manifestation the development of distant metastases. The sites were the lungs and the spine. In all patients, including those with benign teratomas, the diagnosis was made postmortem and no specific treatment had been rendered.

REFERENCES

1. Arshadi, S., and Watson, D.G.: Teratocarcinoma of the heart. Case report and review of primary malignancies in children. *Am J Dis Child* **112:**87, 1966.
2. Cabañas, V.Y., and Moore, W.M.: Malignant teratoma of the heart. *Arch Pathol* **96:**399, 1973.
3. Solomon, R.D.: Malignant teratoma of the heart. Report of case with necropsy. *Arch Pathol* **52:**561, 1951.

40

Chondrosarcoma of the Larynx

CHONDROSARCOMA OF THE larynx represents an uncommon but well-established entity. In general, cartilaginous tumors originate from the laryngeal cartilages and the majority of them are benign in character. The ratio of benign to malignant cartilaginous laryngeal neoplasms is in the range of 4:1.[8] Bang and Nilsen[1] encountered one chondrosarcoma among 707 malignant laryngeal tumors. Earlier, Huizenga and Balogh,[4] reviewing the experience at Massachusetts General Hospital, found eight chondrosarcomas among 5000 primary laryngeal neoplasms. It can therefore be said that chondrosarcomas comprise 0.14–0.16% of the laryngeal malignancies.

Approximately 70% of the patients are males, an observation made in more than one series.[4,5] The majority are in their fifth and sixth decades of life.

PATHOLOGY

Chondrosarcomas originate from the laryngeal cartilages. Although benign chondromas have occurred in the vocal cords, no such a case of malignant chondrosarcoma has been reported. There is a distinct predilection for the cricoid cartilage. In the series by Hyams and Rabuzzi[5] 11 of 16 laryngeal chondrosarcomas (68.7%) were seen in the cricoid cartilage. In the same series four occurred in the thyroid cartilage and one in the arytenoids.[5] In the series by Huizenga and Balogh[4] five were seen in the cricoid and

three in the arytenoid cartilage. In the series by Goethals et al.[3] all but two of the 18 chondrosarcomas arose in the cricoid cartilage. Few cases of epiglotic primaries have been reported.[5]

The tumor presents with a smooth and hard surface and lies submucosally. Usually, diagnostic biopsies are difficult to obtain because of the overlying normal epithelium and because of the hardness of the tumor.[2] Chondrosarcomas arise only from the hyaline cartilage of the larynx and no such tumors were found originating from the elastic cartilage.[5]

The criteria of malignancy, or of benignity for that matter, are those established by Lichtenstein and Jaffe[6] regarding the cartilagenous tumors in general. Thus, many cells with plump nuclei, many cells with two such nuclei, giant cartilage cells with large single or multiple nuclei or with clumps of chromatin are all histological criteria of a malignant lesion. Differentiation further into low-grade chondrosarcomas may be possible; however, additional information from the clinical history at this point is quite helpful in determining the course of the disease.[2,4]

CLINICAL

Because the majority of the tumors arise from the cricoid cartilage, they are subglottic in location and therefore the primary and most common presenting symptom is that of dyspnea. Mild dyspnea might be present for long periods of time until suddenly severe difficulties develop, manifested as episodes of cough with choking or with what appears to be clinically a situation of laryngeal edema accompanied by thick tenacious mucous secretions. Changes in the tone of the voice, such as dysphonia and a whispering voice, may appear. There is no hemoptysis as a rule. Should the tumor be growing toward the surface of the neck, a lump in the neck will be the presenting symptom and complaint.[2–4] Dysphagia has also been encountered due to esophageal narrowing by posterior protrusion of the tumor. A barium swallow will demonstrate a smooth defect at the subglottic level.[4] Tumors arising from the thyroid cartilage will produce primarily a neck mass with minimal airway obstruction.[5]

On physical examination, an external mass in the neck may be palpable. Otherwise indirect laryngoscopy will reveal a submucosal, smooth, round, and nodular, tumor covered by normal mucous membrane. Direct laryngoscopy will prove its hard nature and it is possible that the surgeon manages only to biopsy the overlying normal mucosa.[1,2,7] Radiographic examination is quite helpful in delineating the extent of the tumor. Tomograms and barium swallow examinations have proved their value. Roentgen examination will also give hints as to the possible diagnosis because calcium or osseous formations may be seen within the mass.[1] (Fig. 40-1).

Metastases to the regional lymph nodes are extremely rare and for all practical purposes they will not occur unless local persistent disease is present. Only 1 of 16 patients reported by Hyams and Rabuzzi[5] was found to have at autopsy cervical lymph node involvement that accompanied local recurrence and metastases to the lungs.[5]

TREATMENT AND RESULTS

It is the consensus of all authors, particularly those reporting on larger series,

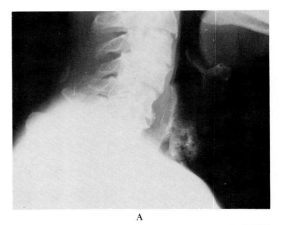

A

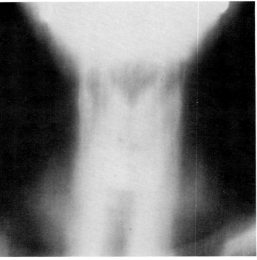

B

FIG. 40-1.   Chondrosarcoma of the larynx in a 68-year-old male. Lateral soft tissue view of the neck demonstrates a large tumor mass in the larynx just below the vocal cords. The tumor contains calcified cartilage (A). Anterior tomogram shows a massive tumor almost completely obstructing the laryngeal lumen (B).

that the proper therapy is surgical. Radiotherapy is not recommended for this neoplasm. In spite of the malignant nature of the lesion the advocated approach is conservative, and actually it is suggested that the initial surgical procedure should be the same for chondromas and chondrosarcomas. Obviously, total removal of the tumor should be done in order to avoid local recurrence, but the procedure should be as conservative as possible in order to accomplish this goal. The neoplasms are slowly growing and rarely spread beyond the larynx or distally. Taking into consideration the age of the patient and the long natural history, a disease-free interval of several years could be provided by a conservative approach and a total laryngectomy could be applied later, if needed.[4,7] A recurrence may require five or more years to become clinically obvious, as was the case in the series by Huizenga and Balogh,[4] at which point further surgery could be performed. In a literature review by the same authors, which included 37 chondrosarcomas, four patients had primary and four had secondary total laryngectomies. None of these eight tumors recurred. Among the 25 patients on whom thyrotomy or laryngofissure was performed, at least nine developed recurrence, the periods of time ranging from six months to eight years postoperatively.[4]

PROGNOSIS AND SURVIVAL

The prognosis is good, especially for patients whose tumor has been removed completely. A number of patients have died because of local recurrence alone or in association with pulmonary metastases.[4,5] Some postoperative deaths have also been recorded.

Our literature review shows that the mortality rate due to the previously mentioned causes is in the range of 20%.

REFERENCES

1. Bang, G., and Nilsen, R.: Chondrosarkom i larynx. En oversikt og rapport av et tilfelle. *Nord Med* **86:**1050, 1971.
2. Brandenburg, J.H., Harris, D.D., and Bennett, M.: Chondrosarcoma of the larynx. *Laryngoscope* **77:**752, 1967.
3. Goethals, P., Dahlin, D., and Devine, K.: Cartilaginous tumors of the larynx. *Surg Gynecol Obstet* **117:**77, 1963.
4. Huizenga, C., and Balogh, K.: Cartilaginous tumors of the larynx. A clinicopathologic study of 10 new cases and a review of the literature. *Cancer* **26:**201, 1970.
5. Hyams, V.J., and Rabuzzi, D.D.: Cartilaginous tumors of the larynx. *Laryngoscope* **80:**755, 1970.
6. Lichtenstein, L., and Jaffe, H.L.: Chondrosarcoma of bone. *Am J Pathol* **19:**553, 1943.
7. Swerdlow, R.S., Som, M.L., and Biller, H.F.: Cartilaginous tumors of the larynx. *Arch Otolaryngol* **100:**269, 1974.
8. Witten, B.R.: The Resident's page. *Arch Otolaryngol* **100:**76, 1974.

41

Extraskeletal Chondrosarcoma

CHONDROSARCOMAS ARE cartilaginous malignant neoplasms primarily associated with the skeletal system. There is evidence to suggest that the majority arise from preexisting, seemingly benign chondromatous tumors. A rare, histologically related tumor originating in the extraskeletal soft tissues was first described by Stout and Verner in 1952.[3] Since then, less than 50 such cases have been reported in the literature.[1,2,4]

The tumors are associated with or actually involve muscle and less often tendons or ligaments. Their primary location is the extremities, particularly the lower where 83% of them have been reported.[1,3] Although most are deep within the muscle, a smaller percentage (approximately 30%) are located in the subcutaneous tissues, remaining separated from the overlying skin.[1]

The average age of the patients has been 46 years.[1–4] However, there is no clear "age peak" and it appears that persons of all ages can develop the tumor. The number of cases available is rather small, but there is a slight male predominance.[1–4]

PATHOLOGY

The gross appearance is that of a lobulated or nodular growth that appears to be well circumscribed and easily detachable from the surrounding tissues. It is somewhat softer in consistency and gelatinous in appearance on the cut surface. Hemorrhages are frequently present within the tumor mass.[1,2] The size has varied from a few to 20 cm or more.[1–4]

Histologically, small uniform cells are to be found rounded or slightly elongated with an eosinophilic cytoplasm and a small hyperchromatic nucleus. Mitotic figures are rarely present and the arrangement of the cells is that of cords, strands, and clusters. Accompanying them is a large amount of myxoid substance whose tinctorial and histochemical characteristics are those of chondroblastic tissue.[1] Fibrous connective tissue surrounds the tumor from which fibrous septa divide the neoplasm into compartments of varying size and shape. The presence of abundant avascular myxoid extracellular matrix is characteristic of these neoplasms and for this reason the term "myxoid chondrosarcoma" has been attached to tumors originating in the soft tissues.[1,3,4]

CLINICAL

The commonest presenting symptom is that of a mass the presence of which has varied from a few weeks to several years. In the series reported by Enzinger and Shiraki[1] the average waiting period prior to seeking medical help was 13 months. Pain or tenderness accompanied the tumor in approximately one-third of the cases.[1,3] Radiographs of the area have failed to show bony involvement and no calcium deposits have been observed within the masses.

On physical examination, apparently the tumors are easily felt, lying deep within the muscle substance and some lying directly below the skin. Their consistency is firm and their margins are easily outlined. The majority of them have a slow growth rate.[1-3]

TREATMENT AND RESULTS

Complete surgical resection is the treatment to be undertaken. This type of management resulted in locally controlling the disease of approximately 75% of the patients. In the remaining further surgery, including amputation, was necessary.[2,3] Recurrence may develop several years following the surgical procedure, indicating that the tumor is of low biological aggressiveness. There are several patients known to have survived for long periods of time following the development of recurrence or metastases. The regional lymph nodes and the lungs have been the commonest metastatic sites.[1,2]

PROGNOSIS AND SURVIVAL

The opinion is expressed that chondrosarcoma of the soft tissues has a better prognosis and a more indolent course than its skeletal counterpart. The five-year-survival rate, as compiled from the series by Enzinger and Shiraki[1] and corrected for deaths from intercurrent diseases, was 68.4%. It is to be said, however, that five-year survival is not synonymous with cure. Actually, a number of patients were living at that time with recurrences present and an even greater number developed local recurrence or distant metastases past the five year point.[2]

REFERENCES

1. Enzinger, F.M., and Shiraki, M.: Extraskeletal myxoid chondrosarcoma. An analysis of 34 cases. *Hum Pathol* **3**:421, 1972.
2. Smith, M.T., Farinacci, C.J., Carpenter, H.A., and Bannayan, G.A.: Extraskeletal myxoid chondrosarcoma. A clinicopathological study. *Cancer* **37**:821, 1976.
3. Stout, A.P., and Verner, E.W.: Chondrosarcoma of the extraskeletal soft tissues. *Cancer* **6**:581, 1953.
4. Weiss, S.W.: Ultrastructure of the so-called "chordoid sarcoma." Evidence supporting cartilagenous differentiation. *Cancer* **37**:300, 1976.

42

Synovial Sarcoma of the Head and Neck

THE TERM "synovioma" was applied by Smith[18] in 1927 to a group of malignant tumors that were primarily located in the extremities and specifically found in association with peripheral joints. Subsequent reviews published on this soft tissue sarcoma pointed out specific clinical features. The tumors comprise approximately 8% of all soft tissue sarcomas. They arise in the region of the joint capsule, being related to articular surfaces, tendons, and bursae. The commonest site is the knee joint. Generally, 50% are to be seen in the lower extremities. There is a male preponderance in the range of 3:2, most of the patients being young adults 20–40 years old.

Due to their distinct histological features, it was assumed that the synovial tissues were directly related in the formation of these neoplasms. This opinion had to be revised, however, for Jernstrom in 1954, reported an increasing number of synovial sarcomas arising in the region of the head and neck.[8] Now it is held that for all synovial sarcomas the tissue of origin is undifferentiated mesenchyme, which has retained the potential of differentiating along synovial lines. This assumption is necessary in order to explain the presence of synovial sarcomas occurring away from joints or articular surfaces, such as the synovial sarcomas found in the head and neck and in the anterior abdominal wall.[2,17]

Since the original report by Jernstrom, 43 cases of synovial sarcoma in the region of the head and neck have been reported. In tabulating the location of these neoplasms we found 50% occurring in the neck and requiring an external approach for their removal, 30% in the laryngopharynx, 10% being of retropharyngeal origin, and the remaining 10% occurring in the oral cavity. The ratio of male to female patients is 2:1 and the average age at the time of the diagnosis is approximately 27 years.[1,2,4,6,7,9,11–14,17]

PATHOLOGY

Generally, the tumors are well-circumscribed solitary masses, at times covered by a thin fibrous membrane. Their size ranges from a few centimeters to growths as large as 10.0 cm in diameter; however, on the average their greatest diameter is 5.0 cm. They may be attached to the surrounding structures rather firmly and this intimate association may require removal of the involved muscles, nerves, or vessels.[6,17] Those located in the oral cavity and oropharynx usually retain an intact overlying mucosa.

Histologically, there are no differences between synovial sarcomas occurring in the head and neck region and those occurring in the extremities. The basic microscopic pattern is that of a biphasic cellular population composed of epithelioid cells arranged in nests, clefts, and acini surrounded by areas of stroma, having an appearance similar to that of fibrosarcoma

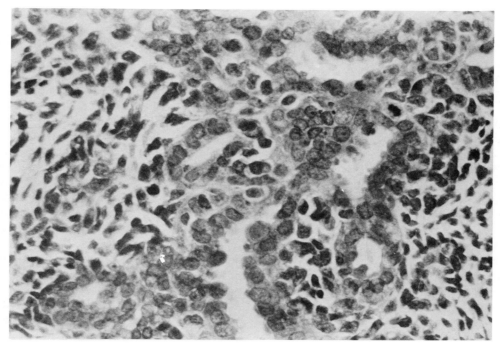

FIG. 42-1. Synovial sarcoma of the head and neck. Biphasic pattern: glandlike areas against a background of sarcomatous stroma.

(Fig. 42-1). The epithelioid cells that form pseudoglandular structures are rather plump, containing pale vesicular and homogeneous nuclei. Amorphous eosinophilic material is often to be found within these structures, which is positive to mucicarmine and periodic and Schiff and alcian blue stains. The stromal component is made up of uniform spindle cells with poorly defined cytoplasm and elongated nuclei.[6,14] Electron microscopic studies have shown the presence of a basement membrane interposed between the pseudoepithelial and the sarcomatous component of the tumor. Roth et al.,[17] reporting on 24 synovial sarcomas of the head and neck studied at the Armed Forces Institute of Pathology, concluded that on the basis of the histological, histochemical, and electron microscopic features these tumors are undoubtedly of synovioblastic origin, indistinguishable from those found in the extremities. It is the opinion of all authors dealing with the subject that synovial structures are not necessarily the tissues giving origin to the neoplasm. Rather, the accepted formation of synovial sarcoma in the head and neck region at least, is the development of a tumor from undifferentiated mesenchyme located among the anatomical structures of the neck. This tissue has retained the potential ability of producing synoviumlike structures.[1,2,4,17]

CLINICAL

The presence of a soft tissue mass, painless in the great majority of cases, is the commonest presenting symptom. The interval between the appearance of the tumor and the time of the diagnosis is in the range of 6–12 months. Those protruding laterally into the neck are otherwise symptomless; however, those located in the region of the oral cavity, oropharynx, and the laryngopharynx have eventually caused swallowing difficulties and respiratory embarrassment.[7,9,11–13] On occasion, lateral neck tumors have caused symptoms related to the brachial plexus.[2,17]

Physical examination has readily revealed the presence of a mass lesion; however, the correct diagnosis, as expected, has never been established preoperatively or intraoperatively, for that matter. Thyroid carcinoma has been the commonest working diagnosis for externally located tumors and very commonly a thyroidectomy has been performed along with the removal of the mass.[2,9] The incidence of regional lymph node involvement is very low. In the present review, which includes 43 patients, we found only one reported as having metastatic lymph node disease.[17] Metastatic lymph node involvement in peripheral synovial sarcomas reportedly occurs in 20% of the cases.

TREATMENT AND RESULTS

Surgical resection should be the primary mode of therapy; however, reports in recent years indicate that there is a definite role to be played by radiotherapy and chemotherapy. Complete resection of the tumor is necessary to achieve cures; however, such an approach might not be always possible in the head and neck region. In addition a number of patients have refused mutilating surgery. The feasibility of complete resection is higher for those lesions appearing in the external surface of the neck because they can be directly approached. The success of resection is reflected best when comparing the rates of local recurrence for lesions of the neck as opposed to those occurring in the oropharynx and laryngopharynx. In the former local recurrences were observed at the rate of approximately 20%, whereas in the latter 53% of the patients returned with recurrent tumors. Because of this high rate, postoperative radiotherapy and systemic chemotherapy should be given stronger consideration. Pack and Ariel[15] reported that all nine of their 60 patients with malignant synovioma who were alive and free of disease for five years or more had been treated with a combination of surgery and radiation therapy.

The value of radiotherapy as a palliative modality has been established by other authors as well.[3,16] Novotny and Fort reported on a 20-year-old male with synovial sarcoma of the base of the tongue. This was treated, following biopsy, definitively by cobalt-60 teletherapy with what can be considered a split course program (3000 rad in two weeks, three-week intermission, 3000 rad in two weeks). There was complete resolution of the tumor and no recurrence occurred during the two years of follow-up.[13] Attie et al.[1] reported on a 15-year-old female with an extensive tumor in the left side of the neck that was only partially resected and postoperatively irradiated to a total dose of 6000 rad. The patient was free of disease 10 years following her treatment. Postoperative radiotherapy has been utilized in many instances following surgery.[6,17]

Gerner and Moore,[5] reporting on 34 cases of peripheral synovial sarcoma, found the antitumor effect of Adriamycin to be encouraging because objective responses were noted in four of seven patients treated. Four patients had disseminated disease. It was noteworthy that reduction of the size of the lesions greater than 75% was observed in one of these four patients and three years elapsed prior to the development of new lesions.[5]

Local recurrence, although a serious sign, does not necessarily imply a hopeless outcome. Several patients have been salvaged following further surgery, either alone or combined with local radiotherapy.[17] Lung metastasis is the commonest development. Metastatic deposits to the bones have also been noted.[9,17]

PROGNOSIS AND SURVIVAL

Synovial sarcoma has a rather slow progress rate and metastases tend to develop late in the course of the disease. It is for this reason that several years are necessary in order to assess treatment results.[5] The five-year-survival rate in the early series reported by Pack and Ariel[15] was found to be 23.5%; however, subsequent reports show improvement perhaps related to both technique and understanding of the disease. Thus, MacKenzie[10] reported 51% disease-free five-year survival. Raben *et al.* reported 33% five-year-survival rate based on 38 cases of malignant synovioma referred to the Bone Service at Memorial Hospital.[16] As far as synovial sarcomas in the head and neck region are concerned, Roth *et al.*[17] found that the clinical behavior was identical to that of synovial sarcomas in other locations. Their five-year-survival rate was 47% and this was based on a follow-up of 24 cases diagnosed at the Armed Forces Institute of Pathology. Prognostically, perhaps, the tumor size is the most crucial factor. Tumors of large size carry the less favorable prognosis.

REFERENCES

1. Attie, J.N., Steckler, R.M., and Platt, N.: Cervical synovial sarcoma. *Cancer* **25**:758, 1970.
2. Batsakis, J.G., Nishiyama, R.H., and Sullinger, G.D.: Synovial sarcomas of the neck. *Arch Otolaryngol* **85**:113, 1967.
3. Berman, H.L.: The role of radiation therapy in the management of synovial sarcoma. *Radiology* **81**:997, 1963.
4. Gatti, W.M., Strom, C.G., and Orfei, E.: Synovial sarcoma of the laryngopharynx. *Arch Otolaryngol* **101**:633, 1975.
5. Gerner, R.E., and Moore, G.E.: Synovial sarcoma. *Ann Surg* **181**:22, 1975.
6. Golomb, H.M., Gorny, J., Powell, W., Graff, P., and Ultmann, J.E.: Cervical synovial sarcoma at the bifurcation of the carotid artery. *Cancer* **35**:483, 1975.
7. Jacobs, L.A., and Weaver, A.W.: Synovial sarcoma of the head and neck. *Am J Surg* **128**:527, 1974.
8. Jernstrom, P.: Synovial sarcoma of the pharynx. Report of a case. *Am J Clin Pathol* **24**:957, 1954.
9. Krugman, M.E., Rosin, H.D., and Toker, C.: Synovial sarcoma of the head and neck. *Arch Otolaryngol* **98**:53, 1973.
10. MacKenzie, D.H.: Synovial sarcoma. A review of 58 cases. *Cancer* **19**:169, 1966.
11. Miller, L.H., Santaella-Latimer, L., and Miller, T.: Synovial sarcoma of the larynx. *Trans Am Acad Ophthalmol Otolaryngol* **80**:448, 1975.
12. Moussavi, H., and Ghodsi, S.: Synovial sarcoma of the tongue, report of a case. *J Laryngol Otol* **88**:795, 1974.
13. Novotny, G.M., and Fort, T.C.: Synovial sarcoma of the tongue. *Arch Otolaryngol* **94**:77, 1971.
14. Nunez-Alonso, C., Gashti, E.N., and Christ, M.L.: Maxillofacial synovial sarcoma. Light- and electron-microscopic study of two cases. *Am J Surg Pathol* **3**:23, 1979.
15. Pack, G.T., and Ariel, I.M.: Synovial sarcoma (malignant synovioma): Report of 60 cases. *Surgery* **28**:1047, 1950.
16. Raben, M., Calabrese, A., Higinbotham, N.L., and Phillips, R.: Malignant synovioma. *AJR* **93**:145, 1965.
17. Roth, J.A., Enzinger, F.M., and Tannenbaum, M.: Synovial sarcoma of the neck: A followup study of 24 cases. *Cancer* **35**:1243, 1975.
18. Smith, L.W.: Synoviomata. *Am J Pathol* **3**:355, 1927.

43

Extramedullary Plasmacytoma

PLASMA CELL neoplasias have a variety of clinical presentations whose basic underlying cause is the same, namely, proliferation of plasma cells. According to Batsakis et al.[1] there is an interrelationship between all the plasma cell dyscrasias. The cells are derived from progenitor reticulum cells existing in their primitive and pleuripotential state in or outside the bone marrow. Thus, solitary myeloma, multiple myeloma, and diffuse myelomatosis arise from progenitor cells of the bone marrow, whereas extramedullary plasmacytoma arises from extramedullary progenitor reticulum cells. Extramedullary plasmacytoma may lead to diffuse myelomatosis or multiple myeloma and reversely diffuse myelomatosis and multiple myeloma may result in extramedullary plasma cell deposits. On pure clinical criteria and on the basis of the extent of the disease at the time of diagnosis, Willis[29] has classified plasmacytomas into three groups. Group I includes patients with typical multiple myeloma having generalized bone disease with characteristic radiographic and biochemical findings. Group II contains solitary plasmacytoma of the bone without signs of generalized disease at the time of the diagnosis. Finally, Group III deals with primary plasmacytomas of the soft tissues; namely, with tumors arising in tissues other than bone without signs of generalized disease at the time of presentation.[29]

The overwhelming majority of ex-tramedullary plasmacytomas arise in the upper respiratory tract and in the region of the oropharynx. In our present review we will deal first with these tumors and in a separate segment we will review the literature with reference to plasmacytomas occurring in other locations.

EXTRAMEDULLARY PLASMACYTOMA OF THE UPPER RESPIRATORY TRACT AND THE OROPHARYNX

The commonest sites of involvement by extramedullary plasmacytomas are the nose, nasopharynx, and paranasal sinuses. This has been the experience of several major United States institutions.[4,14,20,26] Other areas of involvement include the tonsils, the pharynx, and the oral cavity. Virtually every site of the head and neck region has been reported as giving rise to plasmacytomas. The palate, gingiva, the floor of the mouth, the tongue, the larynx, the trachea all have been sites of extramedullary plasmacytomas.[1,8,12,18,19,25] Dolin and Dewar[6] reviewed 161 cases and found that 78.1% of the tumors occurred in the upper respiratory tract and the oral cavity. The quoted incidence of plasmacytomas in these regions in relationship to other malignancies is in the range of 0.5–1.0%.[20]

Most of the patients are older than 50 years of age.[8,14,20] Stout and Kenney[25] reviewed primary plasma cell tumors of the upper respiratory tract in 104 patients.

Three-quarters of the cases developed during the fifth, sixth, and seventh decades of life.[25] In terms of sex all reports point to a definite male predominance. In the series by Stout and Kenney[25] the ratio of male to female was 4:1; however, in subsequent reviews a 2:1 male preponderance was noted.[4,8]

Pathology

The gross appearance is that of a sessile or polypoid growth covered by mucosa. The color is gray-red to deep red because of their increased vascularity. Ulceration may occur. As they grow, lobulation of the surface develops.[1,26] The submucosal location of the tumors is considered an important feature.[20]

Microscopically, differential diagnosis is necessary from the so-called "reactive plasma cell granulomas." The latter are inflammatory conditions of the upper respiratory tract.[1] They have a distinct histological appearance, because they contain a considerable variety of other inflammatory cells, in addition to the plasma cells.

A true plasma cell neoplasm consists of a solid growth of plasma cells in masses that are separated by septa of connective tissue displaying an infiltrative growth.[25] (Fig. 43-1). The morphological features of the plasma cells are related to the maturity of the cell. In any given lesion a mixture of plasma cells of various degrees of maturity may be present. The diagnosis rests upon finding and recognizing the more mature plasma cells. They possess an eccentrically placed dark staining nucleus similar to the one of the normal plasma cell. The more immature forms are composed of larger cells with an increased nuclear size, the position of the nucleus being more central. Mitotic figures are rarely seen.[1] Ewing and Foote[8] found no relationship between histological variations and prognosis.

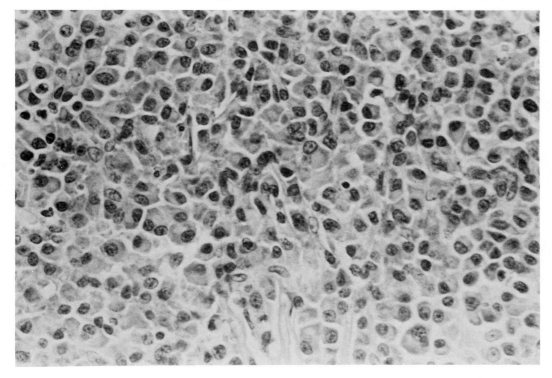

FIG. 43-1. Extramedullary plasmacytoma. Monotonous proliferation of plasma cells, some of them being binucleated. The tumor arose in the nasopharynx.

Atypical cellular properties did not indicate any greater propensity for the disease to become generalized.[8]

Finally, the presence of tumor amyloid detected in a small number of patients does not appear to affect the prognosis. Systemic amyloidosis has not been reported.[1,26]

Clinical

The symptoms are site related. The clinical appearance of the tumor is generally that of an exophytic growth, at times attached to a pedicle and at times broad-based. Those arising in the nasal cavity and paranasal sinuses obstruct the airways. In addition to the obstruction, epistaxis and mucoid rhinorrhea are present.[4,8,14]

For those tumors arising in the oral cavity, a mass, at times ulcerated, and pain are the presenting signs. Laryngeal plasmacytomas manifest themselves with hoarseness of the voice and at times dyspnea. Plasmacytomas of the middle ear present with deafness, otorrhea, and pain.[12,20,26] Lymph node involvement from primary plasmacytoma of the upper respiratory tract has been reported to be in the range of 12–25% and actually this may be the presenting symptom.[9,20,26]

Due to the symptomatology, several patients have been treated for sinusitis or other benign conditions for some time. In a number of cases epistaxis has led directly to the discovery of the tumor.[26] The duration of the symptoms prior to the diagnosis varies from one month to two years.[19] Local bone destruction believed to be secondary to invasion from adjacent soft tissue has been observed. It is the opinion of most authors that this is of prognostic significance because most of these patients have died of their disease.[26] In the series of Kotner and Wang,[14] however, two of four patients with local bone destruction survived longer than five years.

Urine examinations for Bence-Jones protein and serum protein electrophoresis are within normal limits in patients with localized plasmacytomas.[4,14] However, exceptions to this general situation do exist. Fishkin and Spiegelberg[9] described a patient with plasmacytoma originating in the epiglottis whose tumor synthesized IgD, λ myeloma protein (M-protein). This was detected both in the serum and the urine, the abnormal protein disappearing within four months of the completion of radiotherapy to the epiglottic tumor.[9]

Treatment and Results

Surgery and radiation therapy have been used in the management. Resections have been performed because of statements to the effect that the radiosensitivity of plasmacytomas in this region is limited. Indeed, Dolin and Dewar[6] in their review reported failure of local tumor control when the dose levels below 2500 rad were used. The individual physician's preferences have also played a role in treating extramedullary plasmacytoma in this region surgically.[4]

Review of the literature indicates that radiotherapy when appropriately delivered and definitive in character is curative in the majority of the cases. Actually, those patients who fail, do so primarily because of dissemination of their disease. Kotner and Wang[14] used radiation with dosages ranging from 2200 to 6000 rad at the rate of approximately 1000 rad per week. Of the 16 patients treated, 11 survived five or more years, thus yielding a five-year-survival rate of 69%. There was only one patient who developed local recurrence eight years following the original radiation therapy. He was included among the eight survivors. Patients who died did so from unrelated causes or because of disseminated multiple myeloma.[14] Petrovich et al.[19] reported on seven patients with confirmed histological diagnosis of extramedullary plasmacytomas of the upper respiratory tract. All patients were irradiated, five with orthovoltage and two with cobalt-60 modalities. The tumor doses used were in the range of 6000 rad delivered in a period of six weeks. There were no local failures in any of the seven irradiated patients. The patients were followed from 4 to 23 years.[19]

Griffiths and Brown[12] stated that a slow resolution of the tumor might take place following definitive irradiation. This is not to be taken as a sign of failure. The authors reported on a plasmacytoma involving both vocal cords, the arytenoids, and the interarytenoid region, with subglottic extension. The patient was treated by a cobalt-60 unit, receiving 6000 rad to the larynx by opposing fields in a period of six weeks. There was no change in the histological appearance one month following completion of therapy, as demonstrated by biopsy. However, biopsies repeated four months later failed to demonstrate the presence of disease.[12]

A review of the literature shows that systemic chemotherapy has not been used as primary therapy.

Prognosis and Survival

In general, the prognosis is good for localized soft tissue plasmacytomas, certainly far superior than that of multiple myeloma. The following qualifying remarks should be made with regard to prognosis and survival. In a certain number of patients the disease that started as a solitary soft tissue involvement proceeds after a period of several years to become generalized multiple myeloma. This occurs in approximately 25–30% of the cases as described in the series by Ewing and Foote[8] and Kotner and Wang.[14] These patients, although long survivors in terms of several years, eventually succumbed to their disease. Regional lymph node involvement in the area of the neck does not

seem to affect the good prognosis, provided the involved lymph nodes have been included in the irradiation portals. This has been the experience of Poole and Marchetta,[20] Kotner and Wang,[14] as well as Webb et al.[26] and Petrovich et al.[19] All authors have reported patients presenting with metastatic lymph nodes at the time of the diagnosis who have been long-term survivors, beyond the five year point, following definitive radiotherapy. In contrast to this, bone destruction adjacent to the soft tissue tumor carries an ominous prognosis. Whether the lesions begin in the bone and at a later time erupt into the soft tissues or whether they represent primarily soft tissue tumors, it is impossible to determine.[8]

The five-year survival, particularly when reviewing most recent series, has been quite good. Kotner and Wang[14] reported a 69% five-year survival. In the series by Webb et al.[26] 12 of 15 patients (80%) treated five or more years prior to the time of the report were alive and 7 of 11 patients (63%) treated 10 or more years prior to their study were alive and apparently free of recurrence. Finally, all six patients eligible for five-year-survival tabulation were alive (100%) in the series reported by Petrovich et al.[19] The seventh patient from the same series was living four years following treatment without evidence of disease.

EXTRAMEDULLARY PLASMACYTOMA IN OTHER LOCATIONS

LaPerriere et al.[15] in 1973 reported a case of primary cutaneous plasmacytoma and reviewed the literature on the subject. A total of nine cases were thus reviewed. Of these, six were male and three were female. With the exception of a 6-year-old girl, the rest of the patients were all older adults. Three of the lesions were located in the scalp. The tumor size was in the range of 2–4 cm and surgical excision had been the primary form of therapy. Three patients were without signs of recurrent disease for periods ranging from three months to five years. Two were lost to follow-up and the remaining four developed recurrences or dissemination.

Primary plasmacytomas of the central nervous system, according to the majority of the authors, are dural in origin. With the exception of one not well-documented case in which an extraosseous plasmacytoma of the hypothalamus was described—the patient died immediately after the biopsy—all the rest have had as primary site the meninges, existing either alone or extending occasionally to involve adjacent brain tissue. Less than 10 such cases are to be found in the English literature, most of them with well-documented radiographic, surgical, and histological findings.[3,5,10,16,24,27]

Apparently, there is no sex predilection and the majority of the patients were in their fourth and their fifth decades. The symptoms were related to the site of involvement. Radiographically in some instances, thinning of the adjacent cortex of the skull was due to pressure rather than to actual invasion, as shown on histological examination. However, in the majority of the cases no abnormalities from the plain films of the skull were to be identified.[10] Arteriography has been helpful in demonstrating the tumors, most of which have been rather poorly vascularized.[16,27] Ambiguous findings from the cerebrospinal fluid have been reported. In some instances this has been within normal limits, whereas in others malignant cells have been recovered.[3] In the case described by Weiner et al.[27] analysis of the fluid revealed gamma globulin with characteristics of a M-protein, as shown by electrophoresis.

The treatment in the initial phase has been surgery with extirpation of the meningeal tumor and the associated involved parts of the brain. Upon establishing the diagnosis, postoperative radiotherapy has followed in all reported cases. The over-all results have been quite satisfactory.[5,16,24,27] It is primarily the failure to establish the diagnosis that is the main factor that has led to the patient's death.[3,10]

Wile et al.[28] reported on a 40-year-old male with a solitary pulmonary plasmacytoma and reviewed the pertinent literature. Their patient presented with fever and cough and a chest x-ray revealed a very large left intrathoracic mass that during surgery was found to occupy the entire left lower lobe of the lung, surrounding both the pulmonary veins and infiltrating the pericardium. The tumor was associated with the production of M-protein. Histologically, it was composed of sheets of normal-appearing plasma cells that were interspersed with atypical plasma cells. Myeloma of the lung is to be differentiated from plasma cell granuloma, which is a benign lesion. Less than 10 cases of pulmonary plasmacytoma have been reported.[28]

Primary plasmacytomas of the gastrointestinal tract appear to be the most frequently reported lesions outside the head and neck area. They comprise 10% of extramedullary plasmacytomas, whereas those of the upper respiratory tract account for 75–85% of the total. Remigio and Klaum[22] in 1970 and later Godard et al.[11] in 1973 reviewed the published reports on primary gastric plasmacytomas. Approximately 50 such cases have been described of this rare gastric tumor. There is possibly a slight male predominance, the average age of the patients being 52 years.

The commonest presenting symptom that was seen in 70% of the patients is epigastric pain. This was accompanied by weight loss, anorexia, and weakness in several patients. Radiographically, large lesions of the stomach producing appearances similar to those of other lymphomas are to be found (Fig. 43-2). They are rather large masses, infiltrative, nodular, or polypoid in character. Tumor ulceration is present in 60% of patients. The chronic

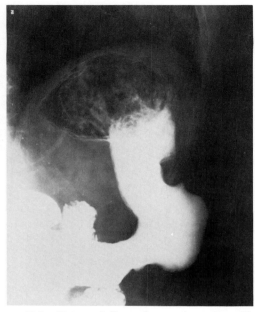

FIG. 43-2. Extramedullary plasmocytoma in a 70-year-old female. Upper gastrointestinal series demonstrates a filling defect of the greater curvature of the stomach.

blood loss results in anemia. Total serum protein levels are within normal limits and only in three cases was serum M-protein identified.

During surgery in the majority of the patients, regional lymph node involvement was recognized as well as invasion of the adjacent organs. Tumor nodules in the omentum, liver, spleen, pancreas, and colon have been found.

It appears that after the surgical procedure radiation therapy alone or in conjunction with chemotherapy is indicated. Following irradiation, there has been a dramatic reduction of the tumor size and regression of the symptoms. All long-term survivors have had radiotherapy as the mainstay of their treatment. The disease carries a serious prognosis and at least 50% of the patients were dead within five years as a result of their tumor. It is possible that this number is higher because long-term follow-up data are incomplete in several cases.[11,22]

Primary plasmacytomas of the small intestine, like those arising in the stomach, tend to present primarily with pain, often associated with a palpable mass. Due to obstruction of the lumen, nausea, vomiting, and diarrhea may be present as well.

Upon laparotomy, the disease as a rule is found to be widespread, involving the mesenteric lymph nodes, adjacent loops of bowel, the omentum, and the abdominal wall.[7] For this reason, surgery alone should be considered inadequate for the management of these patients, and it should be followed by local radiotherapy or by systemic chemotherapy. The disease tends to recur within the abdomen and this is the main mechanism of death in most cases. A change from plasmacytoma to multiple myeloma with all the classical signs is also a possibility.[13]

Ten cases of primary plasmacytoma of the colon have been described in the English literature up to this point.[17,23,30] Nielsen et al.[17] reported a patient of their own and reviewed the clinical findings on the previous seven published cases. Subsequently, Wing et al.[30] and Schweers et al.[23] published individual cases.

The average patient's age has been 48.8 years. Of them three were female and the remaining seven, male. The presenting symptoms included primarily pain, which was associated with abdominal cramps, diarrhea, constipation, and rectal bleeding. The lesions are primarily located either in the region of the cecum and adjacent ileocecal valve or in the rectosigmoid area. The radiographical signs are those of a polypoid tumor protruding into the lumen. Multiple smooth mucosal elevations may be noted. Thus, the diagnosis of polyp at times has been made radiographically.

Surgical resection has been the basic treatment of colonic plasmacytomas. Metastatic disease to the regional mesenteric nodes is a common finding. As in plasmacytomas of the small bowel, the plasma cell infiltrates may be seen through the entire thickness of the bowel wall. Microscopically, the tumors are composed primarily of mature plasma cells; however, more immature forms may be present.[23,30] The patients' follow-up has been either very short or lacking. In a number of cases, symptom-free survival up to one year has been stated.[17]

Proctor et al.,[21] in 1975 reported a primary plasmacytoma occurring in the breast.

Bjørn-Hansen[2] reported a plasmacytoma of the spleen and presented the radiographical findings.

REFERENCES

1. Batsakis, J.G., Fries, G.T., Goldman, R.T., and Karlsberg, R.C.: Upper respiratory tract plasmacytoma. Extramedullary myeloma. *Arch Otolaryngol* **79:**613, 1964.
2. Bjørn-Hansen, R.: Primary plasmacytoma of the spleen. *AJR* **117:**81, 1973.
3. Castleman, B., Scully, R.E., and McNeely, B.U.: Case records of the Massachusetts General Hospital. *N Engl J Med* **288:**150, 1973.
4. Castro, E.B., Lewis, J.S., and Strong, E.W.: Plasmacytoma of paranasal sinuses and nasal cavity. *Arch Otolaryngol* **97:**326, 1973.
5. Clarke, E.: Cranial and intracranial myelomas. *Brain* **77:**61, 1954.
6. Dolin, S., and Dewar, J.P.: Extramedullary plasmacytoma. *Am J Pathol* **32:**83, 1956.
7. Douglass, H.O., Jr., Sika, J.V., and LeVeen, H.H.: Plasmacytoma: A not so rare tumor of the small intestine. *Cancer* **28:**456, 1971.
8. Ewing, M.R., and Foote, F.W., Jr.: Plasma-cell tumors of the mouth and upper air passages. *Cancer* **5:**499, 1952.
9. Fishkin, B.G., and Spiegelberg, H.L.: Cervical lymph node metastasis as the first manifestation of localized extramedullary plasmacytoma. *Cancer* **38:**1641, 1976.
10. Gad, A., Willén, R., Willén, H., and Göthman, L.: Solitary dural plasmacytoma. *Acta Pathol Microbiol Scand [A]* **86:**21, 1978.
11. Godard, J.E., Fox, J.E., and Levinson, M.J.: Primary gastric plasmacytoma. Case report and review of the literature. *Digest Dis* **18:**508, 1973.
12. Griffiths, C., and Brown, G.: Extramedullary plasmacytoma. *Can J Otolaryngol* **3(1):**81, 1974.
13. Harper, T.B., III, Powers, J.M., Russell, H.E.,

Dunn, W.B., III, and Gardner, W.A., Jr.: Primary small bowel plasmacytoma with intracellular fibrils. *Am J Gastroenterol* **64:**200, 1975.
14. Kotner, L.M., and Wang, C.C.: Plasmacytoma of the upper air and food passages. *Cancer* **30:**414, 1972.
15. LaPerriere, R.J., Wolf, J.E., and Gellin, G.A.: Primary cutaneous plasmacytoma. *Arch Dermatol* **107:**99, 1973.
16. Moossy, J., and Wilson, C.B.: Solitary intracranial plasmacytoma. *Arch Neurol* **16:**212, 1976.
17. Nielsen, S.M., Schenken, J.R., and Cawley, L.P.: Primary colonic plasmacytoma. *Cancer* **30:**261, 1972.
18. Noorani, M.A.: Plasmacytoma of middle ear and upper respiratory tract. *J Laryngol Otol* **89:**105, 1975.
19. Petrovich, Z., Fishkin, B., Hittle, R.E., Acquarelli, M., and Barton, R.: Extramedullary plasmacytoma of the upper respiratory passages. *Int J Radiat Oncol Biol Phys* **2:**723, 1977.
20. Poole, A.G., and Marchetta, F.C.: Extramedullary plasmacytoma of the head and neck. *Cancer* **22:**14, 1968.
21. Proctor, N.S.F., Rippey, J.J., Shulman, G., and Cohen, C.: Extramedullary plasmacytoma of the breast. *J Pathol* **116:**97, 1975.
22. Remigio, P.A., and Klaum, A.: Extramedullary plasmacytoma of stomach. *Cancer* **27:**562, 1971.
23. Schweers, C.A., Shaw, M.T., Nordquist, R.E., Rose, D.D., and Kell, T.: Solitary cecal plasmacytoma. Electron microscopic, immunologic, and cytochemical studies. *Cancer* **37:**2220, 1976.
24. Someren, A., Osgood, C.P., Jr., and Brylski, J.: Solitary posterior fossa plasmacytoma. Case report. *J Neurosurg* **35:**223, 1971.
25. Stout, A.P., and Kenney, F.R.: Primary plasma-cell tumors of the upper air passages and oral cavity. *Cancer* **2:**261, 1949.
26. Webb, H.E., Harrison, E.G., Masson, J.K., and ReMine, W.H.: Solitary extramedullary myeloma (plasmacytoma) of the upper part of the respiratory tract and oropharynx. *Cancer* **15:**1142, 1962.
27. Weiner, L.P., Anderson, P.N., and Allen, J.C.: Cerebral plasmacytoma with myeloma protein in the cerebrospinal fluid. *Neurology* **16:**615, 1966.
28. Wile, A., Olinger, G., Peter, J.B., and Dornfeld, L.: Solitary intraparenchymal pulmonary plasmacytoma associated with production of an M-protein. Report of a case. *Cancer* **37:**2338, 1976.
29. Willis, R.A.: *Rathology of Tumors*, 3rd ed. Butterworth, London, 1960.
30. Wing, E.J., Perchick, J., and Hubbard, J.: Solitary obstructing plasmacytoma of the colon. *JAMA* **233:**1298, 1975.

44

Germ Cell Tumors of the Pineal and Suprasellar Region

THE CLASSIFICATION OF these tumors has evolved slowly and it is associated with a long history of confusing and overlapping terminology. Dorothy Russell[16] was the first author to interpret a tumor found in the region of the pineal gland as an atypical form of teratoma. The author stressed the histological similarity between many "pinealomas" and the seminomas of the testis and she suggested that they were indeed teratoid tumors. Friedman[5] in 1947 proposed that the term "germinoma" should be used when referring to these particular neoplasms as a short and descriptive name substituting for such names as "atypical teratoma," "seminoma," and "pinealoma." This proposition has gained acceptance within recent years. Besides seminomas or dysgerminomas, germinomas of the pineal may take the form of embryonal cell carcinoma, choriocarcinoma, adult teratoma, or a combination of these.[5,7,13]

At the present time, the classification of the tumors in the pineal region is that outlined by Rubinstein. The term "germinoma" refers to neoplasms histologically similar to the testicular seminoma, while the terms "teratoma," "choriocarcinoma" and "embryonal carcinoma" correspond to their gonadal counterparts. In the region also exist tumors arising from the pineal parenchyma, which are considerably less common than germinomas and teratomas.[15]

In a literature review performed by McGovern[12] of 236 pineal tumors recorded up to 1946 fewer than one-fifth arose from the pineal parenchyma, the remainder being germinal neoplasms. The pineal parenchymal cells are of a specific type and they cannot be regarded as neurocytes. The term "pinealoma" should be strictly reserved for neoplasms arising from the pineal parenchymal cells. They are subdivided on the basis of their maturation into a primitive form, the pineoblastoma, which is highly malignant, and to a more mature form, the pineocytoma, a tumor that may remain circumscribed and noninvasive or metastasize extensively through the cerebrospinal fluid.[15]

Russell[17] contributed further in the delineation of intracranial germinomas, reporting in 1954 on the so-called "ectopic pinealomas." These tumors were known to occur in the infundibular-suprasellar region, being unrelated to the pineal body itself. Their histological features were similar, however, to those of atypical teratomas, occurring in the pineal gland. At the present time the histological terminology, as described, applies to this group as well. Several publications exist in the literature dealing with germinomas in the suprasellar region.[2,15,19] Kageyama and Belsky[8] analyzed data with regard to germinomas of the infundibular-suprasellar region and divided them into three types on the basis of their origin. The clinical features as well as their relationship with the optic chiasma have been emphasized by Kaglyama in a later report.[9]

Suprasellar germinoma is a relatively rare tumor comprising approximately 2% of all intracranial neoplasms.[20]

Midline tumors of the pineal region are seen primarily in the young. The majority of the patients are in their second decade of life at the time of diagnosis. Germinomas of the suprasellar region show no distinct sex preference.[2,9,14,21] On the other hand, germinomas of the pineal gland occur primarily in males, the male to female ratio being 4:1.[4,21]

PATHOLOGY

The gross appearance of the tumor is that of a lobulated neoplasm white-grayish in color and soft in consistency. As they grow they become poorly circumscribed and they tend to spread in the vicinity. Those arising in the pineal region bring about destruction of the normal pineal gland.[3,15] Often during autopsy examination, no definite statement can be made with regard to the exact point of origin. This is due to their large size that obliterates the pineal region. Commonly, the corpus callosum is invaded by direct extension in the area of the splenium. They tend to extend by means of subependymal implantation within the wall of the third ventricle, eventually entering the lateral ventricles. In a similar manner the cavity of the fourth ventricle may also be invaded through the aqueduct.[4] The tumors of the suprasellar region arise primarily in the vicinity of the floor of the third ventricle and in the region of the hypophyseal stalk and the chiasma. During frontal craniotomy the optic chiasma and on occasion the optic nerves involved appear considerably enlarged and thickened, engulfed by neoplastic tissue that is grayish-white in color. These patients when examined by pneumoencephalography demonstrate defects in the floor of

the third ventricle, an indication that the entire region participates in the neoplastic process.[8,9]

Metastatic deposits, carried by the cerebrospinal fluid, can produce multiple subarachnoidal neoplastic areas. The incidence of this event has been variably reported, the general range being 10–15%.[1,7]

Metastases to the meninges and the cerebral hemispheres have also been reported, occurring with the same mechanism.[3,13] Extracerebral spread of the neoplasm has occasionally taken place, as stated by Dayan et al.[3] in their literature review on the subject.

The histological appearance is quite distinctive, according to Rubinstein.[15] The tumor is composed of two clearly defined cell populations. Thus, large germinal cells polygonal or spheroidal in shape are to be found in association with groups of small, darkly stained cells that presumably are lymphocytes.[15] The larger cells have acidophilic cytoplasm, the nuclei are central in location with distinct borders and frequently they contain large nucleoli. The lymphocytelike cells are distributed along vascular channels and are to be found in abundance at the edge of the advancing tumor[3] (Fig. 44-1).

The histological appearances of choriocarcinoma, embryonal carcinoma, and the mature teratomas are identical to the parallel group of tumors occurring in the gonads.[13,15]

CLINICAL

In germinomas of the pineal region the commonest complaint by which the tumor presents is headache. This eventually is associated with nausea and vomiting. The symptoms are due to increased intracranial pressure. Their duration in more than 50% of the patients, is longer than one year.[1,4]

Visual difficulties, particularly diplopia and blurring, as well as ataxia and somnolence, are also attributable to the increased

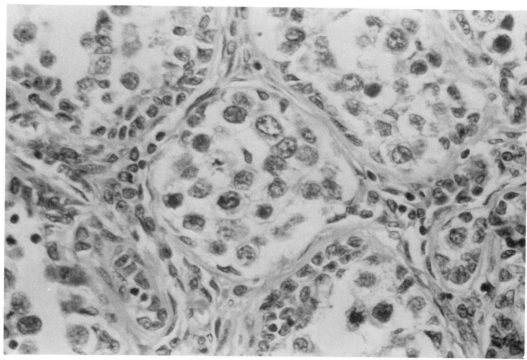

FIG. 44-1.   Pineal germinoma. Clusters of large germinal cells subdivided by connective tissue septae with a few lymphocytes. Appearance similar to seminoma.

intracranial pressure. Invasion of the superior colliculus produces loss of the upward gaze (Parinaud's syndrome) and abnormal pupillary reflexes. Lethargy and unsteady gait are also commonly encountered in approximately 50% of the patients.[21] Papilledema is present in the majority of the cases.

Radiographic examination of the skull is nonrevealing. Calcification of the pineal is seen only in a small number of patients. Arteriography has not been particularly helpful in delineating these tumors. Until recently, pneumoencephalography was the definitive procedure used for the diagnosis. Varying degrees of hydrocephalus were present in practically all patients with dilatation of the third and the lateral ventricles and a tumor located in the posterior part of the third ventricle.[1,21] Extension of the mass into the third ventricle as well as into the lateral ventricles does take place. Similarly, extension

downward into the aqueduct with stenosis has been identified in a number of cases.

The introduction of computerized transaxial tomography (CAT) provides a safe and effective method in assessing the extent of the deep intracranial lesions as well as their effect on the surrounding tissues. Thus Spiegel et al.[20] reported on two patients whose tumors were studied in this manner. Not only were the tumors well identified and the large ventricles promptly visualized, but in addition the subependymal tumor infiltration along the ventricular lining was obvious, especially following contrast enhancement (Figs. 44-2, 44-3).

The suprasellar germ cell tumors— ectopic pinealomas—are characterized by a classical triad of symptoms: diabetes insipidus, visual disturbances, and hypopituitarism. Virtually all patients have diabetes insipidus as the presenting

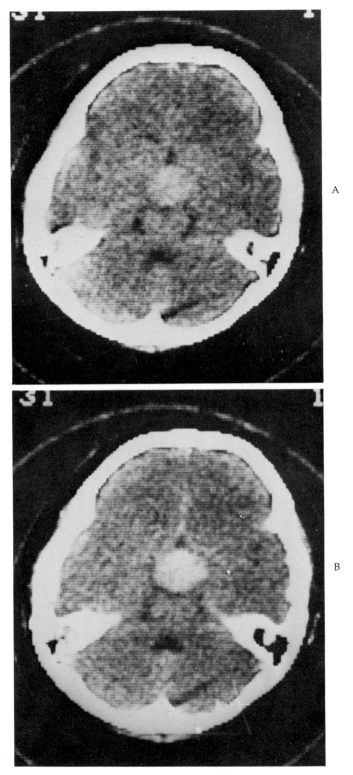

FIG. 44-2.   Suprasellar germinoma. (*A*): Plain CT scan prior to treatment shows a dense mass occupying the suprasellar cistern. (*B*): Administration of contrast medium produces marked enhancement. (Courtesy Y. Onoyama *et al. Radiology* **130:**757, 1979.)

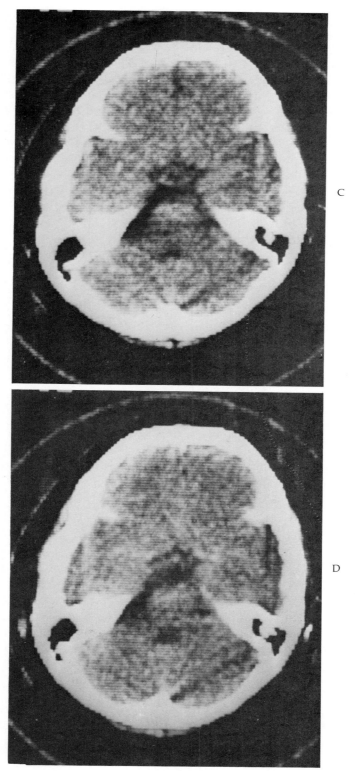

C

D

FIG. 44-3. Same patient, a 14-year-old female, as in Figure 44-2. Plain and contrast CT scans performed after irradiation to 3000 rad (*C, D*). The tumor has completely disappeared. (Courtesy Y. Onoyama *et al. Radiology* **130:**757, 1979.)

symptom. Camins and Mount[2] in a literature review, of 58 patients with primary
suprasellar germ cell tumors, found diabetes insipidus to be present in 95%.
Polydipsia and polyuria may go undiag-
nosed, particularly in young children, for
a considerable length of time.

Visual disturbances, primarily due to
compression and infiltration of the optic
nerves, the optic chiasma, and the optic
tracts, also occur in 95% of the patients.[2,14,19] They are primarily optic atrophy without papilledema and defects in
the visual field usually bitemporal
hemianopia.[19]

Pituitary insufficiency is the most
insidious of all symptoms developing
gradually. Its recognition is important,
since failure to do so in a young patient
will affect the future growth and development.[14,19]

Failure to develop secondary sex characteristics during puberty is manifested by
absence of pubic and axillary hair and
underdeveloped gonads. It is to be mentioned that at times precocious puberty
has been observed as well. Due to the lesion's proximity to the hypothalamus,
hypothalamic manifestations, including
pyrexia, obesity or emaciation, drowsiness, and somnolence, are encountered.
Headaches, mainly during the morning
hours, also occur in a percentage of patients.[14]

Plain skull films are normal in the majority of the cases. Enlargement of the sella
turcica has been found to occur in 20% of
the cases, producing thinning and involvement of the anterior clinoid processes. With tumor extension into the
optic nerves, enlargement of the optic
foramina has been reported.[11,14] Arteriography has not been particularly helpful in
their delineation. Pneumoencephalography shows a filling defect and an elevation of the anterior part of the floor of
the third ventricle with obliteration of that
space.[11,14] The optic and infundibular re-
cesses cannot be identified; instead irregular filling defects are present.

The differential diagnosis of suprasellar
germ cell tumors includes craniopharyn-
giomas, Schüller-Christian disease,
pituitary adenomas, optic gliomas, and
the uncommon entity of infundibuloma, a
tumor arising in the neurohypophysis.[14]

Examination of the cerebrospinal fluid
often shows abnormalities in terms of elevated total protein and pleocytosis. The
monocytes are commonly increased in
those patients with local tumor extension.[21] Sano[18] reported an incidence of
60% of tumor cell present within the cerebrospinal fluid following culture in patients younger than the age of 15 years.[18]
DeGirolami and Schmidek[4] are of the
opinion that positive fluid cytology is an
occasional event. The overall risk of
meningeal seeding in pineal or suprasellar
germinomas is in the range of 10–15%.[7]

TREATMENT AND RESULTS

Surgical therapy for tumors of the pineal
region requires primarily a diversionary
procedure in order to decompress the obstructed ventricular system. Biopsy may
be considered; however, attempts at partial or total removal of the primary are to
be discouraged.[4,7] The decompression
procedure may be a ventriculoperitoneal
shunt, a ventriculoatrial shunt, or a Tor-
kildsen type procedure.[1,4,7,21] Biopsy alone
in this region carried a 33% mortality rate
and subtotal tumor removal resulted in a
60% mortality rate in the series reported
by DeGirolami and Schmidek.[4] In a literature review Jenkin et al.[7] found the operative mortality rate to be in the range of
30–50%; however, it appears that in recent
years biopsy can be performed with considerably lower risk, the mortality being
in the range of 5%.

Histological identification is not absolutely necessary because at this time the
radiosensitivity of pineal germinomas has
been well established. These tumors exhibit the same response as the testicular
seminomas; therefore a definitive course
of radiation therapy will successfully cure

the patient in the majority of the cases. Should the tumor be a resistant variant, such as embryonal cell carcinoma or choriocarcinoma, the response rate obviously will be poorer; however, as the area is inaccessible to surgery, the outlook of the patient will not be affected. For these reasons, in several series the patients have been treated without tissue histology. With the advent of CAT scanning, direct irradiation without craniotomy may be considered.[4,7,20,22]

Germ cell tumors in the suprasellar region (ectopic pinealomas) are easily accessible for exploration and biopsy. Exploratory craniotomy often demonstrates the invasion or the involvement of the optic nerves, the chiasma, the infundibulum, extension into the pituitary fossa, as well as suprasellar extensions into the cerebrum. It is the concensus that radical removal is not justified because no survivors have ever been reported from surgery alone.[2,14] The radiosensitivity of germinomas in this location is a well-established fact (Figs. 44–4, 44–5, 44–6).

Due to the tendency to disseminate along the pathways of the fluid to the meninges and the ventricles, the irradiation fields should be generous enough to encompass not only the tumor but the areas of potential extension. Rubin and Kramer[14] advocate large fields covering the entire cranial contents, ventricles, and subarachnoid space to which 4000 rad should be delivered to the midplane of the brain, followed by localized additional treatment of 1000 rad to the tumor itself, utilizing reduced fields. Bradfield and Perez[1] advocate 4000–4500 rad delivered at a rate of 160 to 180 rad per day, including the entire ventricular system, and follow-

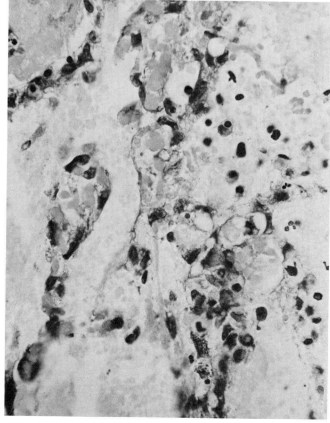

FIG. 44-4. Suprasellar endodermal sinus tumor. The tumor was composed of various histological types. Large round cells with vesicular nuclei, prominent nucleoli, and occasional areas of small lymphocytes constitute the germinoma part (A). Extracellular, periodic acid-Schiff-positive globules are seen in the endodermal sinus tumor part of the neoplasm (B). (Courtesy T.J. Eberts and R.C. Ransburg. *J. Neurosurg* **50:** 246, 1979.)

A

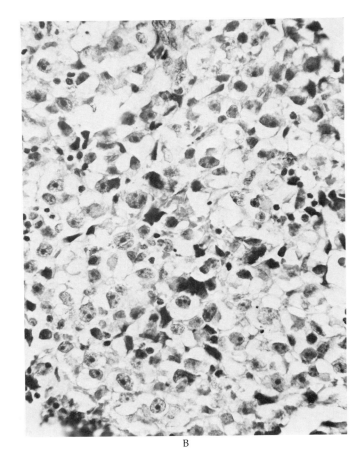

FIG. 44-4
(continued)

B

ing reduction of the portal, an additional 500–1000 rad is delivered to the tumor mass. Jenkin et al.[7] utilized localized fields ranging from 60–100 cm[2]. A total of 5000 rad were delivered in approximately five weeks. Wara et al.[22] reported their experience and reviewed the literature with regard to the effectiveness of irradiation in treating pineal tumors. The total control rate was 64%; however, among the patients with primary tumor failure, not all proved to be germinomas at autopsy.[22] Sung et al.,[21] reviewing the experience at Columbia-Presbyterian Medical Center, showed that dosages in the range of 5000–5500 rad delivered in five to six weeks are superior in terms of tumor control when compared to lower dose levels. Of 32 patients who were given 3800–4500 rad in four to five weeks, 47% presented

with recurrent tumor at the primary site three to seven years following treatment. In contrast, of the 40 patients who received 5000–5500 rad in five to six weeks, only 10% developed subsequent primary tumor recurrence. It is the authors' recommendation that the entire brain be irradiated to 4000 rad in four weeks and the actual tumor be carried to 5000–5500 rad in 5–6.5 weeks.

Metastasis to the cerebral or to the spinal subarachnoid space is known to occur months or years following the treatment to the primary tumor. In the series by Sung et al.[21] 10% of pineal tumors and 37% of suprasellar tumors metastasized to the cerebral or the spinal subarachnoid spaces. In the series by Bradfield and Perez[1] metastases to the spinal axis were demonstrated in 4 of 20 patients (20%).

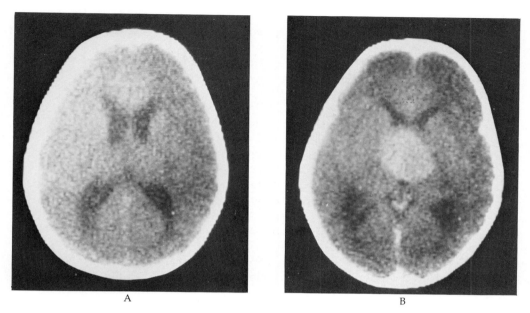

A   B

FIG. 44-5.   Suprasellar endodermal sinus tumor in a 10-year-old female with a two week history of headache and lethargy. CT scans without contrast (A) and with contrast enhancement (B) show an anterior third ventricular tumor producing dilatation of the lateral ventricles (Courtesy T.J. Eberts and R.C. Ransburg. *J Neurosurg* **50**:246, 1979.)

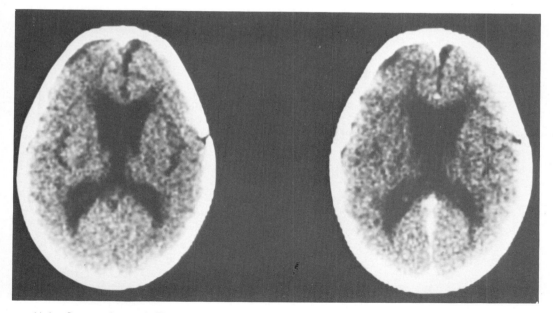

FIG. 44-6.   Same patient as in Figure 44-5. CT scans following 5000 rad. There is no evidence of tumor but the ventricular dilatation remains. (Courtesy T.J. Eberts and R.C. Ransburg. *J Neurosurg* **50**:246, 1979.)

Jenkin et al.[7] state that the risk involved in terms of meningeal seeding is in the range of 10–15%. They favor routine craniospinal irradiation for those patients who have undergone surgical intervention, since their data indicate, a higher risk among patients undergoing some sort of surgical procedure. Others irradiate the entire cranial spinal axis only when cytological examination of the spinal fluid is positive or when clinically subarachnoid metastases are identified.[2] In the series reported by DeGirolami and Schmidek[4] 18 patients survived 5–17 years following treatment to the brain and the spinal cord. A total tumor dose of 4500–5000 rad to the brain over six to seven weeks were delivered, while the spinal cord received 4000 rad. Although no strong statements advocating radiotherapy to the spinal cord are to be found in the literature, it appears that the general tendency is to treat this area rather than not. When one considers that a great percentage of the patients are growing children and that the rate of meningeal involvement is at best an estimate, the physician may choose a more conservative approach, such as periodic cytological cell examinations of the cerebrospinal fluid prior to embarking upon a course of definitive radiotherapy.

Suprasellar germinomas can be well controlled by means of radiation therapy; however, damage to the hypothalamic centers by the neoplasm involving the homeostatic control mechanisms may be complete and irreversible and life threatening in themselves.[7] The rest of the endocrine functions as well remain impaired and panhypopituitarism may be present for several years to come. Therefore, despite the tumor control, proper medical management and hormonal replacement are essential. The requirement of thyroid hormone, steroids, and Pitressin are to be evaluated on each patient.[2,14]

PROGNOSIS AND SURVIVAL

The overall five-year-survival rate in the series reported by Sung et al.[21] was 64%

for patients with verified pineal tumors and 82% for those patients whose tumor was treated without biopsy. The relapse-free survival rate at five years was 57 and 69%, respectively. Patients with verified suprasellar germinomas had a 55% five-year-survival, whereas those with unverified tumors had a survival rate of 100%. The relapse-free survival among these groups of patients was 38 and 75%, respectively.[21] Additional therapy following recurrence of the disease either in the cranial area or along the spinal axis salvaged approximately 50% of them. Most recurrences manifest themselves two or three years following the initial therapy; however, in some patients they were observed beyond the five year point.[21] They were seen primarily among those patients who had received relatively low doses and among those who were treated with small field sizes.

Wara et al.[22] obtained a 76% three-year disease-free survival and a 69% five-year disease-free survival in their group of patients with pineal and suprasellar tumors.[22] The same authors, in reviewing the literature with regard to the effects of irradiation in pineal tumors, found a 64% five-year-survival rate among previously reported series, the patients surviving without evidence of disease for periods ranging from a few months to 14 years. Jenkin et al.,[7] evaluating the results of radiation therapy on pineal and suprasellar tumors at the Princess Margaret Hospital, found the overall 5- and 10-year-survival rate calculated by the actuarial method to be 59 and 55%, respectively. The authors noticed a difference in prognosis for those patients aged 25 years and younger whose five-year-survival rate was 81% compared with 37% for the older patients. From the same series, 10 patients with histologically established diagnosis of pineal germinoma had their primary tumor controlled by irradiation and all survived five years. The patients received dosages close to 5000 rad in 25 fractions and a generous volume around the pineal was included. All had elective cranial irradiation and in five spinal irradiation was added. Among the 15 patients with unbiopsied pineal region tumors, there were 12 survivors. The median survival in this group was eight years.[7]

It is believed that, excluding patients whose germinomas were inadequately treated, those who die of their disease probably have germ cell tumors of different histology or they represent brain gliomas. Embryonal cell carcinomas have been reported occasionally. These represent indeed very uncommon neoplasms.[10,13] Similarly, reports of choriocarcinoma in the pineal and suprapineal regions exist in the literature.[5,6,13] There are no known survivors among them.

Teratomas presenting a microscopic picture similar to that of their counterparts elsewhere in the body, with a wide range of tissue element, have often been reported. Commonly, these tumors contain areas of germinoma. It appears that definitive radiotherapy can be effective in the treatment of pineal and suprasellar teratomas. Four such patients reported by Sung et al.[21] were living for periods ranging from 6 to 10 years following a course of irradiation. This experience, however, is not uniform. Three patients in the series reported by DeGirolami and Schmidek,[4] and patients with teratomas reported in the series by Jenkin et al.[7] and Nishiyama et al.[13] died of their disease following surgery or combination therapy.

REFERENCES

1. Bradfield, J.S., and Perez, C.A.: Pineal tumors and ectopic pinealomas. Analysis of treatment and failures. *Radiology* 103:399, 1972.
2. Camins, M.B., and Mount, L.A.: Primary suprasellar atypical teratoma. *Brain* 97:447, 1974.
3. Dayan, A.D., Marshall, A.H.E., Miller, A.A., Pick, F.J., and Rankin, N.E.: Atypical teratomas of the pineal and hypothalamus. *J Pathol Bacteriol* 92:1, 1966.
4. DeGirolami, U., and Schmidek, H.: Clinicopathological study of 53 tumors of the pineal region. *J Neurosurg* 39:455, 1973.
5. Friedman, N.B.: Germinoma of the pineal. Its identity with germinoma ("seminoma") of the testis. *Cancer Res* 7:363, 1947.
6. Giuffre, R., and Di Lorenzo, N.: Evolution of a primary intrasellar germinomatous teratoma into a choriocarcinoma. Case report. *J Neurosurg* 42:602, 1975.
7. Jenkin, R.D.T., Simpson, W.J.K., and Keen, C.W.: Pineal and suprasellar germinomas. Results of radiation treatment. *J Neurosurg* 48:99, 1978.
8. Kageyama, N., and Belsky, R.: Ectopic pinealoma in the chiasma region. *Neurology* 11:318, 1961.
9. Kageyama, N.: Ectopic pinealoma in the region of the optic chiasm. Report of five cases. *J Neurosurg* 35:755, 1971.
10. Khantanaphar, S., and Bunyaratvej, S.: Embryonal carcinoma in the cerebellum. Case report. *J Neurosurg* 40:657, 1974.
11. Luccarelli, G.: Ectopic pinealomas of the optic nerves and chiasma. Report of two personal cases. *Acta Neurochirurg* 27:205, 1972.
12. McGovern, F.J.: Tumours of the epiphysis cerebri. *J Pathol Bacteriol* 61:1, 1949.
13. Nishiyama, R.H., Batsakis, J.G., Weaver, D.K., and Simrall, J.H.: Germinal neoplasms of the central nervous system. *Arch Surg* 93:342, 1966.
14. Rubin, P., and Kramer, S.: Ectopic pinealoma: A radiocurable neuroendocrinologic entity. *Radiology* 85:512, 1965.
15. Rubinstein, L.J.: *Tumors of the Central Nervous System*. Armed Forces Institute of Pathology, Washington, D.C., 1972.
16. Russell, D.S.: The pinealoma: Its relationship to teratoma. *J Pathol Bacteriol* 56:145, 1944.
17. Russell, D.S.: "Ectopic pinealoma." Its kinship to atypical teratoma of the pineal gland. Report of a case. *J Pathol Bacteriol* 68:125, 1954.
18. Sano, K.: Pinealoma in children. *Childs Brain* 2:67, 1976.
19. Simpson, L.R., Lampe, I., and Abell, M.R.: Suprasellar germinomas. *Cancer* 22:533, 1968.
20. Spiegel, A.M., Di Chiro, G., Gorden, P., Ommaya, A.K., Kolins, J., and Pomeroy, T.C.: Diagnosis of radiosensitive hypothalamic tumors without craniotomy. Endocrine and neuroradiologic studies of intracranial atypical teratomas. *Ann Intern Med* 85:290, 1976.
21. Sung, D.I., Harisiadis, L., and Chang, C.H.: Midline pineal tumors and suprasellar germinomas: Highly curable by irradiation. *Radiology* 128:745, 1978.
22. Wara, W.M., Fellows, C.F., Sheline, G.E., Wilson, C.B., and Townsend, J.J.: Radiation therapy for pineal tumors and suprasellar germinomas. *Radiology* 124:221, 1977.

45

Germ Cell Tumors of the Mediastinum and Retroperitoneum

AN INCREASING number of carefully studied cases of extragonadal germ cell tumors located in the anterior mediastinum and the retroperitoneum has shown that they indeed represent primary neoplasms. Their formation has not been defined. Two theories as to their plausible development are to be found in the pertinent literature. Schlumberger[19] in 1946 put forward the thesis that teratomas occurred in areas where primitive totipotential cells rest. These represent primitive rests left during the blastula or morula stage of the embryonic development. Another hypothesis of embryological origin has been advanced by a number of authors and summarized by Fine et al.[9] Primordial germ cells from the entoderm of the yolk sac or from the urogenital ridge fail to migrate completely into the scrotum during the embryonic development. In the embryo the urogenital ridge extends from the sixth cervical to the second sacral vertebral body and remnants of it left behind give genesis to midline teratomatous lesions during the subsequent adult life.

Extragonadal germ cell tumors were considered by many authors to represent metastases of occult or "burned-out" primary gonadal lesions. Indeed, they are rare when compared to metastases from primary gonadal tumors, involving the thoracic and retroperitoneal lymph nodes. In clinical practice it behooves the physician to rule out a testicular or an ovarian primary before making the diagnosis of mediastinal or retroperitoneal germ cell tumor.

The average age of the patients at the time of the diagnosis is 27–29 years.[11,21] In a series of 30 patients with mediastinal germ cell tumors reported by Martini et al.[12] most patients were 15–35 years of age. Twenty-two patients were male and eight female; however, most reported major series in the literature pertain primarily to male patients.[1,11,12,18,21] Cox[5] reported on 24 cases of primary malignant germinal tumors of the mediastinum of which 22 were men and two were women.

PATHOLOGY

In order to differentiate a primary retroperitoneal neoplasm from that of a metastatic primary testicular tumor, Abell et al.[1] set forward the following criteria in descending order of importance: 1) the tumor should have non-neoplastic gonadal tissue in the capsule or in the immediate vicinity; 2) it should be encapsulated with no lymph node involvement; and 3) a high retroperitoneal neoplasm should have no involvement of the lower aortic, iliac, or pelvic lymph nodes. Under these circumstances, retroperitoneal neoplasms would be unlikely to represent metastasis from an occult gonadal primary.

Theoretically speaking, removal and

128

histological scrutiny of the testicles should be the ultimate proof of a primary retroperitoneal or mediastinal tumor; however, bilateral orchiectomy is not recommendation for a young man whose testicles on clinical or ultrasonic examination are negative for tumor.[1,10] Some of the lesions indeed represent metastasis from primary testicular neoplasms and it is only through thorough examination at autopsy that these patients have been identified. The presence of a well-defined fibrous scar in the testis composed of collagenous tissue often associated with remnants of hyalinized seminiferous tubules as well as the presence of amorphous granular deposits within it (hematoxyphilic bodies) represent, according to Mostofi and Price[13] an adequate proof of the previous presence of a "burned-out" primary testicular tumor.

In the mediastinum approximately 50% of the teratomatous lesions are benign.[14,15] These tumors are grossly well encapsulated and circumscribed and histologically they are composed of mature tissue elements. Synonyms used to describe them are "benign cystic teratomas" or "mediastinal dermoid cysts."[14,15] Malignant teratomas demonstrate either contiguous spread to adjacent structures or distant metastases.[14] On cut surface, multiple cystic areas are seen, as well as calcifications and hemorrhage. On histological examination, epidermoid carcinoma and adenocarcinoma are the malignant elements. In certain cases undifferentiated malignant epithelial cells are to be found.[15]

In addition to malignant teratomas germ cell tumors of the mediastinum and retroperitoneum present appearances histologically identical to those of the primary gonadal tumors. Thus, seminomas, choriocarcinomas, embryonal carcinomas, and admixtures of these pure forms are to occur. On histological examination, there is no difference between primary gonadal and primary extragonadal germ cell tumors.[14,15,18,21]

CLINICAL

The majority are located in the anterior superior mediastinum. Some are found to arise in the superior and middle mediastinum or in the middle mediastinum.[16] In the review by Martini *et al.*[12] the tumor was located in the anterior mediastinum in all 30 of the reported patients.

The patients may be entirely asymptomatic, particularly when the tumor is a benign teratoma or a seminoma.[12,15] In our literature review we have found that in approximately 25–30% of the patients the first sign of disease was an abnormal chest x-ray taken on a routine basis. Seminomas tend to be less invasive than the rest of the malignant germ cell tumors; however, due to their location, they produce substernal pressure and pain radiating to the neck and the arms. They impede upon the venous return, producing swelling of the face and, from pressure on the trachea, hoarseness and dyspnea.[20] The tumors at times could be very large, metastasizing to adjacent lymph nodes. Embryonal cell carcinoma, teratocarcinoma, and choriocarcinoma are more aggressive infiltrating neoplasms, causing pain of variable intensity, pleuritic in character or substernal in location, as the most prominent symptom, accompanied by dyspnea, cough, and hemoptysis. Patients with choriocarcinoma have a positive pregnancy test due to the secretion of chorionic gonadotropins. Urinary chorionic gonadotropins are elevated in all patients with choriocarcinoma; however, breast enlargement—gynecomastia—is present in approximately 40% of the patients at the time of the diagnosis.[4,9,12,15]

Radiographically the borders of the tumors are sharp and in most cases smooth or lobulated in outline. Displacement of the trachea may occur. In patients with aggressive lesions and particularly those with choriocarcinoma and teratocarcinoma metastatic pulmonary nodules may be present at the time of the initial radiographic examination.[16]

Malignant germinal tumors of the mediastinum account for 2–6% of all mediastinal neoplasms.[5]

Retroperitoneal germ cell tumors are located primarily in the upper and mid-retroperitoneal space. Abell *et al.*[1] presented a detailed analysis of 10 patients with retroperitoneal seminoma. In all, the predominant symptom was pain, mostly dull in character, at times recurring, of long-standing duration, which was felt primarily in the upper abdominal regions or in the renal areas. With a few exceptions, palpation will demonstrate the presence of a high abdominal or midabdominal mass representing the neoplasm.[1] Because of this, fullness, nausea, and vomiting can be induced mechanically.[11] An intravenous pyelogram will reveal in most instances displacement of the kidneys or the ureters. It is anticipated that CT scans will provide a very accurate outline of the tumor and its relationship to the surrounding structures.

It is necessary for male patients with mediastinal and retroperitoneal germ cell tumors to undergo a detailed clinical examination of the testicles. At the present time, orchiectomy in the absence of any clinical or radiographic indication of abnormality in the testis is not recommended by most authors.[6,11,18,21]

TREATMENT AND RESULTS

Mediastinal and retroperitoneal seminomas manifest the radiosensitivity of their testicular counterparts. Due to this sensitivity therefore patients whose disease is localized at the time of the diagnosis can be cured. Cox[5] reported on six patients with pure seminoma of the mediastinum, all treated by radiation therapy with dosages ranging from 2000 to 4000 rad. In all individuals there was complete response of the primary tumor and no local recurrence was noted during the follow-up period. Four were alive and well for periods ranging from 2 to 18 years.

In the series by Utz and Buscemi[21] of eight patients with seminomas in the mediastinum and the retroperitoneum treated by radiotherapy, one died of seminoma six and two-thirds years after treatment and another was surviving 10 years later with disease present. The rest were free of tumor. Radiation therapy as the basic treatment modality was utilized in seven patients with retroperitoneal seminomas reported by Abell *et al.*[1] In three additional patients surgical excision was supplemented by radiotherapy. Three patients died of metastatic disease, one patient died several years later due to cardiovascular causes and the remaining seven were alive at the time of the report for periods ranging from 6 months to 24 years free of tumor.[1] Bliss and Barnett[3] in their report presented two patients with large retroperitoneal seminomas treated by biopsy and postoperative radiotherapy, surviving 15 and 6 years without recurrence.

The role of surgical resection in the management of mediastinal and retroperitoneal seminomas need not be excessive. Obviously, surgical exploration is necessary for tissue biopsy and excision of the tumor, if it can be done without undue hardship. However, in view of the radiosensitivity of this particular cell type and because radiotherapy should be always used postoperatively, partial excision can be considered an adequate surgical accomplishment.[20]

Embryonal cell carcinoma, teratocarcinoma, and choriocarcinoma are tumors whose radiosensitivity is limited or nonexistent and therefore the major thrust of therapy remains on their surgical removal. Due to the location however, complete resection is not possible and this is reflected in the poor survival statistics. All but 1 of 20 patients with embryonal carcinoma reported by Martini *et al.*[12] were dead of their disease, the majority within a year from the diagnosis.

Fine *et al.*[9] reviewed the literature and reported on 74 patients with extragenital choriocarcinoma. In the majority of the cases the presenting symptoms were those of pulmonary metastases, namely, hemoptysis, cough, and chest pain. Other symptoms at presentation included hematuria, cerebral disorders, and pain from the primary tumor, all indicating a far-advanced disease at the onset. Once the diagnosis was established, the survival was very short, ranging from days to 15 months. There were no five-year survivors to be found at the time of their reporting.[9] Pachter and Lattes[15] and others[4,11] have encountered similar experience and reported similar poor results in patients with choriocarcinomas. Teratocarcinomas, finally, represent radioresistant tumors that promptly metastasize and that therefore carry a poor prognosis.[5,14,15]

The commonest metastatic sites for seminomatous lesions are the lymph nodes and the bones. Nonseminomatous tumors metastasize widely; primarily, however, to the lungs, pleura, pericardium, heart, and liver.[12] In the majority of the nonseminomatous neoplasms growth at the primary site is persistent and active at the time of the patient's death.[5,16]

The prognosis of testicular tumors has dramatically changed within the last few years, due to recent advents in systemic chemotherapy. Although earlier trials with nitrogen mustard, vincristine, actinomycin D, and cyclophosphamide were occasionally or partially helpful, combination systemic chemotherapy has at the present time established itself as one of the basic therapeutic modalities in the management of these tumors. At the time of this writing, no reports dealing specifically with extragonadal germ cell tumors treated successfully by chemotherapy are to be found in the literature; however, their response should be similar to that of primary testicular cancer. Samuels et al.[17] obtained 32% complete and 44% partial responses in patients with Stage III testicular neoplasms utilizing combination of vinblastine and bleomycin.

Einhorn and Donohue[8] began a study in 1974 utilizing vinblastin, bleomycin, and cis-diamminedichloroplatinum (cisplatin) in the management of disseminated testicular cancer. Reporting their experience with 43 nonseminomatous testicular neoplasms and four seminomas, the authors obtained complete remission in 35 of the 47 patients (74%) and 29 of these complete remissions remained alive and disease-free for periods ranging from 6 to 30 months. The experience has been updated in a later report[7] with particular emphasis to the contribution of cisplatin, vinblastin and bleomycin in conjunction with surgery for patients with Stage C disease (metastases above the diaphragm to the lung or disseminated tumor). Of 50 such patients, 33 (66%) achieved initial complete remission using this drug regimen. Twenty-six remained in continuous complete remission with no evidence of tumor for periods ranging from two to four years. Seven were alive and in partial remission at the time of the report and 17 were dead of their tumor.

PROGNOSIS AND SURVIVAL

Seminomas (germinomas) have the best prognosis. Besznyák et al.[2] reviewed in 1973 the world literature with reference to primary mediastinal seminomas. The overall one-year survival as calculated from their tables is 71%. The three and five-year-survival rates are, respectively, 63 and 54%. The survival for seminomas of the retroperitoneum calculated on the basis of the reports by Abell et al.[1] and by Bliss and Barnett[3] was found to be 70% at the end of the first year and 42.8% at five years.

Embryonal carcinoma has had in the past a poor prognosis. In our literature review we found the survival rate at the end of the first year to be 16% and practically no survivors reported past two years.[5,12,14,21] It is possible that seminomatous elements mixed with embryonal carcinoma afford a better prognosis.[5,16]

Fine *et al.*[9] in their literature review with regard to primary extragonadal choriocarcinomas in male subjects found no survivors at the five-year level. Subsequent reports prior to initiation of present-day systemic combined chemotherapy reflect similar poor prognosis.[5,11,15]

Teratocarcinomas are perhaps the most virulent of all germ cell neoplasms, the average survival time from the diagnosis to their death being four to five months.[5,14,15,21]

At this time, a major change is occurring with regard to the management of seminomatous and nonseminomatous neoplasms. The effectiveness of combined chemotherapy as previously outlined has changed the past prognostications; therefore the survival rates for these tumors most likely will be altered in the future.

REFERENCES

1. Abell, M.R., Fayos, J.V., and Lampe, I.: Retroperitoneal germinomas (seminomas) without evidence of testicular involvement. *Cancer* **18**:273, 1965.
2. Besznyák, I., Sebestény, M., and Kuchár, F.: Primary mediastinal seminoma. A case report and review of the literature. *J Thorac Cardiovasc Surg* **65**:930, 1973.
3. Bliss, W.R., and Barnett, W.H.: Retroperitoneal seminoma (germinoma) without evidence of testicular involvement. *Am J Surg* **120**:363, 1970.
4. Cohen, B.A., and Needle, M.A.: Primary mediastinal choriocarcinoma in a man. *Chest* **67**:106, 1975.
5. Cox, J.D.: Primary malignant germinal tumors of the mediastinum. A study of 24 cases. *Cancer* **30**:1162, 1975.
6. Das, S., Bochetto, J.R., and Alpert, L.: Primary retroperitoneal seminoma. Report of a case and review of the literature. *Cancer* **36**:595, 1975.
7. Donohue, J.P., Perez, J.M., and Einhorn, L.H.: Improved management of non-seminomatous testis tumors. *J Urol* **121**:425, 1979.
8. Einhorn, L.H., and Donohue, J.P.: Chemotherapy for disseminated testicular cancer. *Urol Clin North Am* **4**:407, 1977.
9. Fine, G., Smith, R.W., Jr., and Pachter, M.R.: Primary extragenital choriocarcinoma in the male subject. Case report and review of the literature. *Am J Med* **32**:776, 1962.
10. Gottesman, J.E.: Letter. *J Urol* **119**:298, 1978.
11. Johnson, D.E., Laneri, J.P., Mountain, C.F., and Luna, M.: Extragonadal germ cell tumors. *Surgery* **73**:85, 1973.
12. Martini, N., Golbey, R.B., Hajdu, S.I., Whitmore, W.F., and Beattie, E.J., Jr.: Primary mediastinal germ cell tumors. *Cancer* **33**:763, 1974.
13. Mostofi, F.K., and Price, E.B., Jr.: *Tumors of the Male Genital System.* Armed Forces Institute of Pathology, Washington, D.C., 1973.
14. Oberman, H.A., and Libcke, J.H.: Malignant germinal neoplasms of the mediastinum. *Cancer* **17**:498, 1964.
15. Pachter, M.R., and Lattes, R.: "Germinal" tumors of the mediastinum: A clinicopathologic study of adult teratomas, teratocarcinomas, choriocarcinomas and seminomas. *Dis Chest* **45**:301, 1964.
16. Recondo, J., and Libshitz, H.I.: Mediastinal extragonadal germ cell tumors. *Urology* **11**:369, 1978.
17. Samuels, M.L., Holoye, P.Y., and Johnson, D.E.: Bleomycin combination chemotherapy in the management of testicular neoplasia. *Cancer* **36**:318, 1975.
18. Schantz, A., Sewall, W., and Castleman, B.: Mediastinal germinoma. A study of 21 cases with an excellent prognosis. *Cancer* **30**:1189, 1972.
19. Schlumberger, H.G.: Teratoma of anterior mediastinum in group of military age; study of 16 cases, and review of theories of genesis. *Arch Pathol* **41**:398, 1946.
20. Sterchi, M., and Cordell, A.R.: Seminoma of the anterior mediastinum. *Ann Thorac Surg* **19**:371, 1975.
21. Utz, D.C., and Buscemi, M.F.: Extragonadal testicular tumors. *J Urol* **105**:271, 1971.

PART 2

TUMORS OF UNCOMMON HISTOLOGY

46

Adenoid Cystic Carcinoma of the Nose, Sinuses, and Nasopharynx

ADENOID CYSTIC carcinomas of the upper respiratory passages comprise 18% of such tumors encountered in the head and neck region.[4,6,14]

In the series by Conley and Dingman[4] and by Smith et al.[14] female preponderance was noted. Other authors, however, such as Oppenheim et al.[12] and Eby et al.[6] found no sex related difference.

The tumors occur primarily between the ages of 40 and 60 years.[4,10] Occasionally, they have been seen early in life and reports of patients in advanced age groups can also be found.[12]

Specifically referring to the maxillary antrum, adenoid cystic carcinoma represents no more than 5% of all carcinomas originating at this site.[8]

PATHOLOGY

The gross appearance of the tumors, particularly during their early stages, is quite deceptive. They masquerade as paranasal polyps and it is quite difficult to define clinically their extent. This is particularly true for those arising in the sinuses, where often the disease is quite advanced at the time of the diagnosis.

Grossly, they appear as yellowish-grayish masses with a broad base and incomplete encapsulation. There is relatively little tendency toward cystic degeneration or hemorrhage.[8,12] Histologically, typical cells of cylindromatous appearance, defining areas containing mucin, are encountered (Fig. 46-1). The patterns can be several, depending on the proportions of these two elements.[2,6] They are not encapsulated and they have a distinct tendency for perineural invasion.

CLINICAL

The onset is insidious and the growth slow. Because of this, the disease is usually quite advanced at the time of the diagnosis. Early presenting symptoms for tumors involving the sinuses are nasal obstruction and with it associated mucous discharge, which eventually may become bloody. As the growth progresses and because of the characteristic property to destroy adjacent bone and to infiltrate along the perineural lymphatics, discomfort and pain appear. Oppenheim et al.[12] found, for tumors of the maxillary sinus, irritation of the roof of the mouth, especially when eating and swallowing, to be the main presenting symptom. The patient may also complain of pain similar to that of a toothache or for an ill-fitting dental plate.

Tumors originating in the upper maxillary antrum or in the ethmoids or frontal and sphenoid sinuses may manifest themselves by extension and destruction of adjacent structures, such as the orbit, the base of the skull, and the pterygomaxillary area. Involvement of several cranial nerves

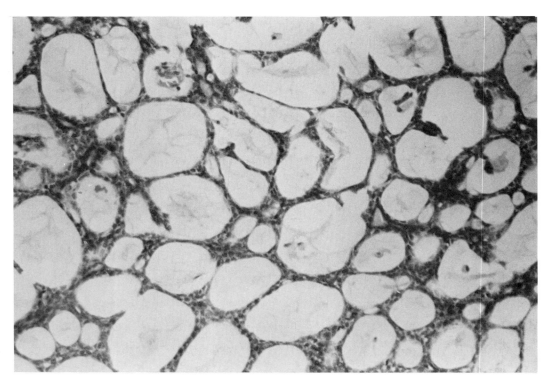

FIG. 46-1.   Adenoid cystic carcinoma of salivary gland. Cribriform formation of tumor cells defining spaces filled with secretory material.

produces facial weakness, diplopia, proptosis, as well as headaches.[3,8,11,12]

Adenoid cystic carcinomas have a slow growth rate. As Horrée[10] notes, an extremely long observation period is necessary in order to appreciate their malignant nature. They tend to recur locally for several times before distant metastases appears. Local recurrences have been encountered in at least 75% of the cases. The metastases are primarily hematogenous, to the lungs and the bones. The regional lymph nodes are seldom involved.[9,10] At the time of the patient's death, local recurrent disease is the rule rather than the exception.

X-ray examination of the sinuses and the nasopharynx is essential in order to define the tumor extent. Plain films of the sinuses, tomograms, and CT scans will more often than not show bony invasion. Dodd and Jing[5] have described in detail the several radiographic manifestations of these particular neoplasms.

TREATMENT AND RESULTS

Prior to any treatment, several factors should be considered. They are: the age of the patient, the long natural history of the tumor, the high recurrence rate, and the inability to define the tumor volume because of the tendency for perineural invasion. Horrée[10] advocates therapeutic classification of the tumors into three categories: inoperable, dubiously operable, and radically operable. Tumors with radiological signs of destruction of bone, particularly when related to the skull, the ethmoids, or sphenoid sinuses, are judged to be inoperable. Dubiously operable are those with clinical or radiological signs of operability but they appear to be large and bulky in character. Radically operable are considered to be those tumors with limited volume which can be removed intact.

Conley and Dingman[4] advocate surgery as the best initial approach. Actually, in their opinion, the procedure should be as extensive as possible. In advanced and grossly incurable tumors they propose radiation therapy or conservative surgical intervention. In older patients, due to the long natural history, the aesthetics of the surgical procedure should be taken into consideration in treatment planning. Unless there are signs of gross extension into the neck lymph nodes, a radical neck dissection is not part of any treatment program. The authors recognize that neoplasms occurring in the nasal cavity, nasal sinuses, and nasopharynx pose a problem in early diagnosis and surgical anatomy. By remaining submucosal, the tumor extends through the periosteum into the marrow spaces of the adjacent bones. The cranial nerves are subsequently involved, and these tumors are inoperable.[4]

Ramsden et al.[13] attempted radical resection in four patients, only to abandon the procedure. The disease had spread beyond the bounds of resectability. Following local excision, however, three of these four patients were symptom-free, without signs of recurrence, two to three years postoperatively. The same authors managed seemingly complete resections, with free specimen margins, in three other patients. Two of them developed local recurrence four and five years postoperatively.[13]

A literature review indicates that, for adenoid cystic carcinomas of the nasal cavity, paranasal sinuses, and nasopharynx, a surgical resection is unable to bring about cure of the patient in the long run.[4,5,10,13,14] On the other hand, a limited surgical resection without mutilation of the face has often resulted in local control for several years.

Adenoid cystic carcinoma is radiosensitive, but it tends to recur. Radiation therapy has a definite role to play in the management of these patients, primarily indicated in bulky tumors, in elderly patients, and in recurrent disease.

Caruso et al.[3] reported on two cases of adenoid cylindroma arising in the sphenoid sinus. In both patients the lesions were very advanced with neurological deficits and with extension into the middle fossa. Radiotherapy was given to both at the level of 6000 rad. Follow-up examination showed complete pain relief and reversal of the neurological deficits in one of them. The second had complete pain relief; however, he developed metastatic disease to the thoracolumbar spine during the interim. This was irradiated locally with good pain palliation.

In his review Snelling[15] concluded that "cylindromas" of the maxillary antrum and the ethmoids were difficult tumors to treat. They invade the orbits and the base of the skull in spite of the surgical attempts at cure. Even worse were the results in tumors of the nasopharynx and the nasal cavity. For this reason he advocated preoperative radiotherapy. Kuhn and Huszár[11] irradiated preoperatively an extensive maxilloethmoidal cylindroma that had produced extensive bone destruction. The patient received 6600 rad following which he underwent a radical resection. There were no signs of recurrence two years later.

Fuchihata et al.[7] used surgery combined with radiotherapy in the management of seven patients with maxillary sinus cylindromas. In their opinion these lesions could be treated by radiotherapy alone, but combination therapy results in better control rates.

Preoperative radiotherapy is advocated by Greenbaum et al.[8] The authors advise that 5000–5500 rad be given in five to six weeks, to be followed by en bloc resection.

Bassilios et al.[1] reported on a case of recurrent maxillary sinus cylindroma. The patient had been treated 21 years earlier by surgery and postoperative radium packing. The recurrence was palliatively irradiated.

In our experience, adenoid cystic carcinoma of the head and neck is a relatively radiosensitive tumor. There has always been tumor regression, lasting for several months, often for more than one year, following the delivery of 4500–5000 rad in 4.5–5 weeks. We have irradiated several patients more than twice, at lesser dosages, at the time of their recurrences. This course of action has been undertaken when surgery is not feasible. In this manner the patient can be kept in comfort for long periods of time.

PROGNOSIS AND SURVIVAL

The course of the disease is very protracted. In spite of the very high incidence of local recurrence and of the poor ultimate prognosis, the patients usually survive for several years prior to their death from uncontrolled disease. For this reason the five-year-survival limit that is applicable in most malignancies does not provide a correct index of cure or survival in adenoid cystic carcinoma. In order to evaluate this tumor, a period of at least 20 years is necessary to appreciate its biological behavior.

Practically, the cause of death is always failure to control the local disease process. Although the rate of recurrence is extremely high, many years may elapse from the initial treatment until recurrence develops.

Tauxe et al.[16] reviewed and reported on 27 adenoid cystic carcinomas arising in the nose and paranasal sinuses. The patients were seen at the Mayo Clinic from the years 1932 through 1950. Twenty-five of the 27 patients were dead at the time of the report. Both of the two survivors had known active disease. One of the deaths was attributed to an unrelated gastric adenocarcinoma. All of the remaining patients died as a result of their tumor, their survival ranging from 2 to 19 years from the onset of the symptoms. The average life-span was 8.8 years. Twelve patients (44.4%) survived for more than 10 years. The five-year survival was 63%.[16]

We have compiled, through a review of the literature, the survival rate from a number of reports related to adenoid cystic carcinoma of the upper respiratory passages. At three years it was found to be 74%, but at five years had decreased to 45%. Patients continued to develop recurrences and die of their disease beyond the five-year level; however, their numbers are too small to derive meaningful percentages. It is certainly true that in this particular location adenoid cystic carcinoma carries a more serious prognosis when compared to tumors of similar histology in the oral cavity or in the major salivary glands.

REFERENCES

1. Bassilios, M.I., Ramm, C., Jarmolych, J., and Goffin, F.B.: Cylindroma of the right maxillary antrum. Case report. *Laryngoscope* **77**:365, 1967.
2. Batsakis, J.G.: *Tumors of the Head and Neck. Clinical and Pathological Considerations.* Williams & Wilkins, Baltimore, 1974.
3. Caruso, V.G., Roncace, E.A., and Brennan, M.T.: Cylindroma of the sphenoid sinus. A study of two cases. *Trans Pa Acad Ophthalmol Otolaryngol* **26**:32, 1973.
4. Conley, J., and Dingman, D.L.: Adenoid cystic carcinoma in the head and neck (cylindroma). *Arch Otolaryngol* **100**:81, 1974.
5. Dodd, G.D., and Jing, B.S.: Radiographic findings in adenoid cystic carcinoma of the head and neck. *Ann Otol Rhinol Laryngol* **81**:591, 1972.
6. Eby, L.S., Johnson, D.S., and Baker, H.W.: Adenoid cystic carcinoma of the head and neck. *Cancer* **29**:1160, 1972.
7. Fuchihata, H., Wada, T., and Inoue, T.: Radiotherapy of adenoid cystic carcinoma of the head and neck. *Oral Surg* **36**:753, 1973.
8. Greenbaum, E.I., Gunn, W., Rappaport, I., and O'Loughlin, B.J.: Cylindroma of the maxillary antrum. A case presentation and review of the literature. *Radiol Clin Biol* **39**:419, 1970.
9. Hair, G.E.: Cylindroma (adenoid cystic carcinoma) of the upper air passages. Two case reports. *Laryngoscope* **77**:1714, 1967.
10. Horrée, W.A.: Adenoid cystic carcinoma of the maxilla. *Arch Otolaryngol* **100**:469, 1974.

11. Kuhn, E., and Huszár, L.: Die kombinierte, radiologisch-chirurgische Behandlung des maxilloethmoidalen Zylindroms. *Z Laryngol Rhinol* **51:**316, 1972.

12. Oppenheim, H., Landau, G.H., Dorman, D.W., Mojsejenko, I., and Sleadd, F.B.: Cylindroma involving the paranasal sinuses. *Eye Ear Nose Throat Monthly* **47:**86, 1968.

13. Ramsden, D., Sheridan, B.F., Newton, N.C., and De Wilde, F.W.: Adenoid cystic carcinoma of the head and neck: A report of 30 cases. *Aust NZ J Surg* **43:**102, 1973.

14. Smith, L.C., Lane, N., and Rankow, R.M.: Cylindroma (adenoid cystic carcinoma). A report of fifty-eight cases. *Am J Surg* **110:**519, 1965.

15. Snelling, M.D.: Histology, natural history and results of treatment of mucous gland tumors. *AJR* **90:**1032, 1963.

16. Tauxe, W.N., McDonald, J.R., and Devine, K.D.: A century of cylindromas. Short review and report of 27 adenoid cystic carcinomas arising in the upper respiratory passages. *Arch Otolaryngol* **75:**94, 1962.

47

Adenoid Cystic Carcinoma of the Oral Cavity, Oropharynx, and Hypopharynx

ADENOID CYSTIC carcinoma of the oral cavity, oropharynx, and hypopharynx represents approximately 30% of all tumors with this histology encountered in the head and neck region.[1,9] Among the various structures of the oral cavity, the palate, according to all series, seems to be the predominant location. Spiro et al.,[8] in a clinicopathological study of 492 cases of minor salivary gland tumors, found that adenoid cystic carcinoma of the oral cavity occurred in the palate with an incidence of 51%. The next most frequent site of occurrence was the tongue, where 21% of the lesions were seen. Other sites include the buccal mucosa, lips, gingiva, floor of the mouth, and tonsil. The oropharynx is infrequently involved, with only 2% of the lesions appearing in this location.[8]

The histological considerations are similar to those described elsewhere for this particular neoplasm.

CLINICAL

In the majority of the cases adenoid cystic carcinomas of the palate occur at the junction of the hard and soft palate.[1] Adenoid cystic carcinoma of the tongue presents as a mass within the tongue and thus it can be contained within this large muscular organ for long periods of time, being the most amenable of adenoid cystic carcinomas to surgical resection. Tumors in the buccal region are always more advanced than originally thought.[1]

The common presenting symptom is that of a mass at the site of origin. Other symptoms, including pain, ulceration, or bleeding, may be encountered; however, they occur only in advanced cases.[9] Examination by inspection or palpation assisted by mirror inspection is feasible for most lesions in this location. Within the oral cavity and oropharynx, a firm mass is palpable covered by an intact mucosa.

Radiographically, involvement of the adjacent bones should be ruled out, particularly for such lesions as those located in the palate, gingiva, or floor of the mouth. Tumors of the tongue will be well outlined by soft tissue, lateral views of the neck, and by barium swallow.[2,8]

Regional lymph node metastases are uncommon, but local recurrences are frequent.[3]

TREATMENT AND RESULTS

Surgery and radiation therapy have been used in the management of these tumors. The surgical measures have varied from local excision of early lesions in the oral cavity, to en bloc resection of advanced neoplasms. In tumors of the palate residual disease has often been seen at the end of the operation. The prognosis in the palate, however, is more favorable when compared to other locations. Snelling[7] found three of nine such cases developing local recurrence and eventually dying of their disease at 3, 5, and 13 years following resection. Radiotherapy was used extensively for local recurrences on the last patient, who died 13 years after resection. Conley and Dingman[1] advocate removal of the major portion of the hard and soft palates, as well as resection of the alveolus, the pterygoid plates and their muscles, and the contents of the nasal cavity.

Three patients with buccal lesions were reported by Ramsden et al.[5] All had complete excision, 2 of them surviving free of recurrence six and two years and a third developing local recurrence two years following the surgery, which was treated with additional surgery, including hemimandibulectomy, and later with radiation therapy. The patient died 7.5 years from the time of diagnosis with lung metastasis. In this region the tumors tend to be more extensive than is apparent clinically. It is thought that the tendency to remove them through the oral cavity enhances the chances for local failure. According to Conley and Dingman[1] a lower lip splitting incision provides better exposure for the resection of the tumor and surrounding fat and musculature. Fuchihata et al.[4] treated one patient with buccal mucosal adenoid cystic carcinoma by means of irradiation. The patient was alive and well three years later.

Tumors of the floor of the mouth similarly require extensive radical resection. Hemimandibulectomy may be necessary in most cases. One such patient reported by Ramsden et al.[5] was living free of disease three years following surgery. Fuchihata et al.[4] report on a patient surviving 5.5 years following his original surgery who was treated by irradiation for local recurrence and with cyclophosphamide for lung metastases. The same authors reported on two additional cases, one treated by surgery who was alive and well four years later and the second treated by radiotherapy having metastases to the lung three years following the original therapy.[4]

Tumors of the base of the tongue render themselves to surgical removal. When unilaterally located, a composite resection of either one-half or all of the tongue, the floor of the mouth, and the adjacent mandible should be contemplated. When a tumor is located in the base of the tongue, total glossectomy is usually necessary. Attention should be given to the resection of the hypoglossal, lingual, and alveolar nerves.[1,5]

Involvement of the peritonsillar region, the pharyngeal walls, and hypopharynx, although reported in the literature, are not too common.[2,3,7,8]

Prognosis and Survival

In most series the survival rate is quoted for all adenoid cystic carcinomas of the head and neck region. We have arrived at the survival percentages for tumors involving the oral cavity, oropharynx, and hypopharynx, combining data from recent series. The survival at five years approaches 70%.

Surviving at five years, however, does not necessarily mean cure of the disease. Actually, local recurrences are the rule rather than the exception. As a result of the natural behavior of adenoid cystic carcinoma, here and at other sites, patients continue to die from their disease several years after the diagnosis. In the present group, the 10-year survival was 30%.[3-7]

References

1. Conley, J., and Dingman, D.L.: Adenoid cystic carcinoma in the head and neck (cylindroma). Arch Otolaryngol 100:81, 1974.
2. Dodd, G.D., and Jing, B.S.: Radiographic findings in adenoid cystic carcinoma of the head and neck. Ann Otol Rhinol Laryngol 81:591, 1972.
3. Eby, L.S., Johnson, D.S., and Baker, H.W.: Adenoid cystic carcinoma of the head and neck. Cancer 29:1160, 1972.

4. Fuchihata, H., Wada, T., and Inoue, T.: Radiotherapy of adenoid cystic carcinoma of the head and neck. *Oral Surg* **36:**753, 1973.
5. Ramsden, D., Sheridan, B.F., Newton, N.C., and De Wilde, F.W.: Adenoid cystic carcinoma of the head and neck: A report of 30 cases. *Aust NZ J Surg* **43:**102, 1973.
6. Smith, L.C., Lane, N., and Rankow, R.M.: Cylindroma (adenoid cystic carcinoma). A report of fifty-eight cases. *Am J Surg* **110:**519, 1965.
7. Snelling, M.D.: Histology, natural history and results of treatment of mucous gland tumors. *AJR* **80:**1032, 1963.
8. Spiro, R.H., Koss, L.G., Hajdu, S.I., and Strong, E.W.: Tumors of minor salivary origin. A clinicopathologic study of 492 cases. *Cancer* **31:**117, 1973.
9. Steinhoff, N.G., Harris, H.S., Jr., and Hori, J.: An analysis of cylindroma of the head and neck. *J Surg Oncol* **5:**17, 1973.

48

Adenoid Cystic Carcinoma of the External Auditory Canal

THE MOST COMMON malignancy arising from the skin of the external auditory canal is undoubtedly squamous cell carcinoma. Adenoid cystic carcinoma has been classified under the collective term of "ceruminomas," which, according to Wetli et al.,[5] include four distinct entities: 1) ceruminous adenoma presenting as well-differentiated benign proliferation of glands, 2) ceruminous adenocarcinoma that, although histologically similar to ceruminous adenoma, exhibits invasion, 3) adenoid cystic carcinoma that histologically and biologically is similar to the counterpart occurring in the minor salivary glands, and 4) pleomorphic adenoma (mixed tumor) in which epithelial cells are seen in a myxoid, pseudocartilaginous, or hyaline stroma containing mucin.

The notion that adenoid cystic carcinoma represents a variety of ceruminomas has been questioned. Batsakis[1] points out that the histology and the natural history of the disease is similar to that of adenoid cystic carcinomas of the head and neck, whereas ceruminous adenocarcinomas have a sweat gland pattern and they are much more aggressive both in terms of local infiltration and of distant metastases.

There is no specific sex predilection and the average age of the patients at the time of the diagnosis has been 44 years. Until 1971, 29 cases of adenoid cystic carcinoma of the external auditory canal had been described.[3,5]

PATHOLOGY

The gross appearance is that of a mass lesion located in the external auditory canal, yellow in color, firm, smooth, having numerous dilated blood vessels stretching over the surface. As the tumor grows, it fills the meatus.[3]

Histologically, the typical "swiss cheese" pattern is encountered. The tumor cells delineate spaces that are cylindrical, some of them empty and others filled with an eosinophilic material. Mitotic figures are relatively few. At times, areas of solid nests or cells without the formation of the cylindromatous pattern are seen. Perineural infiltration by tumor cells is a very common finding. Also, invasion of the fat, the perivascular spaces, as well as involvement of striated muscle and bone can occur.[3,4] Metastatic lesions tend to maintain their primary histological pattern.[2]

CLINICAL

The typical presenting symptom is pain, which is due to the tumor infiltration of the perineural spaces. The pain is deeply seated within the meatus and it can be accompanied by a feeling of a mass being present or by a hearing loss.[2,3,5] The pain occurs relatively early and, as the disease progresses, the pain increases. There is no previous history of ear infection to be found among the patients.

All areas of the external auditory canal may serve as a site of origin. In the early stages mastoid films will be nonrevealing; however, as the disease progresses invasion and destruction in the mastoid regions can be demonstrated radiographically.[2] Erosion of the external auditory canal has also been seen in advanced cases.[3]

The natural history is long. The duration of symptoms varies from 1 to 30 years prior to the time of the diagnosis, the average being six years. In the literature review as compiled by Wetli et al.,[5] among 29 cases, local invasion was found in five and distant metastases, primarily to the lung and regional lymph nodes, were seen in 18 patients. Local recurrence is also a frequent event and may take place as long as 8–10 years following treatment.[3,4]

Distant metastases are a late development and usually appear when the primary has been uncontrolled. These patients suffer from severe relentless pain and the majority die from local extension of the tumor into the brain or from lung metastases.

TREATMENT AND RESULTS

A variety of procedures and methods have been employed in the treatment of adenoid cystic carcinoma of the external auditory canal. These range from local excision to multiple local excisions, wide excisions, radical mastoidectomy, local radiotherapy, and combination techniques.[5] It is readily obvious in reviewing previous reports that local excision has invariably led to recurrence.

Pulec et al.[3] recommend that once the diagnosis of adenoid cystic carcinoma has been established a wide resection of the entire external auditory canal, of the surrounding bone and of part of the pinna be performed. If necessary, extensive radical mastoidectomy with wide excision of the

dura, or total parotidectomy, or a wide excision of any extension to surrounding structures, such as the skin, temporal muscle, or the sternocleidomastoid muscle and the cervical lymph nodes should be performed.[3]

Radiation therapy, although not curative, has much to offer in the way of palliation, particularly by alleviating the excruciating pain experienced by the patients. Turner et al.[4] reported on a recurrent tumor for which radiotherapy was applied at a dose of 6800 rad in 30 fractions. The area of the ear canal remained free of disease for two years, at which point recurrence developed. At that time the patient also developed metastases to the dorsal spine, where excellent relief was obtained by administering radiation at a dose of 3000 rad. Koopot et al.[2] used radiation therapy, for a dose of 2000 rad delivered by a betatron unit, to metastatic lung lesions from primary adenoid cystic carcinoma of the left external auditory canal. There was excellent resolution of disease. The large tumor masses decreased markedly in size.

PROGNOSIS AND SURVIVAL

The prognosis is serious, but survival is long. On the basis of the reported cases and excluding those for whom follow-up is short or lacking, we found the five-year-survival rate to be practically 100%. Although there are patients who developed local recurrences or metastatic disease within the first five years, no patient has been reported as dying from their disease within this time. Even at 10 years, one patient out of a total of 12 died of their disease. At 15 years, however, the survival rate is 50%. The patients continue to die from their disease 20 or 25 years after the diagnosis.[3-5]

REFERENCES

1. Batsakis, J.G.: Tumors of the Head and Neck. Clinical and Pathological Considerations. Williams & Wilkins, Baltimore, 1974.

2. Koopot, R., Reyes, C., and Pifarré, R.: Multiple pulmonary metastases from adenoid cystic carcinoma of ceruminous glands of external auditory canal. A case report and review of the literature. *J Thorac Cardiovasc Surg* **65:**909, 1973.

3. Pulec, J.L., Parkhill, E.M., and Devine, K.D.: Adenoid cystic carcinoma (cylindroma) of the external auditory canal. *Trans Am Acad Ophthalmol Otolaryngol* **67:**673, 1963.

4. Turner, H.A., Carter, H., and Neptune, W.B.: Pulmonary metastases from ceruminous adenocarcinoma (cylindroma) of external auditory canal. *Cancer* **28:**775, 1971.

5. Wetli, C.V., Pardo, V., Millard, M., and Gerston, K.: Tumors of ceruminous glands. *Cancer* **29:**1169, 1972.

49

Adenoid Cystic Carcinoma of the Larynx

ADENOCARCINOMA IN general represents approximately 5% of all laryngeal cancers.[4] Adenoid cystic carcinoma is considered one form of adenocarcinoma and it composes approximately 50% of the entire group. The average age of the patients has been 52 years and there has been no sex predilection, both females and males being affected equally.

PATHOLOGY

The histological appearance is similar to that of adenoid cystic carcinoma in other locations. The lesions were located slightly more frequently in the infraglottic than in the supraglottic area and one patient was described as having a glottic lesion.[3] Cervical lymph node metastases although reported in some instances, are an uncommon development overall.

CLINICAL

In practically all patients hoarseness of the voice associated with some degree of dyspnea and a feeling of a lump in the throat were the most common initial clinical signs. Several patients were symptomatic for many months and actually, on the average, patients experienced symptoms for approximately 16 months prior to their diagnosis.[4] The work-up and the establishment of the diagnosis is the same as in all laryngeal cancers.

TREATMENT AND RESULTS

Total laryngectomy has been the commonest form of applied therapy. In some cases local excision only has been used as the first form of therapy. Local recurrence is a certainty following this type of therapy and a number of patients therefore who were initially treated by one or more local excisions eventually underwent a total laryngectomy.[6]

PROGNOSIS AND SURVIVAL

Patients treated by total laryngectomy have survived the longest. Knowing the natural history of adenoid cystic carcinoma and because in several patients the follow-up is less than five years, the overall prognosis should be viewed with caution. Characteristically, the case described by Leroux-Robert and Courtial[1] dealt with a 62-year-old female surviving for 16 years following a total laryngectomy but died at that time of lung and liver metastases.

We have compiled in the present literature review the survival rates for adenoid cystic carcinoma in this location. At the three-year level, it has been approximately 50%. As stated, the number of cases with long-term follow-up are too few to obtain meaningful figures.

REFERENCES

1. Leroux-Robert, J., and Courtial, C.: Tumeurs mixtes et cylindromas du larynx. *Ann Otol Laryngol (Paris)*, **82:**1, 1965.

2. Putney, F.J., and McStravog, L.J.: Salivary gland type tumors of the head and neck. *Laryngoscope* **64:**285, 1954.

3. Suehs, O.W.: Cylindroma (adenoid cystic car-cinoma) of the larynx and trachea. *Texas State J Med* **54:**934, 1960.

4. Toomey, J.M.: Adenocarcinoma of the larynx. *Laryngoscope* **77:**931, 1967.

50

Adenoid Cystic Carcinoma of the Trachea

CARCINOMA OF THE trachea is rare. It has been estimated that one such tumor corresponds to approximately 180 lung carcinomas or 75 laryngeal carcinomas.[2] Among the various histological types that have been reported as occurring in the trachea, squamous cell carcinoma and adenoid cystic carcinoma are the commonest encountered. In the series reported by Hajdu et al.,[1] of 41 patients with primary tracheal carcinoma, 30 had squamous cell carcinoma; 7, adenoid cystic carcinoma; and 4, mucous-secreting adenocarcinoma. Houston et al.[2] in a review of the material from the Mayo Clinic identified 53 primary neoplasms of the trachea, of which 24 (45.3%) were squamous cell carcinomas, 19 (35.6%) were adenoid cystic carcinomas, and the remaining were mostly single cases of mesenchymal tumors, adenocarcinomas, and undifferentiated carcinomas.

In contrast to patients with squamous cell carcinoma whose age at the time of the onset is around 50 years, patients with adenoid cystic carcinoma are younger and smoking is not to be found in their clinical histories. The average age for both males and females is 42 to 44 years, with several patients to be found younger than the age of 30.[2,4,6]

Adenoid cystic carcinoma occurs with nearly the same frequency among men and women, whereas squamous cell carcinoma, until the present time, has been seen four times more frequently in men than in women, reflecting smoking habits.

PATHOLOGY

The tumor grossly appears as a circumscribed mass presenting in the lumen of the trachea with a smooth surface rarely ulcerated. It may be seen in any tracheal segment. Eleven of 16 patients reported by Pearson[4] had the growth located in the mediastinal and lower trachea, whereas in three patients the lesion involved the cervical part of the trachea extending into the larynx and in two both the mediastinal and cervical segments were involved. Hajdu et al.[1] found five tumors occurring in the upper third of the trachea and only two were located in the distal third. The size of the mass at the time of the diagnosis exceeds 2.0 cm and infiltration of the tracheal wall is the rule.[1] The local invasion is actually a full-thickness penetration of the wall and there is microscopic extension into the submucosa. There is also perineural lymphatic spread far beyond the clinical confines of the tumor.[4]

Microscopically, the lesion is identical to adenoid cystic carcinoma of the salivary glands. The characteristic cords and sheets of fairly uniform cells are seen which outline cystlike spaces of various sizes. The histogenesis of the tumor is attributed to bronchial mucous glands. It is generally agreed that the tracheal epithelium is not implicated in this development, since it usually remains intact.[1,5]

CLINICAL

All patients have been symptomatic prior to the time of the diagnosis. The

148

commonest symptoms are cough, which the patients relate to a tickling sensation in the throat, wheezing respiration, and shortness of breath.[4] Singh and Thomas[7] identified a common complaint among patients with tracheal tumors. It occurs when more than 75% of the tracheal lumen has been occluded and it relates to the manner with which the patient breaths. The respirations are short and sharp, as if the patient is sniffing. The patient says that he breathes this way because he is not certain that he will be able to "breathe all the air out." The authors considered this sign pathognomonic for tracheal occlusion.[7] Hemoptysis, which is frequent with squamous cell carcinoma of the trachea, is uncommonly seen in adenoid cystic carcinomas.[1,4] Hoarseness of the voice is another early, frequently occurring sign.

These complaints regarding the upper respiratory tract are accompanied in most cases by a negative chest radiograph. It is at this time that a tomographic examination of the trachea will be quite helpful in delineating the pathology. The final diagnosis is made by means of bronchoscopy and biopsy. Several patients have been treated for what was considered to be an "allergy" before the diagnosis of tracheal tumor was established.

The tumor extends to the tracheal wall and into the adjacent mediastinal structures. Should the treatment fail to eradicate the disease, extensive destruction of the tracheal cartilage and invasion into the pericardium, the superior vena cava, and the lung will develop. The tumor, when occurring in the trachea, follows its characteristic pattern of behavior, namely, recurring locally, extending beyond the visible margins, and at the same time affording the patient with a long survival in spite of its presence.[8]

Distant metastases to the lungs, bone, liver, and the brain have been reported (Fig. 50-1).[1,2,4] Extension to the regional lymph nodes is not a common finding and was seen only in one patient of the 16 reported by Pearson et al.[4]

TREATMENT AND RESULTS

Surgical resection with reconstruction by primary anastomosis, end tracheostomy, or autologous grafting is the recommended therapy and should be considered as the initial procedure in every patient with the diagnosis of adenoid cystic carcinoma of the trachea unless the tumor appears to be inoperable. During the past 10–15 years, improvement in operative techniques, which have reduced the tension at the anastomotic site, have made extensive tracheal resection and reconstruction by primary anastomosis a feasible procedure. Prior to 1965, these undertakings were accompanied by high mortality.[4]

Postoperative deaths, however, have been noted in patients whose tracheal reconstruction was made with the help of artificial material. Among this group of patients 8 of 12 surviving the postoperative period were alive and clinically free of tumor for periods ranging from 2 to 18 years after resection. One had asymptomatic pulmonary metastases and four patients were dead with recurrent disease. In one of these, extensive metastases were found, and in the remaining three local recurrence occurred.[4]

When the disease is extensive locally, surgical results, as expected, are not permanent. Local recurrence developed in all six cases following partial tracheal resection, as reported by Jajdu et al.[1] Three of the patients were dead of their disease at 1, 12, and 13 years following treatment, and the three survivors were living with active disease present at two, six, and seven years from the time of their treatment.

The role of radiation therapy in the management of this disease has been more or less defined. Although it has failed to control the disease in a definitive manner, several reports exist indicating palliative effects and longer survivals following irradiation. Richardson et al.[6] reported on a 27-year-old female with a large

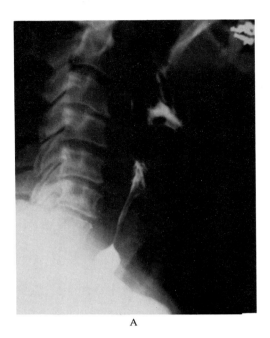

A

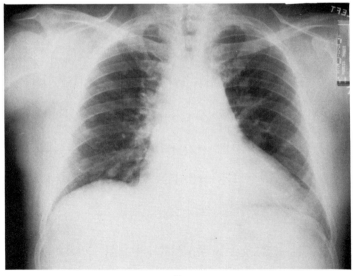

B

FIG. 50–1.   Adenoid cystic carcinoma of the trachea in a 42-year-old
male. *(A):* Lateral view of the neck reveals a soft tissue mass separat-
ing the air column from the cervical esophagus and compressing the
latter. *(B):* In spite of controlling the primary following radiotherapy,
the patient has multiple lung metastases five years later.

mass extending the entire length of the
intrathoracic trachea. The patient received
5000 rad and nine months later an examination by bronchoscopy, tomograms, and
tracheograms failed to reveal any signs of
tumor. Zunker *et al.*[8] reported on a 36-
year-old male whose tumor was found
midway between the larynx and the

carina, presenting as a large mass on the right posterior tracheal wall. The patient received 4650 rad in a one-month period. There was appreciable reduction of the tumor on radiographs 5.5 months later. Enlargement of the mass occurred again 40 months following this therapy and a second course of radiotherapy was delivered for a total of 4900 rad. The patient presented with hemoptysis four years later, at which point again polypoid excressions from the main tumor mass were seen. It was deemed that no further therapy by means of radiation could be delivered. The patient was seen in follow-up visits complaining of gradually increasing respiratory distress. He died two years later, from tumor-related obstruction. On the whole, he had a nine-year survival.

Pearson et al.[4] applied radiation therapy preoperatively using anterior and posterior parallel fields and delivering 3500–4000 rad in 21 days to the tumor. All six patients had definitive surgery with clear resection lines and no patient within this group developed clinical evidence of locally recurrent disease. Because of the good response radiation produces on the gross tumor, the authors are optimistic that this technique offers the best potential for a cure. Due to the long natural history of the disease, however, they are cautious in recommending strongly their management system.

Endoscopic removal of the tumor is a form of effective palliation. Nine patients with adenoid cystic carcinoma received endoscopic removal with or without fulgeration by surgical diathermy. Six lived more than five years. Actually, one patient was alive 10 years following the resection and the rest had survived from 5 to 30 years before dying of their tumor. Although the survival was long, the quality of palliation was poor. The patients underwent multiple bronchoscopic examinations for multiple local recurrences during the course of their disease.[2] Nakratzas et al.[3] reported on a 64-year-old female with adenoid cystic carcinoma of the posterior wall of the trachea. The tumor mass was 8.5 cm long and it was deemed to be inoperable. The patient was treated by bronchoscopic resection under general anesthesia. Following this, the stridor disappeared. The treatment had been repeated six times during a period of three years due to local recurrence, without any complications.

PROGNOSIS AND SURVIVAL

It is obvious that five-year survival is not indicative of cure. On the basis of our literature review, the five-year-survival rate was 64%. In estimating the mortality, deaths related to the tumor or to the treatment were accounted for. The survival at 10 years was 39% and at 15 years, 17%. Actually there are patients who have died of their tumor 25 or 30 years after the diagnosis.[1,2,6,8]

The prognosis is best in small tumors, localized to a small area of the trachea, where complete resection and anastomosis can be performed.[4]

REFERENCES

1. Hajdu, S.I., Huvos, A.G., Goodner, J.T., Foote, F.W., Jr., and Beattie, E.J., Jr.: Carcinoma of the trachea. Clinicopathologic study of 41 cases. *Cancer* **25**:1448, 1970.
2. Houston, H.E., Payne, W.S., Harrison, E.G., Jr., and Olsen, A.M.: Primary cancers of the trachea. *Arch Surg* **99**:132, 1969.
3. Nakratzas, G., Wagenaar, J.P.M., Reintjes, M., Scheffer, E., and Swierenga, J.: Repeated partial endoscopic resections as treatment for two patients with inoperable tracheal tumours. *Thorax* **29**:125, 1974.
4. Pearson, F.G., Thompson, D.W., Weissberg, D., Simpson, W.J.K., and Kergin, D.G.: Adenoid cystic carcinoma of the trachea. Experience with 16 patients managed by tracheal resection. *Ann Thorac Surg* **18**:16, 1974.
5. Reid, J.D.: Adenoid cystic carcinoma (cylindroma) of the bronchial tree. *Cancer* **5**:685, 1952.
6. Richardson, J.D., Grover, F.L., and Trinkle, J.K.: Adenoid cystic carcinoma of the trachea. Response to cobalt-60. *J Thorac Card Surg* **66**:311, 1973.
7. Singh, H.M., and Thomas, D.M.E.: A clinical sign

of adenocystic tumour of the trachea. *Thorax* **28:**442, 1973.

8. Zunker, H.O., Moore, R.L., Baker, D.C., and Lat-tes, R.: Adenoid cystic carcinoma (cylindroma) of the trachea. Case report with 9-year follow-up. *Cancer* **23:**699, 1969.

51

Adenoid Cystic Carcinoma of the Bronchus

MÜLLER[10] FIRST described the bronchial adenoma in 1882. It was not until 1937 when Hamperl[5] identified within the adenoma group two distinct entities, the carcinoid tumors and the cyclindromas. Liebow[7] described the mucoepidermoid tumors and separated them from the cylindromas.

Presently, three tumors are recognized within the group of bronchial adenomas. Carcinoid tumors account for 85–90% of all bronchial adenomas, adenoid cystic carcinomas account for 8–10%, and the remainder are mucoepidermoid tumors of the bronchial tree.[2,11–13]

There is no difference in incidence between males and females, and the average age is 45 years at the time of the diagnosis. The tumors have therefore appeared in a younger age group, compared to patients with carcinoma of the lung.[4,12,13]

PATHOLOGY

Characteristically, adenoid cystic carcinomas are located centrally. They arise from the mucous bronchial glands and their histological pattern is similar to that of adenoid cystic carcinomas of the head and neck. They are centrally located, involving the major bronchi or extending to the trachea. Actually, adenoid cystic carcinoma can occur as a primary tracheal tumor.[2,3]

Grossly, adenoid cystic carcinomas of the bronchus present as polypoid infiltrating tumors that partially or completely obstruct the bronchus. They have a nodular and polypoid appearance extending in a tubular fashion. This propagation along the bronchial lumen can be seen on microscopic examination.[12] On cross section, the tumor often extends through the wall, so that extraluminal infiltration of adjacent mediastinal structures or into the nearby lung tissue is a a distinct possibility.[14] The tumor is often covered with necrotic material and it may bleed easily on manipulation. When bronchial obstruction occurs, particularly in small bronchi, atelectasis associated with infection may develop distally. Histologically, arrangement of small dark-stained cells anastomosing in solid or cystic formations delineating between them collections of relatively acellular connective tissue, which thus gives the typical "swiss cheese" appearance of adenoid cystic carcinoma, is to be found.[12]

Local invasion beyond the bronchial wall apparently is quite high. Goldstraw *et al.*[3] presented four cases of adenoid cystic carcinoma of the bronchus and reviewed the literature. They placed the incidence of local invasion at 75–80%. On the other hand, regional lymph node metastases are to be found in approximately 25% of the patients.[2,3] The tumors are capable of metastasizing distally. Three of five patients reported by Goodner *et al.*[4] and 3 of 13 patients reported by Payne *et al.*[12] developed metastases.

CLINICAL

The leading symptoms are cough, hemoptysis, and recurring bouts of pul-

153

monary infection. It is significant that the average duration of the symptoms in patients with adenoid cystic carcinoma can be very long. In most patients they have been present for two to three years. Other clinical signs include a wheezing and stridor or dyspnea, particularly when extension into the trachea is present. Radiographs of the chest may be within normal limits, especially in small centrally located tumors. Larger tumors produce pneumonitis as a result of bronchial narrowing, and later on atelectasis of a segment, a lobe, or the entire lung.[12,13] Tomograms are very helpful in depicting these intrabronchial tumors.

The definitive method of diagnosis is bronchoscopy and biopsy. This is well achieved for adenoid cystic carcinomas because of their central location, which permits an easy access to the lesion.[14]

Distant metastases when they occur may involve primarily the lungs, the skeletal system, and the liver.[4,12]

TREATMENT AND RESULTS

The term "bronchial adenoma," which denotes a benign more or less clinical course, is indeed a misnomer when it comes to adenoid cystic carcinoma— cylindroma—of the lung, particularly considering the problems encountered in therapy. A significant number of patients are actually nonresectable by standard clinical criteria at the time of the diagnosis due to the fact that the disease exhibits local invasiveness, making complete resection impossible. Some authors have advocated local resection, whereas others feel that radical resection is more appropriate. There is no question that if cure is to be the aim radical removal is in order; however, it is equally important to recognize that many of these lesions are incurable and for this reason palliative procedures, although not definitive, may provide considerable prolongation of life. Along these lines, radiation therapy lo-

cally associated with endoscopic removal of obstructive tumors has been found useful and applicable in nonresectable cases.[2,6]

Should definitive resection be undertaken, the main problem with which the surgeon is faced is the location of the tumor. Because they arise in the main bronchi, they frequently extend to the carina or the trachea. For this reason, tracheoplastic and bronchoplastic procedures are necessary in order to preserve pulmonary function and actually to preserve the life of the patient.[2,8] Payne et al.[12] considered pneumonectomy the only presumably curative procedure, acknowledging, however, that only a few patients with adenoid cystic carcinoma have tumors potentially curable. Vieta and Maier[14] underlined the fact that, because of the central location and frequent extension into the trachea and the longer clinical course that is exhibited in many instances by these neoplasms, it is proper to balance the risks of pneumonectomy plus tracheal reconstruction versus a smaller palliative resection in combination with local radiotherapy. It is generally agreed that some form of tumor removal is necessary in order to avoid suppurative complications which develop distally to the obstructed bronchus. Local radiotherapy has been helpful in bringing about regression of the tumor and affording a worthwhile palliation in several patients.[2,4,14]

Of seven patients with tracheal or tracheobronchial cylindroma who underwent resection and reconstruction reported by Mathey et al.,[8] three died of their disease two months, two years, and 5.5 years after operation. The remaining were well 1, 2, 10, and 11 years from the time of the surgery. Reviewing the experience at the Mayo Clinic, Payne et al.[12] found the average survival at the time of their review to be 4.8 years for patients who underwent surgical resection as opposed to 2.8 years for those who were treated by conservative management. As with cylindromas in other locations, local recurrence and metastases may develop several years following therapy. Meffert and Lindskog[9] reported on such a patient, who died 13 years and 9 months after middle and lower lobectomy for a cylindroma of the bronchus intermedius. Local recurrence and metastases to both lungs had occurred.

Local recurrence is the main problem in managing this neoplasm. This is a frequent event and is due to the fact that extension or metastasis at the time of the initial examination or operation is very high. Donahue et al.[2] found it to be 46%, although others raise this figure even higher. Goldstraw et al.[3] stated that detailed examination of the specimens suggests that the incidence of local invasion may be nearer 100%. This is where the difficulty in controlling the tumor lies.

PROGNOSIS AND SURGICAL

Although the prognosis more often than not is doubtful regarding the cure of the disease, the life-span may be expected in terms of years. Because of the location, however, and the accompanying difficulties in terms of handling the recurrences the overall survival is less, compared to that of adenoid cystic carcinomas in other sites. The five-year-survival rate in the study by Goldstraw et al.[3] was found to be 25%. This sharply contrasts with an 82% five-year survival of carcinoid tumors of the lung and it clearly demonstrates the necessity for subdividing the entities included in the general term "bronchial adenoma." We have compiled from several literature series the survival rates for 5 and 10 years found them to be 40% and 26% respectively.[1,4,6,8,9,11,12,14]

REFERENCES

1. Burcharth, F., and Axelsson, C.: Bronchial adenomas. *Thorax* **27**:442, 1972.

2. Donahue, J.K., Weichert, R.F., and Ochsner, J.L.: Bronchial adenoma. *Ann Surg* **167**:873, 1968.

3. Goldstraw, P., Lamb, D., McCormack, R.J.M., and Walbaum, P.R.: The malignancy of bronchial adenoma. *J Thorac Cardiovasc Surg* **72**:309, 1976.

4. Goodner, J.T., Berg, J.W., and Watson, W.L.: The non-benign nature of bronchial carcinoids and cylindromas. *Cancer* **14**:539, 1961.

5. Hamperl, H.: Über gutartige Bronchialtumoren (Cylindrome and Carcinoide). *Arch Pathol Anat* **300**:46, 1937.

6. Heilbrunn, A., and Crosby, I.K.: Adenocystic carcinoma and mucoepidermoid carcinoma of the tracheobronchial tree. *Chest* **61**:145, 1972.

7. Liebow, A.A.: *Tumors of the Lower Respiratory Tract.* Armed Forces Institute of Pathology, Washington, D.C., 1952.

8. Mathey, J., et al.: Tracheal and tracheobronchial resections. Technique and results in 20 cases. *J Thorac Cardiovasc Surg* **51**:1, 1966.

9. Meffert, W.G., and Lindskog, G.E.: Bronchial adenoma. *J Thorac Cardiovasc Surg* **59**:588, 1970.

10. Müller, H.: Quoted by Engelbreth-Holm, J.: Bnign bronchial adenomas. *Acta Chir Scand* **90**:383, 1945.

11. O'Grady, W.P., McDivitt, R.W., Holman, C.W., and Moore, S.W.: Bronchial adenomas. *Arch Surg* **101**:558, 1970.

12. Payne, W.S., Ellis, F.H., Jr., Woolner, L.B., and Moersch, H.J.: The surgical treatment of cylindroma (adenoid cystic carcinoma) and mucoepidermoid tumors of the bronchus. *J Thorac Cardiovasc Surg* **38**:709, 1959.

13. Wilkins, E.W., Jr., Darling, R.C., Soutter, L., and Sniffen, R.C.: A continuing clinical survey of adenomas of the trachea and bronchus in a general hospital. *J Thorac Cardiovasc Surg* **46**:279, 1963.

14. Vieta, J.O., and Maier, H.C.: The treatment of adenoid cystic carcinoma (cylindroma) of the respiratory tract by surgery and radiation therapy. *Dis Chest* **31**:493, 1957.

52

Adenoid Cystic Carcinoma of the Breast

ADENOID CYSTIC CARCINOMA is an unusual form of breast cancer. The incidence was found to be 0.4% (4 among 1000 cases of breast cancer) in the series reported by Fisher et al.[2] Among 910 cases of breast carcinoma operated on at Scripps Hospital, Hopkins and Tullis[5] identified and reported on three adenoid cystic carcinomas. This uncommon tumor of the breast exhibits the characteristic microscopic pattern seen in the salivary gland counterpart. It has a better prognosis than adenoic cystic carcinoma in other locations and far better than carcinoma of the breast.

The age of most patients at the time of the diagnosis is in the range of 50–55 years.[1,3,4,13] Two male patients with this histological variety of breast tumors have been reported.[12]

PATHOLOGY

The gross appearance is that of a well-defined but not encapsulated tumor.[1,4] The size ranges from 1.0 to 5.0 cm, being 2.5 cm on the average. There are no differentiating signs from adenocarcinoma of the breast.[1,4] Skin involvement can take place, but it is rare. Microscopically, there is a cystic glandular pattern. The cells are small with scanty cytoplasm and small hyperchromatic nuclei. They are arranged in masses or cords delineating spaces filled with amorphous pink-staining material, which occasionally is hyalinized[4] (Fig. 52-1). The material is stained posi-

tively with mucicarmine stain. Cavanzo and Taylor[1] in an analysis of 21 cases found a high tendency for perineural infiltration, which had no bearing on the prognosis. The authors stress the importance of distinguishing adenoid cystic carcinoma from intraductal carcinoma of the breast with cribriform pattern, which superficially may resemble the adenoid cystic pattern.

Koss et al.[6] studied the ultrastructural feature of five adenoid cystic carcinomas of the breast. The similarity between them and their salivary gland counterpart was further strengthened. It was shown that the cystic spaces were not duct or glandular spaces but extracellular compartments enclosed by tumor cells. The compartments were lined by an uninterrupted basement membrane from which the contents of the cyst appeared to be derived. It was concluded that the most likely site of origin are the small ducts of the breast.

CLINICAL

The commonest symptom is the presence of a mass in the breast. This at times is tender and at times painless. It is well defined on palpation. Skin retraction has been reported in a few cases. The duration of its presence has varied from a few days to several years.[1,3,13]

Most authors conclude that regional lymph node metastases rarely occur. This is exemplified in the case reported by Lerner et al.[7] The patient presented with a

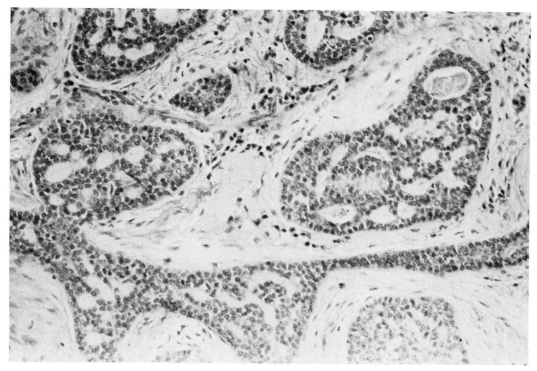

FIG. 52-1.   Adenoid cystic carcinoma of the breast. Irregular islands of tumor cells with cribriform pattern.

large mass replacing the right breast, measuring 8.0 by 10.0 cm. There was ulceration of the skin in the areolar region. There was even invasion of the local lymph vessels. In spite of the extensiveness of the disease, no lymph node involvement was found following a modified radical operation. The lack of nodal involvement and the slow growth of the primary tumor account for the good prognosis. The tumors also rarely metastasize distantly; however, local recurrences in the chest wall can occur. Wilson and Spell[14] reported on a 54-year-old patient whose primary tumor measured 2.8 cm and was removed by simple mastectomy. A recurrent nodule on the scar was excised along with the pectoral muscles and axillary contents five years later. Ten years after the second operation, another recurrent mass was removed from the chest

wall. The patient was surviving without signs of dissemination 15 years from the diagnosis.

Nayer[9] published a report on a 39-year-old female who underwent a radical mastectomy for adenoid cystic carcinoma of the breast. All the lymph nodes were free. Lung metastases were detected eight years later. The patient eventually died of her disease 13 years after the original operation and five years after the diagnosis of pulmonary metastases.

Similarly Cavanzo and Taylor[1] identified two patients remaining alive and well 9 and 14 years after treatment of their recurrent disease. Verani and Bel-Kahn[12] in their report of a 78-year-old man with adenoid cystic carcinoma stated that the patient was aware of the tumor being present 10 years prior to the diagnosis. Soon thereafter, he developed lung metastases; however, he had enjoyed a symptom-free life with active disease for 10 years.

Most authors emphasize the long natural history, the paucity of lymph node involvement, and the favorable prognosis.

TREATMENT AND RESULTS

Simple mastectomies and radical mastectomies have been performed. Due to the fact that local recurrences have occasionally appeared following simple mastectomy, some of the authors advocate radical approach. It is true that following radical mastectomy no local recurrence has taken place; however, it is also true that lymph node involvement was not found in any of those cases.[1,14] Some patients have been treated only by local tumor excision and have shown no local recurrence or distant metastasis several years thereafter.[4,11]

The general opinion is that a simple mastectomy is an adequate procedure for the management of this lesion provided that histologically the diagnosis has been established and provided that the tumor has been differentiated from cribriform ductal carcinoma on frozen section examination.[1,5]

The patient described by Nayer[9] whose tumor metastasized to the lungs failed to respond to hormonal therapy.

PROGNOSIS AND SURVIVAL

Unlike adenoid cystic carcinomas in other locations where, in spite of their often prolonged course, local recurrences and distant metastases are commonplace, the tumor when present in the breast pursues a much more benign course and affords a favorable outlook. The five-year survival is virtually 100%. Actually review of the literature reveals only two patients dying of their disease.[3] Those are the patients reported by Nayer[9] and by O'Kell.[10]

They developed metastatic disease, dying 14 and 3.6 years, respectively, from the time of the diagnosis. Both were treated initially with radical mastectomies.

There are several patients whose follow-up periods have been longer than 10 years, surviving without signs of local recurrence or distant metastases.[1,5,6,8,11]

REFERENCES

1. Cavanzo, F.J., and Taylor, H.B.: Adenoid cystic carcinoma of the breast. An analysis of 21 cases. *Cancer* **24:**740, 1969.
2. Fisher, E.R., Gregorio, R.M., and Fisher, B.: The pathology of invasive breast cancer. A syllabus derived from findings of the National Surgical Adjuvant Breast Project (Protocol No. 4). *Cancer* **36:**1, 1975.
3. Friedman, B.A., and Oberman, H.A.: Adenoid cystic carcinoma of the breast. *Am J Clin Pathol* **54:**1, 1970.
4. Galloway, J.R., Woolner, L.B., and Clagett, O.T.: Adenoid cystic carcinoma of the breast. *Surg Gynecol Obstet* **122:**1289, 1966.
5. Hopkins, G.B., and Tullis, R.H.: Adenoid cystic carcinoma of the breast. *Calif Med* **117:**9, 1972.
6. Koss, L.G., Brannan, C.D., and Ashikari, R.: Histologic and ultrastructural features of adenoid cystic carcinoma of the breast. *Cancer* **26:**1271, 1970.
7. Lerner, A.G., Molnar, J.J., and Adam, Y.G.: Adenoid cystic carcinoma of the breast. *Am J Surg* **127:**585, 1974.
8. Lusted, D.: Structural and growth patterns of adenoid cystic carcinoma of the breast. *Am J Clin Pathol* **54:** 419, 1970.
9. Nayer, H.R.: Cylindroma of the breast with pulmonary metastases. *Dis Chest* **31:**324, 1957.
10. O'Kell, R.T.: Adenoid cystic carcinoma of the breast. *Mo Med* **61:**855, 1964.
11. Schulenburg, C.A.R., and Pepler, W.J.: Adenoid cystic carcinoma of the breast. *Br J Surg* **56:**395, 1969.
12. Verani, R.R., and van der Bel-Kahn, J.: Mammary adenoid cystic carcinoma with unusual features. *Am J Clin Pathol* **59:**653, 1973.
13. Weitzner, S., Chaney, G.C., and Bass, H.L.: Adenoid cystic carcinoma of the breast: Report of a case and review of the literature. *Am Surg* **36:**571, 1970.
14. Wilson, W.B., and Spell, J.P.: Adenoid cystic carcinoma of breast: A case with recurrence and regional metastasis. *Ann Surg* **166:**861, 1967.

53

Adenoid Cystic Carcinoma of the Uterine Cervix

THE FIRST CASES of adenoid carcinoma in this location were described by Paalman and Counseller[11] in 1949 and by Tchertkoff and Sedlis[13] in 1962. Although it is a rare tumor, 33 cases being reported thus far, its existence is well established and review of the files at the Armed Forces Institute of Pathology showed it to represent 3% of all primary adenocarcinomas of the cervix.[9,12]

The lesion is to be found in patients older than those with squamous cell carcinoma or adenocarcinoma of the cervix. The age range has been from 39 to 89 years; however, the average age at the time of the diagnosis is 66 years. All of the patients, with the exception of two, were postmenopausal. Of the 30 for whom parity was reported, 24 had had two or more children.[4,6,9,12]

PATHOLOGY

Grossly, the tumor is exophytic in character, presenting as a hard or friable mass and sometimes as an endocervical polypoid lesion. Cytology was reported in 17 of 18 cases as being positive for various degrees of cellular atypia.[12] The size of the neoplasm has ranged from less than a centimeter to masses greater than 5.0 cm in diameter.[9] Microscopic examination reveals cells forming cords only a few layers thick or solid masses that contain punched-out areas filled with hyalinelike eosinophilic acellular material, providing thus the appearance of cylinders.[9,12] The cells are uniform in character, with darkly stained nuclei and relatively little cytoplasm. The mitotic activity is usually minimal. The contents of the cylinders stain positive for hyaline and mucin.[9] Often other patterns of carcinoma coexist. In 22 of 33 cases analyzed of carcinoma in situ, invasive squamous carcinoma and adenocarcinoma are to be found mixed within the histological pattern of adenoid cystic carcinoma.[1,2,5,9,13] The presence of neoplasias with varying histology perhaps indicate that the histogenesis of adenoid cystic carcinoma of the cervix can be ascribed to a basal or reserve cell within the cervical epithelium, from which this particular histological pattern through the process of a sideline differentiation develops. It appears that these mixtures of histology derive their origins from a relatively multipotential reserve cell. These cells lie beneath the columnar mucinous epithelium of the endocervix and they are those from which the squamous and the glandular epithelium in these locations are replenished.[4,9,10]

CLINICAL

The most frequent presenting symptom is vaginal bleeding. This is usually in the form of spotting; however, overt bleeding has been occasionally reported. There is no clinical sign that distinguishes this lesion from the rest of the cervical carcinomas. As stated, cytology of the vaginal smears has been positive.

Most patients had disease confined to the cervix at the time of the diagnosis in the series reported by Miles and Norris.[9] Cases reported by other authors had larger tumors with parametrial or vaginal extension. Pelvic extension has been documented in six of the reported cases and distant metastases in five. Metastatic sites include the liver, lung, bones, and peritoneal cavity. Adenoid cystic carcinoma in this location retains the characteristic property of invading lymphatic channels and this was seen in 11 of the 12 cases studied by Miles and Norris.[9] It is this biological behavior that accounts for the aggressiveness of the tumor, aggressiveness similar to the salivary gland counterpart.[5]

TREATMENT AND RESULTS

Both surgery and radiation therapy have been used for the management of these patients. The commonest surgical procedure has been total hysterectomy, with bilateral salpingo-oophorectomy. In some cases, pelvic lymphadenectomy has been performed.[2,7,8,9,13] The radiation therapy techniques have been similar to those employed for squamous cell carcinoma of the cervix. A combination of external beam radiotherapy by which 5000–6000 rad delivered to the pelvis was supplemented by cervical radium placements by which additional 3000–6000 rad were delivered in the vicinity of the tumor.[4–6,9,12,14] No clear superiority of either technique has been demonstrated.

In the case of Ramzy et al.[12] the patient was surviving without signs of recurrence two years following radiation therapy.

Gallagher et al.[5] reported on a patient surviving three years free of disease following radiotherapy and eventually dying of a cerebrovascular accident. Miles and

Norris[9] in their review found three patients surviving 2.4, 4, and 5.2 years following radiation therapy, whereas two other patients died at 0.8 and 3.3 years with tumor after administration of radiation therapy. Genton[6] encountered massive local recurrence following a definitive program of radiotherapy for a Stage III carcinoma. The patient not only had extensive local disease but, in addition, distant metastasis with involvement of the pericardium, myocardium, and the liver. The patient described by Dahlin[3] was initially treated by radiotherapy, showing recurrent disease three years later, at which point anterior pelvic exenteration was performed.

Of the five patients treated exclusively by surgery in the series by Miles and Norris,[9] four were alive and well for 0.8–2.5 years. This, of course, is a short time to evaluate results in adenoid cystic carcinomas.

Baggish and Woodruff[1] reported long-term survivals on three patients with adenoid cystic carcinoma of the cervix in situ. All were treated surgically and all were living and well 5,7, and 13 years later.

PROGNOSIS AND SURVIVAL

The biological behavior of adenoid cystic carcinoma of the cervix is similar to that shown by this particular neoplasm in other locations. In spite of early good results caution is required because of the tendency of the tumor to recur locally. This is due to the tendency to infiltrate along the lymph vessels. There are many cases in which recurrence was noted several years after treatment. De la Maza et al.[4] reported diffuse abdominal recurrence with involvement of the serosal surfaces and the omentum, producing bowel obstruction. There were no signs of recurrence in the cervix. The patient had been treated three years earlier by radiation therapy. Gallagher et al.[5] reported liver and chest metastases two years following treatment of the primary.

With a few exceptions, practically all reported patients survived for two years. However, as follow-up reveals, the survival rate was approximately 50% between the third and the fourth year from the time of the diagnosis.[4,6,9,12–14]

REFERENCES

1. Baggish, M.S., and Woodruff, J.D.: Adenoid basal lesions of the cervix. *Obstet Gynecol* **37**:807, 1971.
2. Benitez, E., Rodriguez, H.A., Rodriguez-Guevas, H., and Chavez, G.B.: Adenoid cystic carcinoma of the uterine cervix. Report of a case and review of 4 cases. *Obstet Gynecol* **33**:757, 1969.
3. Dahlin, D.C.: Case No. 9 Proceedings from the seminar of the Houston Society of Clinical Pathologists, 1966.
4. De la Maza, L.M., Thayer, B.A., and Naeim, F.: Cylindroma of the uterine cervix with peritoneal metastases: Report of a case and review of the literature. *Am J Obstet Gynecol* **112**:121, 1972.
5. Gallagher, H.S., Simpson, C.B., and Ayala, A.G.: Adenoid cystic carcinoma of the uterine cervix. Report of 4 cases. *Cancer* **27**:1398, 1971.
6. Genton, C.: Adenoid cystic carcinoma of the uterine cervix. *Obstet Gynecol* **43**:905, 1974.
7. Gordon, H.W., McMahon, N.J., Agliozzo, C.M., Rao, P.R., and Rogers, J.: Adenoid cystic (cylindromatous) carcinoma of the uterine cervix: Report of two cases. *Am J Clin Pathol* **58**:51, 1972.
8. McGee, J.A., Flowers, C.E., and Tatum, B.S.: Adenoid cystic carcinoma of the cervix. Report of a case. *Obstet Gynecol* **26**:356, 1965.
9. Miles, P.A., and Norris, H.J.: Adenoid cystic carcinoma of the cervix. An analysis of 12 cases. *Obstet Gynecol* **38**:103, 1971.
10. Moss, L.D., and Collins, D.N.: Squamous and adenoid cystic basal cell carcinoma of the cervix uteri. *Am J Obstet Gymecol* **88**:86, 1964.
11. Paalman, R.J., and Counseller, V.S.: Cylindroma of the cervix with procidentia. *Am J Obstet Gynecol* **58**:184, 1949.
12. Ramzy, I., Yuzpe, A.A., and Hendelman, J.: Adenoid cystic carcinoma of uterine cervix. *Obstet Gynecol* **45**:679, 1975.
13. Tchertkoff, V., and Sedlis, A.: Cylindroma of the cervix. *Am J Obstet Gynecol* **84**:749, 1962.
14. Van Velden, D.J.J., and Chuang, J.T.: Cylindromatous carcinoma of the uterine cervix. A case report. *Obstet Gynecol* **39**:17, 1972.

54

Carcinoid Tumors of the Gastrointestinal Tract

CARCINOID TUMORS have been described in all parts of the gastrointestinal tract, with the exception of the esophagus. Sanders and Axtell[12] reviewed 2502 cases of gastrointestinal carcinoids and tabulated them by region. Their incidence was as follows: stomach, 3.4%; duodenum, 2.3%; jejunum and ileum, 32.2%; appendix, 45.5%; rectum, 12%; the remainder of the colon, 2.6%, carcinoids in Meckel's diverticulum, 1.3%, and carcinoids of the gallbladder, approximately 0.5%.

The tumors occur in all age groups.[4] Carcinoids of the appendix appear in younger patients, the average age at the time of the diagnosis being 40 years.[7] Patients with carcinoids in the remaining parts of the gastrointestinal tract are in the 60 to 65 year age group.[4]

There is no sex predilection except in carcinoids of the appendix, where the tumor occurs three times more frequently in females than in males.[4,7,12]

Ryden et al.[11] reported 30 cases of carcinoid tumors involving the appendix in children younger than 15 years of age. Of them, 23 were girls and seven were boys.

Gastrointestinal carcinoids may be asymptomatic or they may produce symptoms that relate to the site of their origin. As such, abdominal pain, diarrhea, intestinal obstruction, and rectal bleeding may be encountered.

CARCINOID SYNDROME

Carcinoids are hormone-secreting neoplasms. Therefore in addition to their local manifestations symptoms related to their endocrine activity may occur, constituting the so-called "carcinoid syndrome." The manifestations of it can be classified clinically as follows: 1) flushing of the skin and cyanosis, the so-called "vasomotor disturbances"; 2) gastrointestinal symptoms, which include diarrhea, nausea, vomiting, and intermittent coliky abdominal pains; 3) respiratory symptoms in the form of wheezing, cough, and difficulty in breathing due to bronchial constriction; 4) anatomical changes in the heart, predominately on the right side involving the endocardium covering the valves and the cardiac chambers. The development of fibrous tissue leads to pulmonic stenosis and tricuspid insufficiency.[9,10,12]

The syndrome is usually seen only after metastatic deposits of considerable size to the liver have developed. Even so, it is not common, occurring in less than 5% of the patients.[12] Most often, it is observed in association with carcinoids of the small intestine, being extremely rare or practically nonexistent in carcinoid of the appendix.

The secretory products responsible for the syndrome include serotonin, histamine, bradykinin, and possibly other, yet undetectable substances. Chemically, serotonin is 5-hydroxytryptamine, a product of metabolism of tryphophan. In the presence of monoamine oxidase it is metabolized to 5-hydroxyindoleacetic acid and excreted in the urine. It is believed that serotonin is responsible for the gastrointestinal symptoms and histamine may account for the vasomotor manifestations. With regard to the cardiac changes, the most recent literature indicates that bradykinin may be implicated. Certainly their development has not been clearly defined.[4,9,12,13]

PATHOLOGY

Grossly, the tumors appear as submucosal growths, round or in the form of flat plaques. The overlying mucosa may ulcerate but this is not seen often.[9]

They are composed of small uniform cells that are polygonal or cuboidal in shape. They form primarily nests and strands and occasionally glandtype configurations. The cells contain granules within their cytoplasm, which give a positive argentaffin reaction (Fig. 54-1). It is because of this reaction that carcinoids are called argentaffinomas.[9]

They are thought to arise from gastrointestinal endocrine cells and as such they belong to the APUD system. They are classified as orthoendocrine apudomas producing hormones similar to those of the cells of their origin.[13] The concept of the APUD system is discussed in the chapter on pancreatic insulinomas.

CARCINOID OF THE STOMACH

The clinical symptoms of gastric carcinoids are similar to those seen in patients with carcinoma of the stomach or with peptic ulcer disease. They include epigastric pain, heartburn, nausea, and vomiting. Melena, hematemesis, anemia, and weight loss may also occur. In the absence of signs related to the carcinoid syndrome the diagnosis made is never that of carcinoid of the stomach. Radiographically, the lesion appears to be a sharply circumscribed polypoid filling defect, usually covered by a normal mucosa. Ulceration of the mucosa may be found in those cases with bleeding.[12] They are most commonly located in the antral region of the stomach and, of course, the diagnosis requires histological proof.[2]

Godwin[4] in his review article found the percentage of carcinoids of the stomach with regional or distant extension to be 55% at the time of diagnosis. Similarly, Hajdu et al.[5] found that among 10 patients with carcinoid of the stomach seen at Memorial Hospital, five had superficially invasive disease and the remaining five, deeply invasive disease that resulted in metastases.

The treatment is surgical, requiring wide excision of the lesion, which in most instances results in a total gastrectomy. Metastatic deposits to the liver or the regional lymph nodes should be excised if technically feasible, since their removal may decrease considerably the intensity of the carcinoid syndrome or delay its appearance.[12]

The prognosis for carcinoid of the stomach is good, provided the disease was localized in character at the time of the diagnosis. For these patients, the five-year survival is about 93%. Patients with regional extension of the disease have a 23% five-year survival, whereas no patient with distant metastases survived for five years. The overall survival figure for carcinoid of the stomach, thus, is approximately 52%[4]

CARCINOID OF THE DUODENUM

Approximately 80% of the duodenal carcinoids are symptomatic, whereas the remaining represent incidental findings.[12] Sanders and Axtell[12] in their collective review of carcinoids of the gastrointestinal

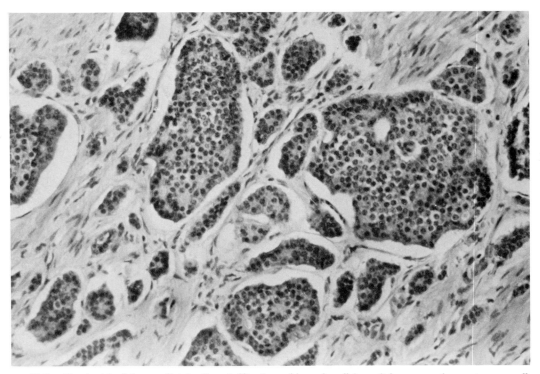

FIG. 54-1.   Carcinoid of the small intestine. Infiltration of bowel wall by solid masses of monotonous cells with central small round nuclei.

tract have identified three groups of symptoms: duodenal obstruction caused by protrusion of the tumor within the lumen, jaundice caused by compression and obstruction of the common bile duct, and duodenal ulceration. In general, the tumors are rather small and the largest reported size has been 4.0 cm. They are covered by an intact mucosa in most instances. This is depicted in the radiographs.

Carcinoid is a possibility when obstructing duodenal lesion is found with an intact mucosa. Penetration and involvement of the muscularis is estimated to occur in 36% of the cases and distant metastases in 22%.

Resection of carcinoid tumor located in the duodenal bulb as well as of those lesions located in the third and fourth part of the duodenum could be performed relatively easily in early lesions with end-to-

end anastomosis for the latter and a gastroduodenostomy or gastrojejunostomy for the former. Patients with carcinoid of the second portion of the duodenum in the region of the ampulla of Vater represent a special problem. A partial excision of the lesion might be attempted. This, however, will lead to local recurrence a few years later. The alternative is radical pancreatoduodenectomy from which some mortality should be anticipated. Considering the fact that carcinoids are slowly growing tumors, the age and overall health of the patient should be considered prior to selecting the method of therapy.

The prognosis of duodenal carcinoids is similar to that of carcinoids of the small intestine in general. When the tumor is small and not deeply penetrating, the prospects of cure by surgical resection are very high.[7]

CARCINOID OF THE JEJUNUM AND THE ILEUM

After the appendix, the small intestine is the commonest site of carcinoid tumors. Although the natural history of the disease is similar in tumors occurring in the jejunum and the ileum, carcinoids are very uncommon surgical lesions of the jejunum when compared to those of the ileum. In the series by Moertel et al.[6] the ratio was 1:10. The same authors noted a tendency for multicentricity. In 29% of the patients multiple primary lesions were present.

The incidence of a second unrelated primary malignant tumor in patients with carcinoids of the small intestine has also been high. In several reported series a second neoplasia was diagnosed in 15–30% of these patients.[6,9]

In the literature review by Godwin[4] 60% of the tumors in the small intestine and ileocecum were extending beyond the confines of the bowel. In the series reported by Hajdu et al.[5] from the Memorial Hospital, 17 of 43 cases of small intestine carcinoid were superficially invasive and 26 were deeply invasive tumors. Of the latter group, 23 had metastasized.

In general, carcinoid tumors of the small intestine are the commonest neoplasms in that area, most of them remaining asymptomatic. Many are incidental findings during autopsy examination. In the series by Moertel et al.[6] of 209 cases only 56 patients (27%) had symptoms related to their carcinoid tumors; in the remaining the diagnosis was an incidental finding at autopsy or during laparotomy for other reasons.

When symptomatic, the patient presents with abdominal pain, which is associated with intermittent bowel obstruction. Bleeding with melena is rather infrequent. On clinical examination, there is a palpable mass associated with gasseous distention of the abdomen.

Radiographically, submucosal nodules protruding into the bowel lumen are encountered and these, when multiple, must be differentiated from such processes as lymphoma of the bowel, diffuse metastatic disease of other origin, neurofibromatosis, and the Peutz-Jeghers syndrome. Carcinoid tumors provoke a fibroplastic reaction as they extend beyond the bowel wall (Fig. 54-2). Through the mesentery, they enter and involve the lymph nodes at the root of this structure. The fibrous reaction involves primarily the mesentery in the form of scar tissue, which pulls and buckles the bowel, creating a kinking of its lumen. This is quite evident radiographically and quite characteristic of this condition (Fig. 54-3). Due to the abundant scar tissue formation, there is a diffuse luminal narrowing and asymmetry of the mucosal folds develops.[1]

Arteriographically, irregularity and obstruction of the distal intramesenteric arteries are to be found associated with obstruction of the mesenteric veins (Fig. 54-4). The tumors themselves are not significantly hypervascular; however, injection of epinephrine reportedly accentuates their vascularity. It is this fibrotic reaction that produces a bending of the bowel lumen and compromises the vascularity of the bowel, which is responsible for most of the symptoms with which the patients present.

The incidence of lymph node involvement and that of metastatic disease depends upon the kind of patient population examined. Thus, while in the series of Goodwin[4] 60% of the patients had disease involving the lymph nodes or distant metastases present at the time of the diagnosis, in the series by Moertel et al.[6] the corresponding rate was 31.5%. The difference is due to the fact that the former series included patients with symptomatic disease only and the latter included all cases of carcinoid tumors diagnosed by pathological examination of small bowel specimens.

The mass of mesenteric lymph nodes may lead to vascular compromise of the bowel and to volvulus.[6]

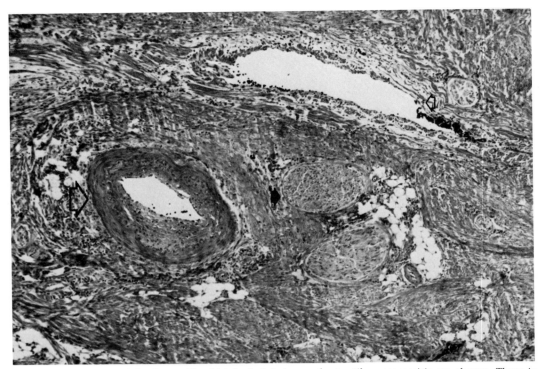

FIG. 54-2.   Carcinoid of the ileum. The histological features of retractile mesenteritis are shown. There is marked fibrosis surrounding the arteries (open large arrow), nerves, (closed small arrow), and veins (small open arrow). (Courtesy R.S. Seigel *et al.* Radiology **134**:437, 1980.)

Common metastatic sites are the peritoneal cavity and the liver. Carcinoid symdrome is seen in 6% of patients with metastases.

The treatment is surgical for the operable lesions. It should include resection of the tumor with adequate margins on either side, as well as resection of the mesentery associated with that part of the bowel because this represents the anatomical pathway for regional metastases. Tumors in the region of the terminal ileum are treated best by a right hemicolectomy.[12] Surgery is the primary form of treatment in the majority of cases (85%). Patients with inoperable tumors are considered for chemotherapy or radiation therapy. Of the chemotherapeutic agents, Cytoxan, methotrexate, and actinomycin D have been mentioned without prolonged remissions. With reference to the carcinoid syndrome, agents blocking serotonin synthesis or serotonin action have been used, such as methysergide and parachlorophenylalanine. The results have been variable. Certainly there is no direct antitumor effect.

Ecouraging results of long-term control or even cure of carcinoid tumors by radiation were published by Gaitan-Gaitan *et al.*[3] The authors treated nonresectable carcinoid tumors with radiation therapy, delivering doses in the order of 2500 rad fractionated over four to six weeks. The entire peritoneal cavity was included in the field of treatment. Among the results, three patients with inoperable small bowel carcinoid with lymph node or liver metastases were alive and well 33, 51, and 18 months following such a treatment program.

The disease has a slow progression and

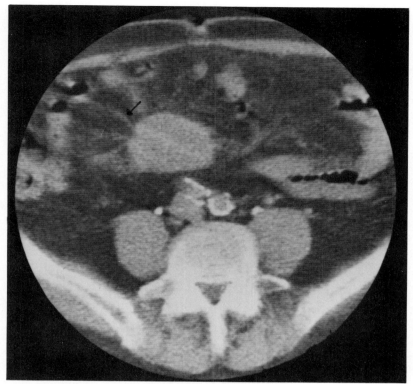

FIG. 54-3.   Carcinoid of the ileum in a 74-year-old male. CT scan demonstrates the tumor as a soft tissue mass 5.0 cm in diameter, in the right lower quadrant. Radiating from it are linear densities, which represent the fibrosed and retracted mesenteric bundles (arrow). (Courtesy R.S. Seigel *et al. Radiology***134**:437, 1980.)

even when metastatic in character it allows a reasonably comfortable survival for several months or even years. The overall prognosis is quite good, considering the fact that the majority of small bowel carcinoids are incidental findings. In the series from the Mayo Clinic the five-year-survival rate for patients with inoperable nodal or peritoneal metastases was 38% and for those with hepatic metastases, 21%[6] In this context it is important to consider palliative resection of carcinoid masses during the surgical intervention in patients with carcinoid syndrome because the removal will minimize or delay the hormonal toxic effects.

As with carcinoids in other locations, the size of the primary lesion and the depth of invasion within the bowel wall are the main prognostic factors. The five-year-survival rate for patients with local disease is 75%. Patients with regional extension had a rate of 59%.[4]

CARCINOID OF THE APPENDIX

This is the commonest location of carcinoid tumors. As stated, there is a female predominance, the ratio of female to male patients being in excess of 2:1. The patients with appendiceal carcinoid are younger than the rest, most of them between 20 and 40 years of age.[7,12] Ryden *et al.*[11] published a report on carcinoid tumors involving the appendix in children. A total of 30 patients were included whose ages ranged from 9 to 14 years. In the series by Moertel *et al.*[7] the youngest patient was 6 years old.

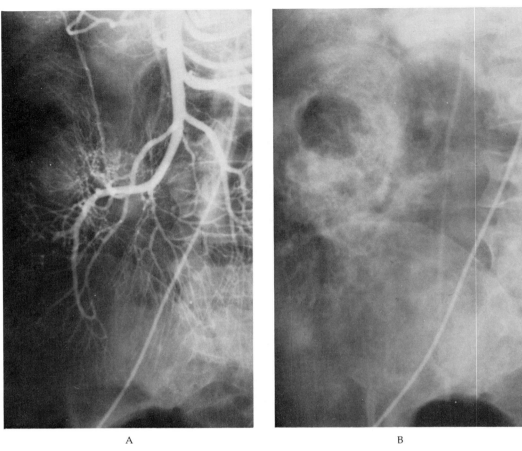

A   B

FIG. 54-4. Carcinoid of the ileum in a 50-year-old male. Superior mesenteric arteriogram shows crowding and kinking of the ileocolic branches (A). In the capillary phase an abnormal tumor stain is well shown (B). (Courtesy R.S. Seigel *et al. Radiology* **134**:437, 1980.)

The majority of appendiceal carcinoids are asymptomatic and they represent an incidental laboratory finding in appendices submitted during the course of another abdominal procedure. A small number, approximately 10% however, present as an inflammatory process due to obstruction of the appendiceal lumen by the tumor.[12] This is particularly true for carcinoids in children. Twenty-nine of the 30 patients reported by Ryden *et al.*[11] presented with signs or symptoms of acute appendicitis. The tumors have a great predilection for the tip of the appendix,

71% arising in this location. On palpation during the operation, the appendix carries a bulbous enlargement at the tip or thickening of the body is found, findings suggesting fecalith. The size of the tumor rarely exceeds 2.0 cm in diameter.

Histologically, the appearance is similar to that of carcinoids in other locations and evidence of extension to the peritoneal surface can be demonstrated in two thirds of all cases. Actually, lesions proximally located near the base of the appendix have a 98% microscopic evidence of lymph vessel permeation.[7] In spite of these micro-

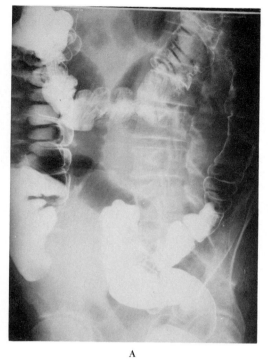

A

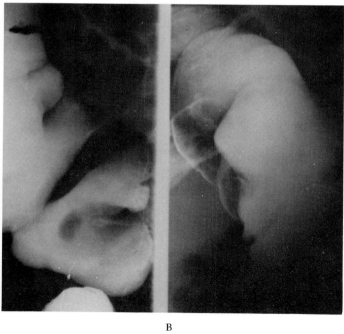

B

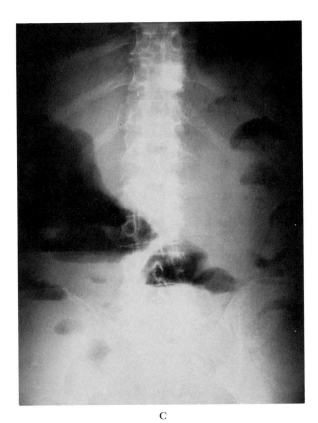

C

FIG. 54–5. Carcinoid of the cecum in a 64-year-old
male. Incomplete filling of the medial aspect of the
cecum on barium enema *(A)*. Spot film reveals the tumor
as a filling defect *(B)*. Five years later the patient has
developed local recurrence and distant metastases.
There is intestinal obstruction due to a tumor mass present in the right lower quadrant. Osteoblastic metastases can be seen in the left aspect of the T11 vertebral
body *(C)*.

scopic findings, the disease macroscopically remains localized and metastases are
quite rare. In the review article by Godwin,[4] less than 1% of appendiceal carcinoids had distant metastases. The same
is the experience of Moertel et al.,[6] who
found two patients with metastasizing
disease among 144 cases reviewed. It
seems, as is true for the rest of the gastrointestinal tract, that the main prognostic factor is the size of the tumor. No
tumors smaller than 2.0 cm exhibited
signs of malignancy.

On the basis of several hundred appen-

diceal carcinoids reported in the literature,
the appropriate treatment for the majority
of them is simple appendectomy. This
recommendation is based on the fact that
no recurrences have been observed and no
metastatic disease has been shown following such therapy, in spite of the fact that
histological signs of tumor extension into
the lymphatics are quite common. Exception could be made for tumors larger than
2.0 cm for which right hemicolectomy may
be appropriate.[2,4,7,12]

The prognosis in general is excellent.
Moertel et al.[6] comment on the fact that

these tumors are seen in younger patients, whereas appendices are removed in all age groups during laparotomies performed for other causes. This observation combined with the indolent clinical course raises the question about the neoplastic nature of appendiceal carcinoids. The authors feel that argentaffin cell collections may represent developmental abnormality rather than neoplasia which degenerates with the passage of time.[7]

CARCINOID OF THE CECUM AND COLON

These are the most aggressive carcinoid tumors of the gastrointestinal tract. In the review by Sanders and Axtell[12] 26 of 39 cecal carcinoids, or 67%, develop metastases and 10 of 26 colonic tumors, or 38%, have positive lymph nodes Godwin[4] in his review found 71% of colonic carcinoids to have regional or distant metastases. Hajdu et al.[5] have demonstrated the importance of deep invasion into the bowel wall.

There was no metastasis in four patients with superficially invasive tumors, whereas metastases were seen in four other patients, all of whom had deeply invasive disease.

The presenting symptoms are similar to those of colonic carcinoma. Most cecal lesions presented with pain in the right lower quadrant associated with a mass lesion in that area. Obstruction at the ileocecal valve level is also among the clinical findings (Fig. 54-5). Similar symptoms ware to be found for carcinoids in the remainder of the colon.

Because of the high propensity for regional lymph node metastases and because colonic carcinoids are potentially lethal tumors, the surgical resection should be adequate and hemicolectomy is the recommended procedure. In our experience the tumor is radioresponsive but not radiocurable.

The five-year-survival rate in a composite literature review was found to be 52%.[4]

CARCINOID OF THE RECTUM

The majority of rectal carcinoids are asymptomatic. This is concluded from an earlier literature review by Sanders and Axtell[12] as well as by subsequent authors.[2] The carcinoids are found primarily during routine rectal examinations or during sigmoidoscopy. They are submucosal in location and bleed only occasionally, due to mucosal interruption. Many of them are superficial lesions, and as such they do not develop lymph node metastases or distal spread. When deeply invasive, however, such a clinical course is the rule.[4,5] Metastatic disease correlates also with the size of the tumor. In the review by Peskin and Orloff[8] lesions greater than 2 cm metastasized to the regional lymph nodes in 90% of the cases and gave distant metastases in 60%. On the other hand, none of the 20 cases with superficially invasive carcinoid of the rectum reported by Hajdu et al.[5] had regional or distant metastases.

Based on the size of the lesion and the extent of invasion within the bowel wall, it appears that superficial rectal carcinoids smaller than 2.0 cm in diameter can be treated adequately by local excision only. However, if there is evidence of deep invasion or if the size of the tumor is greater than 2.0 cm, a greater surgical procedure is necessary and that should include lymph node resection. An anterior rectosigmoid resection or a combined abdominoperineal resection is recommended for these tumors.[12]

The overall five-year-survival rate is 83%.[4]

CARCINOID IN MECKEL'S DIVERTICULUM

Most of these tumors are incidental findings at autopsy or at surgery. The presenting symptom can be that of volvulus of a Meckel's diverticulum.[6,12] Approximately 30 such cases have been reported. Sanders and Axtell[12] in their review of the literature found that most carcinoids arising in Meckel's diverticula tended to behave more like carcinoids of the small intestine rather than like appendiceal carcinoids. For this reason, it is their recommendation that these patients undergo a wide resection of the intestine with large wedge removal of the adjacent mesentery.

CARCINOID OF THE GALLBLADDER AND BILIARY TRACT

These structures represent a rare site for carcinoid tumors. Godwin[4] in his literature review found one tumor present in the gallbladder and another in the biliary tract. Sanders and Axtell[12] found five case reports of gallbladder carcinoids. It appears that carcinoids in this location show a benign course and cholecystectomy is an adequate treatment.

REFERENCES

1. Bancks, N.H., Goldstein, H.M., and Dodd, G.D., Jr.: The roentgenologic spectrum of small intestinal carcinoid tumors. *AJR* 123:274, 1975.
2. Cunningham, P.J., Norman, J., and Cleveland, H.R.: Malignant carcinoid associated with thoraco-abdominal aneurysm and analysis of thirty-one case of gastrointestinal carcinoid tumors. *Ann Surg* 176:613, 1972.
3. Gaitan-Gaitan, A., Rider, W.D., and Bush, R.S.: Carcinoid tumor—cure by irradiation. *Int J Radiat Oncol Biol Phys* 1:9, 1975.
4. Godwin, J.D., II: Carcinoid tumors. An analysis of 2837 cases. *Cancer* 36:560, 1975.
5. Hajdu, S.I., Winawer, S.J., and Myers, W.P.L.: Carcinoid tumors. A study of 204 cases. *Am J Clin Pathol* 61:521, 1974.
6. Moertel, C.G., Sauer, W.G., Dockerty, M.B., and Baggenstoss, A.H.: Life history of the carcinoid tumor of the small intestine. *Cancer* 14:901, 1961.
7. Moertel, C.G., Dockerty, M.B., and Judd, E.S.: Carcinoid tumors of the vermiform appendix. *Cancer* 21:270, 1968.
8. Peskin, G.W., and Orloff, M.J.: A clinical study of 25 patients with carcinoid tumors of the rectum. *Surg Gynecol Obstet* 109:673, 1959.
9. Robbins, S.L., and Cotran, R.S.: *Pathologic Basis of Disease.* W.B. Saunders Co., Philadelphia, 1979.
10. Roberts, W.C., and Sjoerdsma, A.: The cardiac disease associated with the carcinoid syndrome (carcinoid heart disease). *Am J Med* 36:5, 1964.
11. Ryden, S.E., Drake, R.M., and Franciosi, R.A.: Carcinoid tumors of the appendix in children. *Cancer* 36:1538, 1975.
12. Sanders, R.J., and Axtell, H.K.: Carcinoids of the gastrointestinal tract. *Surg Gynecol Obstet* 119:369, 1964.
13. Webourn, R.B.: Current status of the apudomas. *Ann Surg* 185:1, 1977.

55

Carcinoid Tumors of the Thymus

THIS IS AN uncommon location for a neo-plasm of this histological type; how-ever, at least 19 well-documented mi-croscopically-established cases can be found in the literature.[1,2] It has been shown by means of histochemical and ul-trastructural studies that enterochromaffin cells—Kulchitsky—are present in the thymus of some animals and electron mi-croscopy has revealed the presence of occa-sional cells along similar lines in the nor-mal human thymus.[1] It is therefore sug-gested that thymic carcinoids arise from these structures in a manner similar to that of carcinoids in the lung and the gastroin-testinal tract.

Both the histology and the natural his-tory of the disease are similar to that of carcinoid tumors in other locations. It has been stated by all authors that these tumors resemble bronchial adenomas and that they bear no similarity to thymomas. There is a male predominance, the median patient age at the time of the diagnosis being 43 years. Of the 19 reported pa-tients, 15 were male. Approximately one-third of the cases occurred as part of a multiple endocrine adenomatosis syn-drome.[1,2]

CLINICAL

The presenting symptoms are usually respiratory. Dyspnea and pain in the chest are the commonest, occurring a few weeks to a few months prior to the diagnosis.

Other signs include shoulder pain, edema of the face or the upper extremities, cough, and a sensation of pressure. Fi-nally, about 25% of the patients were asymptomatic, the diagnosis being made by means of chest radiographs.

Radiographically, a superior, anterior irregular mediastinal mass is to be seen. There has been no patient presenting or developing myasthenia gravis.

TREATMENT, RESULTS, AND PROGNOSIS

Complete or partial resection following thoracotomy has been the mainstay of treatment. In six patients who underwent incomplete resection the treatment was combined with radiation therapy.[1,2] In one patient no therapy was rendered due to advanced age. The tumor was found in the anterior, superior mediastinum as a large, slightly irregular mass measuring approximately 10 cm. In another case the mass was located in the posterior medias-tinum.

At the time of surgery gross invasion was reported to be present in 10 cases. In three patients metastases were found. These were primarily to the regional cervi-cal, supraclavicular, and intrathoracic lymph nodes.

Recurrent disease developed in four pa-tients who underwent combined partial resection and radiotherapy treatment. The fifth patient in combined therapy died, reportedly of complications of his treatment eight years later without signs of recurrent disease. Patients developing recurrence or metastasis lived for a number of years with their disease and this is exemplified by the untreated patient reported by Salyer et al.[2] who survived for four years without therapy.

Tabulating the five-year-survival rate among the patients reported thus far, we found it to be 85%. This, however, does not reflect necessarily freedom from the disease. Patients have died 6, 9, and even 18 years later of their tumor.

REFERENCES

1. Rosai, J., and Higa, E.: Mediastinal endocrine neoplasm of probable thymic origin related to carcinoid tumor. Clinicopathologic study of 8 cases. *Cancer* **29**:1061, 1972.
2. Salyer, W.R., Salyer, D.C., and Eggleston, J.C.: Carcinoid tumors of the thymus. *Cancer* **37**:958, 1976.

56

Carcinoid Tumors of the Bronchus

UNDER THE COLLECTIVE name of "bronchial adenoma," a term used in the past to differentiate this group of tumors from carcinomas of the lung, three distinct histopathological entities have been defined. Weiss and Ingram[8] and Goodner et al.[3] analyzed the literature on "bronchial adenomas" and demonstrated the incorrectness the term conveys with regard to the biological activity and the nonspecificity of the histological diagnosis.

It has now been accepted that the group of bronchial adenomas includes: carcinoid tumors of the bronchus, adenoid cystic carcinoma of the bronchus, and mucoepidermoid carcinoma. Bronchial adenomas as a whole comprise 6–10% of all primary lung tumors. Of the bronchial adenomas, carcinoids are the most common, representing 80–85% of the entire group. Adenoid cystic carcinomas comprise 10–12% and mucoepidermoid carcinomas, 2–3%.[1–3]

There is no sex predominance as to the occurrence of bronchial carcinoid. The average mean age of the patients at the time of the diagnosis is 45 years. The age range, however, extends from the late teens to the seventh decade of life.[2,3,7,9]

PATHOLOGY

The majority of the tumors, approximately 70%, are centrally located within the reach of the bronchoscope. The remaining are peripheral, at the level of the segmental bronchi or in the region of the

more distal bronchioles.[2,7] There is no predilection for any particular lobe or segment and the tumors occur with an equal frequency in the right and the left lung.[3,7] They are broadly based, usually covered by bronchial epithelium and submucosa. Endobronchial presentation, at least in part, is seen in 90% of the cases.

Histologically, they are made of sheets of rather uniform small cells arranged in cords and nests. They are similar to islet cell tumors or oat cell carcinoma.[4]

Salyer et al.[7] pointed out that a histological distinction could be made between the centrally located carcinoids and those in the peripheral parts of the lung. Central tumors are composed of uniform cells in a rather orderly arrangement with absent or rare mitoses. Peripheral carcinoid tumors were often found to be associated with hyperplasia of the basal cells of the normal bronchiolar epithelium. The arrangement is more disorderly, the cells being more pleomorphic with frequent spindle cells. Centrally located carcinoids are presumed to arise from the main stem bronchus and the segmental bronchi, where Kulchitsky cells are known to be present. It is presumed that peripheral carcinoids arise from precursors of Kulchitsky cells located in the peripheral bronchial epithelium.[7]

Due to the fact that the tumor is covered by the overlying mucosa, pathologists have emphasized that misleading information may be obtained by bronchoscopy.[5]

Goldstraw et al.[2] in a retrospective literature analysis of 71 bronchial carcinoids found the incidence of local invasion to be reported from 10–94%, the median figure being 50%. Regional lymph node metastasis has been variously reported from 0–30% and blood-borne metastases from 0–42%. Metastatic sites include the liver, skeleton, chest wall, and brain.[2]

CLINICAL

The commonest clinical presentation is chronic cough, productive in character, accompanied by frequent bouts of pneumonia. Hemoptysis occurs in one-third of the patients.[2,3,7]

The duration of the symptoms is rather long, often more than one year.[2] In approximately 20% of the patients, no symptoms are present. Their diagnosis is made following an abnormal chest radiograph.[2,7]

Chest X-ray examination will reveal a distinct mass in one-third of the cases, and in the remainder the superimposed atelectasis, bronchitis and pneumonitis may mask the tumor[1,3] (Fig. 56-1, 56-2).

On physical examination, two-thirds of the patients will have abnormal findings. Included are decreased breath sounds and dullness to percussion over the involved area.[5]

Carcinoid syndrome has been observed in lung carcinoids, but infrequently, occurring in about 3% of the patients.[1,2,4,7] Bronchial carcinoids have been shown to produce not only serotonin, but also insulin, glucagon, gastrin, ACTH, and ACTH-like hormones.[1] Their products enter directly into the systemic circulation and thus carcinoid syndrome is possible.

On bronchoscopic examination, the typical polypoid mass will be seen as an exophytic growth within the lumen in most of the patients.[3,6] They tend to bleed during manipulations and biopsies.[5]

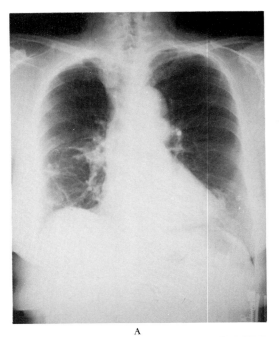

A

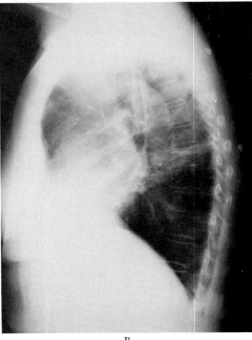

B

FIG. 56-1. Bronchial carcinoid in a 78-year-old female. There is a round density in the region of the right hilum (A). On bronchoscopy the tumor was present in the right main stem bronchus, producing atelectatic changes in the superior segment of the right lower lobe, as seen on the lateral view (B).

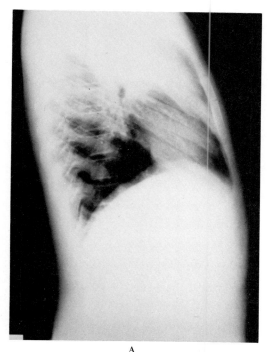

A

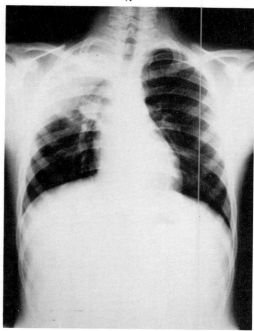

B

FIG. 56-2. (A)(B) Carcinoid of the bronchus in a 12-year-old male. Radiographs of the chest show a right hilar mass, which produces atelectasis of the right upper lobe. Clinically, this was associated with pneumonitis.

TREATMENT AND RESULTS

Surgery is the basic form of therapy. The procedure can be a segmental resection, a lobectomy, or a pneumonectomy, depending on the location and the size. The commonest approach, in 60% of the patients, has been lobectomy. At times two lobes were resected. Twenty-five percent of the patients require pneumonectomy and the remaining 10–15%, segmental resection.[1,3,6,7] Radiation therapy and endobronchial resection have been occasionally employed.

Unless the disease is too advanced at the time of the diagnosis, resection will result in cure in most instances. Radiation therapy should be used if surgery is not feasible. Irradiation can stabilize the tumor and provide many years of survival.[3]

Postoperative recurrences do take place, but, according to most authors, infrequently.[6,7]

PROGNOSIS AND SURVIVAL

The prognosis, generally, is considered to be good. Salyer et al.[7] in their series encountered a mortality rate of 7.4%. The patients were observed for periods ranging from 1 to 21 years, with a median follow-up period of five years. All patients who were alive at the time of the report, 92.6%, were free of disease.[7]

In the series reported by Meffert and Lindskog,[5] of 32 patients with carcinoid of the bronchus with an average follow-up period of 11 years, 23 were known to be in excellent health, four were lost to follow-up, and five were dead of their disease. O'Grady et al.[6] found in their review of 29 patients with bronchial carcinoids the survival rate to be 95%. Finally, the report by Goodner et al.[3] presents a less optimistic view. Of 21 evaluable patients with bronchial carcinoids, 12, or 57%, were surviving at five years. In addition, only seven (33%) were free of disease.

REFERENCES

1. Donahue, J.K., Weichert, R.F., and Ochsner, J.L.: Bronchial adenoma. *Ann Surg* **167:**873, 1968.
2. Goldstraw, P., Lamb, D., McCormack, R.J.M., and Walbaum, P.R.: The malignancy of bronchial adenoma. *J Thorac Cardiovasc Surg* **72:**309, 1976.
3. Goodner, J.T., Berg, J.W., and Watson, W.L.: The nonbenign nature of bronchial carcinoids and cylindromas. *Cancer* **14:**539, 1961.
4. Hajdu, S.I., Winawer, S.J., and Myers, W.P.L.: Carcinoid tumors. A study of 204 cases. *Am J Clin Pathol* **61:**521, 1974.
5. Meffert, W.G., and Lindskog, G.E.: Bronchial adenoma. *J Thorac Cardiovasc Surg* **59:**588, 1970.
6. O'Grady, W.P., McDivitt, R.W., Holman, C.W., and Moore, S.W.: Bronchial adenomas. *Arch Surg* **101:**558, 1970.
7. Salyer, D.C., Salyer, W.R., and Eggleston, J.C.: Bronchial carcinoid tumors. *Cancer* **36:**1522, 1975.
8. Weiss, L., and Ingram, M.: Adenomatoid bronchial tumors; consideration of carcinoid tumors and salivary tumors of the bronchial tree. *Cancer* **14:**161, 1961.
9. Wilkins, E.W., Jr., Darling, R.C., Soutter, L., and Sniffen, R.C.: A continuing clinical survey of adenomas of the trachea and bronchus in a general hospital. *J Thorac Cardiovasc Surg* **46:**279, 1963.

57

Carcinoid Tumors of the Testis

CARCINOID OF THE testis is an infrequent tumor, representing a clinical curiosity. To the present time, 15 such cases have been reported, the average age of the patients at the time of the diagnosis being 48 years.[2] These are older men, compared to those with gonadal tumors.

In all cases the diagnosis has been made following histological examination.[3] The tumors exhibit large irregular-shaped masses of epithelial cells, which are columnar in type and demonstrate distinct palisading. Mitotic activity is present in the nucleus and the cytoplasm contains argentaffin-positive granules.[1-3]

The clinical appearance is that of a slow, painless testicular enlargement. Of the 15 cases hitherto reported, four were metastatic in character and therefore should be excluded. Of the 11 primary tumors arising in the testis, two were associated with teratomas and nine were pure carcinoids.[2]

No patient with testicular carcinoid has presented with, or has subsequently developed, carcinoid syndrome. These neoplasms, although they have a histological appearance of low-grade malignancy have not metastasized and no patient is known to have died from them.

The prognosis is excellent following orchiectomy. Contrary to primary testicular carcinoid, metastasis to the testicle from carcinoid elsewhere in the body carries a poor prognosis, indicating generalized disease.[1-3]

58

Carcinoid Tumors of the Ovary

MOST PRIMARY OVARIAN carcinoids are part of an ovarian teratoma. Approximately 73% of them belong in this group and the remaining are histologically pure carcinoids arising *de novo* in the ovary.[6] Altogether, they are uncommon tumors, comprising less than 1% of all ovarian teratomas; conversely, they account for less than 1% of all carcinoids.

Carcinoid elements may coexist with thyroid tissue, thus being part of a struma ovarii.[3]

The pure form is considered to be either a single-sided development of a benign teratoma or a tumor arising from argentaffin cells in the ovary. These cells could possibly be present within the ovary or they could have colonized the ovary in the form of migratory APUD cells.[8–10]

The average age of the patients at the time of the diagnosis is 55–60 years.[2]

CLINICAL

Due to the rarity of the tumor, the diagnosis cannot be made preoperatively, unless a carcinoid syndrome is present. The venous drainage of the ovary is to the inferior vena cava. In this way the liver is bypassed and detoxification of the serotonin and related substances does not take place.[1] Ovarian carcinoids, for this reason, can produce carcinoid syndrome with smaller tumor volumes and in a greater percentage of cases than those of the gastrointestinal tract. It is estimated that the syndrome is present in 33% of patients with ovarian carcinoid.[6] The median diameter of the hormonally active tumors is 9.0 cm, as opposed to 3.0 cm diameter for those not exhibiting the syndrome.[6]

When associated with a teratoma, the carcinoid element appears as a nodule on the wall of a cyst, which is otherwise filled with hair and sebum. When alone, ovarian carcinoids present as solid masses.[2,6]

Hot flashes are the commonest manifestations of the carcinoid syndrome, followed by diarrhea and cardiac murmurs. The hot flashes have often been attributed to the patients' menopause.[1] In patients without the syndrome abdominal enlargement associated with discomfort is the usual presenting sign. Other ways of detection have included vaginal bleeding, routine pelvic examinations, and hysterectomy for uterine fibroids.[6] Tricuspid valvular disease and pulmonary valvular stenosis was reported by Chatterjee and Heather[2] in four patients with ovarian carcinoids, associated with heart failure. Three patients became symptom-free following removal of the tumor and the fourth was untreated, the tumor being found at autopsy.[2]

Generally the flushes and the diarrhea cease in the immediate postoperative period, usually the next day after the tumor removal.[6] By following the levels of 5-hydroxyindoleacetic acid, carcinoid recurrences can be verified.

For the most part, ovarian carcinoids pursue a benign course. Qizilbash *et al.*[5] in reviewing 47 previously documented cases of ovarian carcinoids found four that were malignant.[4,7] Robboy et al.[6] reported two additional cases. The patients developed pelvic or abdominal recurrence and liver metastases. The patient reported by Koven et al.[4] recurred with mediastinal and left supraclavicular adenopathy.

TREATMENT AND RESULTS

Unilateral salpingo-oophorectomy is considered to be adequate therapy of ovarian carcinoid in the premenopausal patient. If the patient is postmenopausal, then bilateral salpingo-oophorectomy and hysterectomy is recommended. During surgery, the gastrointestinal tract should be thoroughly searched for a primary carcinoid. The opposite ovary, if it is to be preserved, should be biopsied.[6]

Systemic chemotherapy and local radiotherapy have a role to play palliatively in the patient with disseminated disease and for prolonging the survival.

PROGNOSIS AND SURVIVAL

Both the survival and the prognosis of ovarian carcinoids is good because very few of them are malignant. Robboy et al.[6] estimated the actuarial survival to be 95% at five years and 88% at 10 years.

REFERENCES

1. Brown, P.A., and Richart, R.M.: Functioning ovarian carcinoid tumors. Case report and review of the literature. Obstet Gynecol 34:390, 1969.
2. Chatterjee, K., and Heather, J.C.: Carcinoid heart disease from primary ovarian carcinoid tumors. A case report and review of the literature. Am J Med 45:643, 1968.
3. Dikman, S.H., and Toker, C.: Strumal carcinoid of the ovary with masculinization. Cancer 27:925, 1971.
4. Koven, B.J., Dollinger, M.R., and Nadel, M.S.: Response to actinomycin D of malignant carcinoid arising in an ovarian teratoma. Am J Obstet Gynecol 101:267, 1968.
5. Qizilbash, A.H., Trebilcock, R.G., Patterson, M.C., and Lamont, K.G.: Functioning primary carcinoid tumor of the ovary. A light- and electron-microscopic study with review of the literature. Am J Clin Pathol 62:629, 1974.
6. Robboy, S.J., Norris, H.J., and Scully, R.E.: Insular carcinoid primary in the ovary. A clinicopathologic analysis of 48 cases. Cancer 36:404, 1975.
7. Saunders, A.M., and Hertzman, V.O.: Malignant carcinoid teratoma of the ovary. Can Med Assoc J 83:602, 1960.
8. Toker, C.: Ovarian carcinoid. A light and electron microscopic study. Am J Obstet Gynecol 103:1019, 1969.
9. Torvik, A.: Carcinoid syndrome in a primary tumor of the ovary. Report of a case with extensive peritoneal fibrosis resembling Pick's syndrome. Acta Pathol Microbiol Scand 48:81, 1960.
10. Trevenen, C., Banerjee, R., and Laughlan, S.C.: The ovarian carcinoid. Cancer 31:1482, 1973.

59

Mucoepidermoid Carcinoma of the Salivary Glands

STEWART et al.[10] in 1945 were the first to describe a group of salivary gland tumors with distinct histological and clinical characteristics, which are substantial enough to warrant separation of these tumors from the rest of the salivary glands neoplasms. The authors formulated the term "mucoepidermoid" to denote the two principle histological characteristics, namely, the presence of areas of mucous cells adjacent to areas of epidermoid and squamous cells. Due to the great differences with regard to aggressiveness, the term "tumor" rather than carcinoma has been often applied.

Mucoepidermoid carcinomas comprise approximately 6–8% of all salivary gland tumors. More specifically, those occurring in the parotid gland represent 6% of all tumors in the organ and 27% of all malignant tumors.[11] With reference to the minor salivary glands, mucoepidermoid carcinomas account for 22% of the malignant tumors found in the oral cavity. The commonest location is the palate, where 36% occur, followed by the buccal mucosa (29%), the floor of the mouth (21%), and the lips (14%).[5] They also have been reported in the tongue, the paranasal sinuses, the nasal cavity, the retromolar triangle region, and in the submaxillary gland.[9] Mucoepidermoid tumors of the re-

spiratory tract are dealt with in a separate chapter.

In spite of the fact that in some series a male predominance occurred, a later analysis of a large number of cases revealed no sex predilection for tumors occurring in the major salivary glands.[2,6,9] As far as mucoepidermoid carcinoma of the minor salivary glands is concerned, a slight female predominance may exist.[6]

Several of the patients are young, although 50% of the tumors occur during the third, fourth, and fifth decades of life. Twenty-two percent of the reported cases of mucoepidermoid carcinomas of the major salivary glands were seen in the 20–30 age group. Those occurring in the minor glands exhibit a more even distribution being encountered from the first to the eighth decade.[6]

PATHOLOGY

Stewart et al.[10] in tracing the origin of these neoplasms pointed out that scattered mucous cells can be found within the duct epithelium of the major salivary glands. Although difficult to demonstrate, this happens also in the minor salivary glands. In addition to the mucous cells the salivary gland ducts include rounded basal cells, elliptical or rounded intermediate cells, and columnar cells. The authors express the opinion that the site of origin of mucoepidermoid tumors are the ducts of the salivary glands.[10] Subsequent authors have agreed with this view.[3,4] Batsakis[2] emphasizes the multifaceted histological appearances of these tumors. Bhaskar and Bernier[3] identified on the basis of histology and staining characteristics mucous cells responsible for the production of mucous pools, clear cells, and columnar cells. In addition maternal cells, intermediate cells, and, of course, epidermoid cells are found. The combination, in various proportions, of these six cell types accounts for the individual appearance of each tumor.[2]

On the basis of histology, an attempt to separate benign and malignant variants was made by Stewart et al.[10] In their view, benign tumors contained a wide range of individual cell types, their main characteristic feature being overproduction of mucus with prominence of mucous elements and columnar cells. Malignant forms contained predominately epidermoid or intermediate cell types. Subsequent experience with the disease suggested that a distinction between benign and malignant variants on the basis of histology requires some degree of reservation. It was shown that in a broad sense mucoepidermoid tumors could be considered malignant. On the basis of their histology, a differentiation to "low grade," "intermediate grade," and "high grade" of malignancy can be established. This classification is of prognostic value to a certain extent.[2,4,8,9]

The gross appearance of the low-grade mucoepidermoid tumors is that of a relatively well-defined tumor similar to a pleomorphic adenoma. The neoplasm is circumscribed but unencapsulated, with average diameter of 2–3 cm. Cystic changes, particularly in the well-differentiated variants, are commonly observed.[4,11] High-grade tumors are diffuse in their presentation and infiltrating in character.[4]

CLINICAL

Mucoepidermoid carcinoma of the major salivary glands presents itself as a mass lesion. This may be mobile in character; however, in later stages it may ulcerate and become fixed to the overlying and underlying structures. Facial paralysis and salivary fistulas occur, particularly in tumors of high grade.[3]

When arising in the minor salivary glands, they are more prone to develop ulceration and fixation to the underlying structures. A typical example is mucoepidermoid carcinoma of the hard palate, where bony destruction may be observed associated with the ulceration. Bleeding or nasal discharge can be present in tumors of the maxillary sinuses.[3,9]

The duration of the symptoms prior to the diagnosis varies. By some patients, they were perceived as being present a few days only, whereas in others it was a matter of several years. In the series by Thorvaldsson et al.[11] a well-differentiated tumor of the major salivary gland was diagnosed within 12 months of its presentation, whereas those of high grade were diagnosed on the average 18 months from the presenting symptoms.[11]

Local recurrences following surgical resection are common. The overall recurrence rate is estimated to be approximately 30%.[2] High-grade tumors recur more often. Their rate is in the range of 35–65%. Low-grade lesions can also recur but they do so less frequently. Their reported recurrence rate is 15–28%.[8,11]

Metastases to the regional lymph nodes are relatively infrequent. They have been reported as occurring in 4–18% of the patients; however, most of them were seen in high-grade tumors.[8,9,11]

Distant metastases are uncommon. For practical purposes, they appear only in patients with high-grade tumors and they occur in approximately 5% of the patient population.[3,7] They have been seen in several organs, including the brain, lungs, skin, and bones.

TREATMENT AND RESULTS

Major Salivary Glands

The basic therapy is surgical resection. The extent of the procedure has varied. The most common form has been local excision. This indeed may be adequate therapy for Grade I or Grade II tumors provided that margins free of tumor can be established.[6,9] In the series by Bhaskar and Bernier[3] of 96 patients who were free of disease for more than 3 years, 80 (83.3%) had local excision as their only therapy.[3]

High-grade tumors require total parotidectomy in the opinion of most authors.[6,8,9,11] Jakobsson et al.[8] and Thorvaldsson et al.[11] advocate radical parotidectomy accompanied by radical neck dissection for high-grade lesions. It is in these tumors that high recurrence rate has been observed, resulting in the lowest survival rate of all patients with mucoepidermoid tumors.[8,11]

The presence of tumor at the margins of the resection is an important prognostic sign, as expected. Healey et al.[9] observed a 68% recurrence rate in those patients who had involved surgical margins, as opposed to 3% recurrence rate for those who did not demonstrate tumor at the margin of the resection.

Radiotherapy has been an adjuvant form of therapy, primarily for those patients whose tumor margins were found to be involved at the time of the resection. Three such patients with low-grade tumors were reported surviving without recurrent disease two, five, and six years after treatment. In contrast, three patients with high-grade tumors developed recurrences in spite of radiotherapy one, four,

and eight years later.[9] In another series four patients with Grade III mucoepidermoid carcinoma had postoperative radiotherapy following total parotidectomy. Three of these were alive and well 5, 6, and 15 years later, the fourth patient dying of both local and distant metastases in four months.[11] From data supplied by Jakobsson et al.,[8] it is obvious that no effect on the tumor is to be expected from radiotherapy if only modest doses are applied. There are no data on the use of chemotherapy.

Minor Salivary Glands

Surgery alone or in combination with radiation therapy has been the major form of treatment, adapted according to the location of the tumor. Lesions in the region of the lip can be excised with adequate wide margins of normal tissue around them. Those of the floor of the mouth require a wider excision and so do those in the region of the buccal mucosa. Should regional lymph node metastasis be clinically suspected, ipsilateral neck dissection is in order. More difficult to treat, because of the extensive surgery needed, are tumors occurring in the palate. A limited maxillectomy or hemimaxillectomy can be performed initially and consideration to postoperative radiotherapy should be given.[5] Frable and Elzay[7] reported on 11 patients with mucoepidermoid carcinoma of the minor salivary glands, seven occurring in the palate, one in the epiglottis, and three in the oral cavity. All were treated by surgical excision successfully. One patient was lost to follow-up, the remainder being followed from 1 to 15 years. The experience of Bardwil et al.[1] was somewhat disappointing. Of 17 patients, 15 were treated by surgery alone and 2 by a combination of surgery and radiotherapy. Nine patients died from the lesion and the three-year survival was 30%, approximately.

PROGNOSIS AND SURVIVAL

The histological grading represents a moderately reliable prognostic factor. In the series by Healey et al.[9] the overall five-year survival was 90% for Grade I lesions, 80% for Grade II, and 31% for grade III. In 44 patients with low-grade tumors the five-year-survival rate was 94% in the series by Jakobsson et al.[8] For those with high-grade tumors, it was 56%. Similar results have been published by others as well.[3,11]

REFERENCES

1. Bardwil, J.M., Reynolds, C.T., Ibanez, M.L., and Luna, M.A.: Report of one hundred tumors of the minor salivary glands. *Am J Surg* **112**:493, 1966.
2. Batsakis, J.G.: *Tumors of the Head and Neck. Clinical and Pathological Considerations.* Williams & Wilkins, Baltimore, 1974.
3. Bhaskar, S.N., and Bernier, J.L.: Mucoepidermoid tumors of major and minor salivary glands. Clinical features, histology, variations, natural history, and results of treatment for 144 cases. *Cancer* **15**:801, 1962.
4. Chaudhry, A.P., Vickers, R.A., and Gorlin, R.J.: Intraoral minor salivary gland tumors. An analysis of 1,414 cases. *Oral Surg* **14**:1194, 1961.
5. Epker, B.N., and Henny, F.A.: Clinical, histopathologic, and surgical aspects of intraoral minor salivary gland tumors: Review of 90 cases. *J Oral Surg* **27**:792, 1969.
6. Eversole, L.R.: Mucoepidermoid carcinoma: Review of 815 reported cases. *J Oral Surg* **28**:490, 1970.
7. Frable, W.J., and Elzay, R.P.: Tumors of minor salivary glands. A report of 73 cases. *Cancer* **25**:932, 1970.
8. Jakobsson, P. A., Blanck, C., and Eneroth, C.: Mucoepidermoid carcinoma of the parotid gland. *Cancer* **22**:111, 1968.
9. Healey, W.V., Perzin, K.H., and Smith, L.: Mucoepidermoid carcinoma of salivary gland origin. Classification, clinical-pathologic correlation, and results of treatment. *Cancer* **26**:368, 1970.
10. Stewart, F.W., Foote, F.W., and Becker, W.F.: Mucoepidermoid tumors of salivary glands. *Ann Surg* **122**:820, 1945.
11. Thorvaldsson, S.E., Beahrs, O.H., Woolner, L.B., and Simons, J.N.: Mucoepidermoid tumors of the major salivary glands. *Am J Surg* **120**:432, 1970.

60

Mucoepidermoid Carcinoma of the Respiratory Tract

THERE ARE FEW reported cases of laryngeal mucoepidermoid carcinoma and even fewer tumors of this histological pattern have been encountered in the trachea. Fechner[3] found in 1975 nine reported cases of laryngeal mucoepidermoid carcinoma. Cady et al.[1] in reviewing 31 patients with nonepidermoid carcinoma of the larynx found two patients with mucoepidermoid tumors.

The average patient's age is 60 years and the majority are males. The treatment programs have included laryngectomy and definitive radiotherapy.[1,9]

Larson et al.[4] reported one patient with mucoepidermoid tumor of the supracarinal region of the trachea. This created airway obstruction and was successfully treated by segmental resection via a transthoracic approach, which was followed by primary anastomosis of the lower part of the trachea. The patient was well nine months later.

Mucoepidermoid tumors of the bronchial tree are an established clinical entity, representing the third tumor group, which, with adenoid cystic carcinomas and carcinoids of the lung, comprise the so-called "bronchial adenomas." The incidence of mucoepidermoid carcinoma is far less than that of the other two, for only 2–3% bronchial adenomas are mucoepidermoid tumors.

A review of the literature on the subject reveals contrasting information with regard to the age, sex, smoking habits, extent of the disease, prognosis, and, finally, survival. Sniffen et al.,[8] Meffert and Lindskog,[6] Meckstroth et al.,[5] and Wilkins et al.[11] are of the opinion that mucoepidermoid carcinoma is a low-grade noninvading tumor with good prognosis following resection. In these reports both male and female patients are included and it appears that the symptoms have been present long before the diagnosis; in the series by Wilkins et al.[11] the symptoms were present for six years prior to the diagnosis. On the other hand, Turnbull et al.,[10] Dowling et al.,[2] and Ozlu et al.[7] in reviewing mucoepidermoid lung tumors describe an aggressive tumor that exhibits a tendency for prompt metastatic spread to the hilar lymph nodes and beyond, invasion of the great vessels, and a lethal outcome in a short period of time. A smoking history was elicited in all patients described by Turnbull et al.[10] and there was a male predominance. The average patient's age was 60 years. An exception to this, however, is the patient described by Dowling et al.[2] Their patient was a 32-year-old female.

CLINICAL

Chest pain associated with shortness of breath has been the commonest presenting symptom, particularly in those cases that pursued a malignant course. Associated are generalized cachexia and weakness as well as pain associated with metastatic bone disease. Chest x-rays show a mass lesion or atelectasis resulting from bronchial obstruction.[2,7,10] The bronchial obstruction may be manifested clinically as a wheezing.

The diagnosis is to be established by bronchoscopy, biopsy, or cytology.[11]

TREATMENT AND RESULTS

Patients whose disease followed an aggressive course often presented with an extensive tumor both locally and in terms of distant metastasis; therefore operative intervention could be contemplated in less than 50%. Of those patients explored, less than 50% were considered resectable and underwent pneumonectomy or lobectomy. The remainder, following the diagnosis, received radiotherapy or chemotherapy or remained untreated. Regardless of mode of therapy, all patients died from their disease, including those who underwent pneumonectomies. The average survival time from diagnosis until death is in the range of six to eight months.[2,7,11]

Six patients with mucoepidermoid tumor reviewed by Wilkins et al.[11] were followed from 1 to 16 years after their tumor resection. One patient died seven months postoperatively following hemorrhage due to local recurrence. The remaining five were alive and well with only one patient developing a local recurrence 10 years after a right upper lobectomy.

PROGNOSIS

It is obvious that two distinct groups of mucoepidermoid bronchial tumors exist, one affording a lengthy survival and the other representing an aggressive tumor that results in the patient's death in a manner similar to that seen in bronchogenic lung carcinoma. It is possible that this different biological behavior is due to the different histological grading. It is also possible, according to Wilkins et al.,[11] that the highly malignant mucoepidermoid tumor may actually be a mucous-secreting bronchogenic carcinoma.

REFERENCES

1. Cady, B., Rippey, J.H., and Frazell, E.L.: Nonepidermoid cancer of the larynx. *Ann Surg* **167**:116, 1968.
2. Dowling, E.A., Miller, R.E., Johnson, I.M., and Collier, F.C.D.: Mucoepidermoid tumors of the bronchi. *Surgery* **52**:600, 1962.
3. Fechner, R.E.: Adenocarcinoma of the larynx. *Can J Otolaryngol* **4**:284, 1975.
4. Larson, R.E., Woolner, L.B., and Payne, W.S.: Mucoepidermoid tumor of the trachea. Report of a case. *J Thorac Cardiovasc Surg* **50**:131, 1965.
5. Meckstroth, C.V., Davidson, H.B., and Kress, G.O.: Mucoepidermoid tumor of the bronchus. *Dis Chest* **40**:652, 1961.
6. Meffert, W.G., and Lindskog, G.E.: Bronchial adenoma. *J Thorac Carciovasc Surg* **59**:588, 1970.
7. Ozlu, C., Christopherson, W.M., and Allen, J.D., Jr.: Muco-epidermoid tumors of the bronchus. *J Thorac Cardiovasc Surg* **42**:24, 1961.
8. Sniffen, R.C., Soutter, L., and Robbins, L.L.: Mucoepidermoid tumors of the bronchus arising from surface epithelium. *Am J Pathol* **34**:671, 1958.
9. Thomas, K.: Mucoepidermoid carcinoma of the larynx. *J Laryngol Otol* **85**:261, 1971.
10. Turnbull, A.D., Huvos, A.G., Goodner, J.T., and Foote, F.W., Jr.: Mucoepidermoid tumors of bronchial glands. *Cancer* **28**:539, 1971.
11. Wilkins, E.W., Jr., Darling, R.C., Soutter, L., and Sniffen, R.C.: A continuing clinical survey of adenomas of the trachea and bronchus in a general hospital. *J Thorac Cardiovasc Surg* **46**:279, 1963.

61

Verrucous Carcinoma

FRIEDELL AND ROSENTHAL[11] in 1941 reported on eight patients with lesions of the buccal mucosa and lower gingiva which were attributed to tobacco chewing, a habit all patients had. The growths had a verrucous appearance and indeed Ackerman[1] subsequently included them in the clinical entity of verrucous carcinoma, a tumor whose features were fully analyzed by him.

The neoplasm is considered to be variant of squamous cell carcinoma; however, the differences between the two, both in terms of histology and of natural history, far exceed their similarities. Early reports emphasized the importance of tobacco chewing as an etiological factor in producing verrucous carcinoma of the oral cavity; however, as subsequent publications have shown, poor oral hygiene and ill-fitting dentures should be included in the causative factors.[9,17] Smoking is to be found in the clinical history of patients with verrucous carcinoma of the larynx and poor personal hygiene in patients with verrucous carcinoma of the perineal region.

VERRUCOUS CARCINOMA OF THE ORAL CAVITY

The typical patient who develops this tumor is a male in his sixth or seventh decade of life with poorly fitting dentures, poor oral hygiene or carious, partially broken teeth, and most probably a tobacco chewer. It is to be said, however, that ver-rucous carcinoma of the oral cavity has been reported in younger patients and in females.[9,17] The ratio between males and females is in the range of 5:1.[1,14,23] The oral cavity is by far the commonest site of occurrence. In the series by Kraus and Perez-Mesa[17] 73% of the tumors occurred in the oral cavity, 11% in the larynx, 4% in the nasal cavity, and 11% involved the genitalia and the perineum.[17] Within the oral cavity, the overwhelming majority of tumors favor the buccal mucosa and the gingival ridges.[14,17] The incidence of verrucous carcinoma of the oral cavity is small when compared to the overall number of malignancies occurring in this region. In the series by Goethals et al.[14] 55 patients fulfilled the histological criteria for verrucous carcinoma among 1217 cases of carcinoma of the oral cavity seen at the Mayo Clinic. Verrucous carcinoma therefore accounted for 4.5% of all oral cancers.[14]

Pathology

The gross appearance of the tumors is quite characteristic. Their color is light white or gray. They are exophytic in character with irregular shaggy or warty surfaces growing in a pattern resembling a cauliflower. Their consistency is firm and their size varies according to the time elapsed between the onset and the diagnosis. Certainly sizes in excess of 5.0 cm are common. There is no bleeding encountered and at times the superficial layers can be shed.[14,17] The often extensive lesion is piled up, producing rugal folds and between them deep cleft spaces exist, associated particularly in the deeper layers with considerable infection. The gross appearance corresponds well to that seen microscopically. There is a piling up of keratin on the surface and there is a down growth of fingers of epithelium that push rather than infiltrate into the deeper tissues (Fig. 61-1). Typically and characteristically, the epithelium is well differentiated and the impression on examination is that the basement membrane remains intact. Spaces containing degenerating keratin are to be seen and as the epithelium grows the central portion of the projecting fingerlike formations undergo cystic degeneration.[1] There is inflammatory reaction associated with the tumor, composed of plasma cells, lymphocytes, and early small abscesses. The evo-

lution is slow, occurring over several years; however, there is a relentless and gradual invasion of local tissues and structures. The cheek, the floor of the mouth, the mandible and the antrum are gradually invaded and directly penetrated by this advancing process of neoplasia and inflammation.

Since these developments take place at depth, what does a biopsy of the tumor reveal? Indeed the undulating densely keratinized outer layer covers large papillary projections that are composed of large well-differentiated squamous epithelial cells. Anaplasia is lacking and the individual cells are uniform in character, containing vesicular nuclei and abundant cytoplasm.

Confronted with this picture, the pathologist will diagnose such entities as hyperkeratosis, parakeratosis, well-differentiated keratinizing papillary

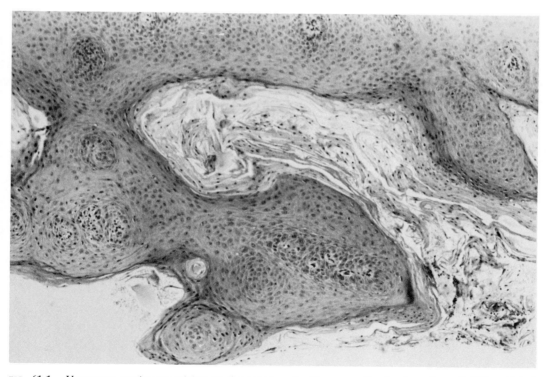

FIG. 61-1.   Verrucous carcinoma arising in the gingiva. Papillary growth of extremely well-differentiated squamous cells. The tumor clinically eroded the mandible.

squamous cell tumor, or acanthosis. The comment will be included that, because of the intact basement membrane and the well-differentiated nature of the tumor, no malignancy can be diagnosed.[3,4,22] It is often possible for several biopsies to be performed with the clinician insisting that indeed a great lesion is present and the pathologist persisting in the judgment that there is no histological sign of malignancy. Elliott *et al.*[7] in their excellent diatribe on the problems encountered with this particular tumor express the view that the intactness of the basement membrane, a generally accepted criterion for lack of invasion, is subject to certain limitations. It has been shown that primitive ectoderm can initiate the production of collagen in the underlying dermis, thus producing an epithelial basement membrane that therefore should be viewed as a functional product and not as a passive barrier. Verrucous squamous carcinomas induce or produce their own basement membrane around some of the tongues that already have invaded deeply into adjacent structures. Therefore the intactness of the basement membrane is not a reliable criterion of noninvasion. Obviously in order to diagnose the lesion the clinical information must be furnished to those studying the histological sections. If the impasse between the clinician and the pathologist continues, then the latter should be asked to visit the patient and then, to quote Kraus and Perez-Mesa,[17] "he will discover that the lesion he regards as benign half fills the mouth and has destroyed the mandible" (Fig. 61-2).

Clinical

The initial phase of the tumor seems to be that of a flat leukoplakia of long duration in terms of several years. Gradually from this the warty lesion arises, simultaneously invading deeper and expanding laterally. Actually, leukoplakia can be seen adjacent to, or surrounding the tumor

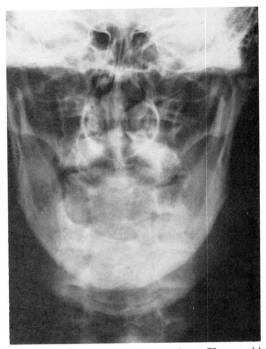

FIG. 61-2. Verrucous carcinoma in a 72-year-old male. Posterioanterior view of the mandible demonstrates erosion and lack of cortical continuity at the superior margin of the mandible at a point corresponding to the left lateral incisor, canine, and first premolar. The patient had an extensive tumor involving the left gingiva and floor of the mouth.

mass in approximately 60% of the patients who present with large invasive tumors.[7,14] As mentioned earlier, the buccal mucosa and the gingival regions are the predominant sites; however, the hard palate, the tongue, and the tonsillar area occasionally have been the primary sites.[1,17]

In the early stages with the exception of the visual change no symptoms can be ascertained; however, as the tumor increases, a sensation of soreness or burning sets in. Due to the poor oral hygiene of the patients, the early symptoms are disregarded for a considerable length of time or they are ascribed to ill-fitting dentures or to bad teeth. Eventually, they will all present with a painful mass that they will describe as a swelling, a lump, or a rough spot.[1,14,17] The average duration of the symptoms prior to the patient seeking medical advice is approximately one year and a half.[14] Bleeding, unlike squamous cell carcinoma of the oral cavity, is rarely seen with verrucous carcinoma.[1,17] The continuous tumor growth produces difficulties with mastication and the pain increases as the wave of inflammation and tumor occupies the adjacent mandible or maxilla. This invasion is orderly in fashion, with a more or less uniform radiographic pattern. One sees an eroded broad area of the mandible starting from the alveolar border and gradually extending toward the inferior margin of the bone. The advancing tumor border also may extend toward the adjacent soft tissues, namely, the tongue, the floor of the mouth, or, most commonly, the cheek, eventually protruding massively through the skin in an ulcerated cauliflowertype mass of respectable size.

Lymph node enlargement is a common finding with large bulky tumors; however, this is due practically always to inflammatory reaction and not to metastasis. In 19 patients who underwent node dissections reported by Kraus and Perez-Mesa[17] no metastatic disease was found. In the experience of Goethals et al.[14] enlarged ipsilateral lymph nodes were inflammatory in character and in those patients who underwent lymph node dissection no metastatic disease was present. The enlarged lymph nodes are invariably tender and this clinical appearance further perplexes the discrepancy between the histological examination and the clinical. The large tumor associated with greatly enlarged regional lymph nodes gives the clinical impression of an advanced malignancy, contrasting with the pathological report of "epithelial hyperplasia."

Distant metastases are not a consideration; however, as we will discuss later, following radiotherapy, both regional lymph node involvement and distant disease have been described.[23]

Treatment and Results

Since Ackerman[1] described the tumor, a continuous controversy has existed with regard to the role of radiation therapy. In his initial report of 14 patients irradiated, eight developed local recurrence. The report by Goethals et al.[14] followed with more or less similar results. Of 10 lesions irradiated, seven recurred. Kraus and Perez-Mesa[17] and Perez et al.[23] pointed out the failure of radiation to control sizable tumors and in addition they reported anaplastic transformation in verrucous carcinomas following radiotherapy. Eight patients with verrucous carcinoma of the oral cavity were presented, all treated by radiation therapy at levels ranging between 5000 and 7000 rad in five to seven weeks. In spite of the fact that there was excellent regression at the completion of the therapy, subsequent local recurrence of the primary tumor was observed in all cases. In three patients a rapid anaplastic transformation was seen histologically and the authors raised the question that ionizing radiation may have accounted for this biological change.[23] Similar experiences are to be found in the reports of Cardo and Stratigos[3] and Fonts et al.[9]

Our own experience has been similar. We recently saw and irradiated a 71-year-old male with verrucous carcinoma involving the left buccal mucosa and the left lower gingival ridge. He received a total of 7000 rad as a calculated tumor dose by means of a cobalt-60 modality in 35 treatment sessions. At the completion of the course, there was marked regression but no disappearance of the tumor. One month following the end of therapy, regrowth was obvious and the tumor eventually destroyed the mandible and penetrated through the skin of the face. This rapid recrudescence is not unusual, although recurrence may be seen some years following the completion of therapy.

Support for radiotherapy is to be found in the reports by Rider[24] and Schwade *et al.*[25] The former wrote on verrucous carcinoma of the larynx, which we will review later. The latter report presented five patients with verrucous carcinoma of the oral cavity who received tumor dosages ranging from 5580 to 7000 rad. Two patients were followed for 4.5 years without signs of recurrence, one for two years, similarly doing well, and the remaining two died in less than a year from the time of their treatment, one with and the other without signs of local recurrence.[25] Elliott *et al.*[7] reported on 33 patients with verrucous carcinoma. The authors provide analytical data for nine of their patients with oral cavity tumors. Of these, five developed recurrences following radiation therapy and four apparently had their tumor controlled. The follow-up time was extremely short in one patient, whereas in the rest it was 7.5, 5, and 2 years.

Obviously radiation is capable of controlling the disease in a certain number of individuals, particularly those with small tumors; however, a literature review convinces us that the chances of failure far exceed those of success. It is for this reason that surgical approach should be recommended. Obviously, this approach is not feasible at all times, since the patients are in the older age group, presenting with far-advanced locally extensive tumors. However, due to the fact that both regional lymph node and distant metastases, for practical purposes, never take place, complete surgical resection will offer cure. In the series by Kraus and Perez-Mesa,[17] of 64 patients whose oral cavity verrucous carcinoma was treated by surgery, control of the disease was achieved in 55. Recurrence at the site of the primary developed in nine patients. Of these, five remained well in excess of four years following reexcision of their tumor. Death from the disease occurred in only four patients. This represents a failure rate of approximately 6.5%. In the series by Goethals *et al.*[14] there was a 33% recurrence rate (9 of 28) among patients whose primary tumor was removed by diathermy and 5% recurrence rate (1 of 17) among patients whose tumor was resected.

Prognosis and Survival

The delayed diagnosis, which is due to the long indolent natural life of the tumor, the socioeconomical status of the patient, and the lack of prompt histological identification on the initial biopsy result in many patients having sizable tumors before treatment starts. This has rendered a number of them suboptimal operative candidates because of the extent of mutilating surgery required to resect the lesion. For this reason, the decision for irradiation has been made and this combination of circumstances often results in failure. The tumor persists locally, causing pain and creating mechanical problems with its volume. The associated infection and drainage further hinder the ability for food and fluid intake. The patient enters a status of inanition, which eventually leads to his death.

The prognosis should be excellent and the life-span should be unchanged if total resection can be done. In tabulating the five-year-survival rates we must take into account the fact that these are elderly individuals in poor health and indeed death from intercurrent disease nonrelated to their malignancy has been quite common.[1,14,17] The results in the series by Goethals *et al.*[14] illustrate this point. Of 55 patients whose cases were reviewed, 36 were dead at the time of the publication. The authors established that deaths from unrelated causes occurred in 25 patients, and the remaining 11 were believed to have died from their oral carcinoma.

VERRUCOUS CARCINOMA OF THE LARYNX

As is the case with the oral cavity, this is considered here to be a variant of squamous cell carcinoma and comprises 1–2% of all laryngeal carcinomas. In the series by Rider,[24] 16 cases were found in a little more than 1000 laryngeal cancers, an incidence of about 1.6%. In the series by Kraus and Perez-Mesa 12[17] laryngeal verrucous carcinomas were identified among 600 patients with laryngeal carcinoma treated at the McMillan Hospital, an incidence of 2%. Males outnumber females with a ratio of 5:1 and practically all patients have been heavy smokers.[2,8,24]

Pathology

The characteristic difficulties due to the delayed pathological confirmation in diagnosing carcinoma are encountered in this location as well. The gross appearance of the tumor is that of a grayish-white exophytic growth with filiform projections.[15]

In the series by Biller et al.[2] it took two to seven biopsies to establish the diagnosis of verrucous carcinoma in 12 patients. The initial diagnosis was hyperkeratosis in 10 patients and squamous cell carcinoma was diagnosed erroneously in the remaining two. The histological appearance is that of an orderly maturation with prominent Malphighian layer covered by thick parakeratotic superficial layer. The tumor produces bulbous rete pegs that push and penetrate by compression the surrounding stroma. Inflammatory reaction composed of lymphocytes and plasma cells surrounds the tumor margins. Keratin debris produces an intense leukocytic reaction with the formation of micro- or even macroabscesses.[2] If neglected, the tumor by means of pressure necrosis and extension invades the thyroid cartilage, giving rise to a painful soft tissue mass in the anterior neck. Lymph node metastases rarely occur; however, inflammatory reactive lymphadenopathy is common.[2,8,17,24]

Clinical

Hoarseness of the voice has been the presenting symptom in all instances. Bulky tumors may produce dysphagia and in several patients respiratory difficulty was present. In some tracheostomy was necessitated. Obviously this is not a fast-growing neoplasm, since the great majority of the patients had symptoms of more than one year's duration, some as long as six years prior to seeking advice.[2,17] Basically, there is an even distribution in terms of location, with an equal number of tumors occurring in the supraglottic, glottic, and infraglottic regions.[8] The initial clinical impression, apparently, can be quite suggestive of the diagnosis. The clinician is obliged to advise the pathologist of the findings so that both can arrive at the correct conclusion.

Treatment and Results

In two of the three major series on the subject laryngeal surgery is the clear recommendation. Partial resection was applied in two supraglottic and in eight glottic lesions in the series by Biller et al.[2] and in the remaining five patients total laryngectomy was performed. Local recurrence occurred in two patients eight months and three years following supraglottic resection and total laryngectomy respectively.[2] In the series by Kraus and Perez-Mesa[17] all 12 cases were treated surgically, with none of the patients developing local recurrence during the follow-up period, which ranged from 3 to 13 years. The extent of the surgical procedures has not been delineated by the authors; however, obviously the approach should be such that complete removal be achieved. This will be dictated by the extent of tumor involvement. Rider[24] presented the experience at Princess Margaret Hospital, which included 16 cases. Six were treated surgically, all of them successfully. Laryngeal fissure was performed in two, hemilaryngectomy in two, and total laryngectomy in the remaining two. One of the patients died two years later because of a second primary. Of the remaining 10 patients, definitive radiotherapy was applied in seven. The patients were treated by a cobalt-60 modality, receiving 5500 rad as a calculated tumor dose in five weeks. Control of the tumor was achieved in all seven patients. of the remaining three, one received palliative radiation due to the presence of a second primary, and the remaining two had squamous cell carcinoma prior to the development of verrucous tumor. On the basis of these results, the author recommends radiotherapy as the first modality to be applied because of the superior function and results derived from preservation of the laryngeal anatomy.[24]

Prognosis and Survival

This tumor is highly curable and indeed, among the patients of the three major series we have reviewed, only 2 of 40 patients were known to develop local recurrence during the follow-up period.[2,17,24]

VERRUCOUS CARCINOMA OF THE PERINEAL REGION

In the recent years the concept of verrucous carcinoma of the penis, vulva, and anus increasingly merged with that of the giant condyloma acuminatum. A synonymous term is "tumor of Buschke-Loewenstein" after the names of the authors who reported on this entity.[16]

Giant condyloma acuminatum of the penis is to be differentiated from the benign and much more common condyloma acuminatum. The former has a predilection for the prepuce and a pronounced tendency to grow deeply into the underlying tissues, displacing them in a fashion similar to that of verrucous carcinoma. They do not respond to podophyllum therapy, a therapy most effective in the removal of simple condylomas.

The clinical appearance is similar to that described for verrucous carcinomas, namely, a warty, exophytic tumor that on microscopic examination shows occasional pearl formation, elongated papillae penetrating deeply; associated with it frequently is an inflammatory infiltrate composed of lymphocytes, plasma cells, histiocytes, and eosinophils.

Clinically, most patients give a history of previous venereal disease and most of them are uncircumcised. No metastases to the regional lymph nodes or distantly have been reported.

The treatment requires complete surgical excision. Anything short of total removal will result in recurrence. Fistulous formations and abscesses are common following recurrence.[5,13,18,21]

Verrucous carcinoma of the female genital tract in the opinion of most authors conforms, as does the penile counterpart, to the original descriptions by Buschke and Loewenstein. Lucas et al.[20] in 1974 reported three examples and reviewed the literature on the subject. The authors were able to identify 14 additional cases that qualified as invasive verrucous carcinomas of the female genital tract. The majority of the lesions involve the vulva; verrucous carcinoma involving the cervix has been described as well.[15,20] The histology is that of verrucous carcinoma and the clinical symptomatology is that of a granular mass invariably recurring following attempted local excision. The natural life of the tumor is usually long; however, once deep structures are involved due to the inflammatory component fistulas and abscesses develop that invite secondary infections and present as acute clinical problems. In the early periods a verrucous, small, innocuous wart is seen progressively enlarging over several months. Deep extensions into the ischiorectal and gluteal regions as well as involvement of the rectum have been described.[12] Lymph node metastasis and distant metastasis are practically unknown. Radiotherapy in general has failed to control the disease;

actually lack of response to radiation has been reported.[10,20] The procedure of choice is vulvectomy, which most authors have performed in a radical fashion supplemented by lymph node dissection. The regional lymph nodes remain free of disease unless they have been engulfed by the advancing neoplastic wave.

In the anorectal region similar reports have appeared in the literature, indeed with an increasing frequency during the last few years. Here, too, it is gradually being recognized that verrucous carcinoma and giant condylomas of the rectum represent the same entity.[6,19,26] A chronic history of drainage accompanied eventually by fistulous formation, progression, and expansion of the tumor by pressure into the adjacent tissues and lack of response to conventional therapy are the hallmarks of the disease in this region as well. The gross and microscopic appearance of the tumor is similar to that already described. Due to failure to recognize the malignant process, recurrences following partial resection have been quite frequent.[6] It behooves therefore the clinicians of the future to recognize this entity and treat it swiftly by complete surgical resection.

The prognosis for verrucous carcinoma involving the penis, the vulva, and the rectum should be excellent, provided the diagnosis is made on time and that the tumor removal is complete. This requires awareness of this capricious tumor entity.

REFERENCES

1. Ackerman, L.V.: Verrucous carcinoma of the oral cavity. *Surgery* **23**:670, 1948.
2. Biller, H.F., Ogura, J.H., and Bauer, W.C.: Verrucous cancer of the larynx. *Laryngoscope* **81**:1323, 1971.
3. Cardo, V.A., Jr., and Stratigos, G.T.: Verrucous carcinoma of the palate: Report of case. *J Oral Surg* **31**:61, 1973.
4. Demian, S.D.E., Bushkin, F.L., and Echevarria, R.A.: Perineural invasion and anaplastic transformation of verrucous carcinoma. *Cancer* **32**:395, 1973.
5. Dreyfuss, W., and Neville, W.E.: Buschke-Löwenstein tumors. (Giant condylomata acuminata). *Am J Surg* **90**:146, 1955.
6. Drut, R., Ontiveros, R., and Cabral, D.H.: Perianal verrucose carcinoma spreading to the rectum: Report of a case. *Dis Colon Rectum* **18**:516, 1975.
7. Elliott, G.B., MacDougall, J.A., and Elliott, J.D.A.: Problems of verrucose squamous carcinoma. *Ann Surg* **177**:21, 1973.
8. Fisher, H.R.: Verrucous carcinoma of the larynx—a study of its pathologic anatomy. *Can J Otolaryngol* **4(2)**:270, 1975.
9. Fonts, E.A., Greenlaw, R.H., Rush, B.F., and Rovin, S.: Verrucous squamous cell carcinoma of the oral cavity. *Cancer* **23**:152, 1969.
10. Foye, G., Marsh, M.R., and Minkowitz, S.: Verrucous carcinoma of the vulva. *Obstet Gynecol* **34**:484, 1969.
11. Friedell, H.L., and Rosenthal, L.M.: The etiologic role of chewing tobacco in cancer of the mouth. *JAMA* **116**:2130, 1941.
12. Gallousis, S.: Verrucous carcinoma. Report of three vulvar cases and review of the literature. *Obstet Gynecol* **40**:502, 1972.
13. Gersh, I.: Giant condylomata acuminata (carcinomalike condylomata of Buschke-Löwenstein tumors) of the penis. *J Urol* **69**:164, 1953.
14. Goethals, P.L., Harrison, E.G., Jr., and Devine, K.D.: Verrucous squamous carcinoma of the oral cavity. *Am J Surg* **106**:845, 1963.
15. Jennings, R.H., and Barclay, D.L.: Verrucous carcinoma of the cervix. *Cancer* **30**:430, 1972.
16. Knoblich, R., and Failing, J.F.: Giant condyloma acuminatum (Buschke-Löwenstein tumor) of the rectum. *Am J Clin Pathol* **48**:389, 1967.
17. Kraus, F.T., and Perez-Mesa, C.: Verrucous carcinoma. Clinical and pathologic study of 105 cases involving oral cavity, larynx and genitalia. *Cancer* **19**:26, 1966.
18. Lepow, H., and Leffler, N.: Giant condylomata acuminata (Buschke-Lowenstein tumor): Report of two cases. *J Urol* **83**:853, 1960.
19. Lock, M.R., Katz, D.R., Samoorian, S., and Parks, A.G.: Giant condyloma of the rectum: Report of a case. *Dis Colon Rectum* **20**:154, 1977.
20. Lucas, W.E., Benirschke, K., and Lebherz, T.B.: Verrucous carcinoma of the female genital tract. *Am J Obstet Gynecol* **119**:435, 1974.
21. Machacek, G.F., and Weakley, D.R.: Giant condylomata acuminata of Buschke and Löwenstein. *Arch Dermat* **82**:41, 1960.
22. Mason, D.A.: Verrucous carcinoma of the mouth. *Br J Oral Surg* **10**:64, 1972.
23. Perez, C.A., Kraus, F.T., Evans, J.C., and Powers, W.E.: Anaplastic transformation in verru-

cous carcinoma of the oral cavity after radiation therapy. *Radiology* **86:**108, 1966.

24. Rider, W.D.: Toronto experience of verrucous carcinoma of the larynx. *Can J Otolaryngol* **4(2):**278, 1975.

25. Schwade, J.G., Wara, W.M., Dedo, H.H., and

Phillips, T.L.: Radiotherapy for verrucous carcinoma. *Radiology* **120:**677, 1976.

26. Sturm, J.T., Christenson, C.E., Uecker, J.H., and Perry, J.F., Jr.: Squamous-cell carcinoma of the anus arising in a giant condyloma acuminatum: Report of a case. *Dis Colon Rectum* **18:**147, 1975.

62

Carcinosarcoma of the Lung

THE FIRST CASE of pulmonary carcinosarcoma was described in 1908. It is a rare tumor and up to 1977 42 cases had been reported in the literature.[3-5] It has definite sex predilection, the ratio of male to female being 5:1.[4,5] In the so-called "endobronchial carcinosarcoma" the ratio is even higher (11:1), as reported in the series by Ludwigsen.[5] The majority of patients are in their late fifties or early sixties at the time of the diagnosis. Cigarette smoking may be implicated as an etiological factor.[2]

PATHOLOGY

Moore[6] identified two groups of carcinosarcomas of the lung on the basis of their location: central and peripheral. The former arise in the major bronchi and the latter in the periphery of the lung.[6] Histologically, the commonest carcinomatous component has been squamous cell carcinoma; however, other types, such as adenocarcinoma and undifferentiated carcinoma, have been encountered. The sarcomatous components with which the carcinomas intermingle are for the most part fibrosarcomas or spindle cell sarcomas. Less commonly, however, chondrosarcomas or osteogenic sarcomas have been identified.[5,6,8]

CLINICAL

Cough and hemoptysis are the common presenting symptoms. The central tumors cause bronchial obstruction, creating atelectasis with secondary infection.[2,4] Radiographically, bronchography has identified these lesions well.[6] The peripheral tumors infiltrate into the adjacent pleura or mediastinum and show a higher propensity for metastasis, both to the regional hilar nodes and to distant sites.[2,6,7] Radiographically, they present as mass lesions, at times cavitating.[8]

TREATMENT AND RESULTS

Most of the patients with endobronchial central tumors are potential surgical candidates. In a review of 24 such patients, Ludwigsen[5] found 19 who underwent surgery (14 lobectomy and five pneumonectomy). Of these 19, one survived without disease for six years, and there were seven patients surviving for periods ranging from three months to three years postoperatively. The remaining 11 died, most of them as a result of their tumor. Parenchymal lesions, even if successfully resected, have a great tendency for distant metastases.[2]

With the exception of one case in which postoperative radiotherapy was given to the level of 5000 rad and in which subsequent autopsy showed persistent disease, there are no data available on the effectiveness of radiation and chemotherapy in the treatment of this tumor.[2]

The regional hilar and mediastinal nodes represent the first metastatic site.

Distant metastases, hematogenous in character, may be seen in such organs as the liver, brain, adrenals, intestine, kidneys, and heart.[1,2]

PROGNOSIS AND SURVIVAL

The endobronchial lesions carry a relatively better prognosis. This is primarily because only a small percentage of them (15–30%) metastasize to the regional lymph nodes in the early period of the disease.[4–6] The one-year-survival rate for this group, as a whole, is 36%. The one-year survival for those who actually underwent surgical resection was 42%.[5] Patients with peripheral tumors have a very poor prognosis.[2,6]

REFERENCES

1. Bergmann, M., Ackerman, L.V., and Kemler, R.L.: Carcinosarcoma of the lung. Review of the literature and report of two cases treated by pneumonectomy. *Cancer* 4:919, 1951.
2. Bull, J.C., and Grimes, O.F.: Pulmonary carcinosarcoma. *Chest* 65:9, 1974.
3. Diaconiță, G.: Bronchopulmonary carcinosarcoma. *Thorax* 30:682, 1975.
4. Kakos, G.S., Williams, T.E., Jr., Assor, D., and Vasko, J.S.: Pulmonary carcinosarcoma. Etiologic, therapeutic and prognostic considerations. *J Thorac Cardiovasc Surg* 61:777, 1971.
5. Ludwigsen, E.: Endobronchial carcinosarcoma. *Virchows Arch [Pathol Anat]* 373:293, 1977.
6. Moore, T.C.: Carcinosarcoma of the lung. *Surgery* 50:886, 1961.
7. Razzuk, M.A., Urschel, H.C., Race, G.J., Arndt, J.H., and Paulson, D.L.: Carcinosarcoma of the lung. Report of two cases and review of the literature. *J Thorac Cardiovasc Surg* 61:541, 1971.
8. Stackhouse, E.M., Harrison, E.G., and Ellis, F.H.: Primary mixed malignancies of the lung. Carcinosarcoma and blastoma. *J Thorac Cardiovasc Surg* 57:385, 1969.

63

Carcinosarcoma of the Thyroid

IN THE GENESIS of these tumors the carcinomatous part, which may be follicular, papillary, mixed, or undifferentiated carcinoma, combines with either fibrosarcomas or osteogenic sarcomas. They are very rare and have a poor prognosis due to their tendency to metastasize extensively. The overall survival is less than one year.[1,2]

REFERENCES

1. Arean, V.M., and Schildecker, W.W.: Carcinosarcoma of the thyroid gland. Report of two cases. *South Med J* **57**:446, 1964.
2. Rube, J., Cabrera, A., and Pickren, J.W.: Carcinosarcoma of thyroid gland. *NY State J Med* **67**:716, 1967.

64

Carcinosarcoma of the Breast

UNTIL 1974, 16 cases of primary breast carcinosarcoma had been reported.[3] The usual symptom is a mass in the breast. The size of the tumors varied from 1.8 to 13.0 cm and on the average was 8.0 cm, measuring the surgical specimen.[1-3]

The histological pattern is that of an infiltrating ductal adenocarcinoma or squamous cell carcinoma combined with sarcoma. The sarcomatous part has been spindle cell sarcoma, fibrosarcoma, or osteogenic sarcoma.

The primary mode of treatment has been mastectomy, simple or radical. Some patients have received postoperative radiotherapy. Carcinosarcoma of the breast has a relatively better prognosis and therefore offers a better chance of survival than carcinosarcomas in other locations. The axillary lymph nodes were found to be involved only in 35.0% of the cases and distant metastatic disease, primarily to the lung, was found in 50.0% of the patients.

Harris and Persaud[3] tabulated previously reported cases and added two of their own. In that review it is shown that approximately 60.0% of the patients were alive and well from periods ranging from a few months to five years following surgery. In general, carcinosarcomas are tumors persistent locally and it is conceivable that specifically in the breast a complete tumor removal is possible by means of mastectomy.

REFERENCES

1. Budd, J.W., and Breslin, F.J.: Carcino-osteogenic sarcoma; malignant mixed tumor of the chest wall: Report of a case. Am J Cancer 31:207, 1937.
2. Curran, R.C., and Dodge, O.G.: Sarcoma of the breast with particular reference to its origin from fibroadenoma. J Clin Pathol 15:1, 1962.
3. Harris, M., and Persaud, V.: Carcinosarcoma of the breast. J Pathol 112:99, 1974.

65

Carcinosarcoma of the Esophagus

STOUT et al.[9] in 1949 reviewed the literature with reference to esophageal carcinosarcomas. They uncovered 18 cases and added one of their own. Until 1973 an additional 28 such tumors had been reported in the literature.[1,4] Most of the patients are males and the ratio of male to female is in the range of 3:1. The patients are in the older age bracket, the average age at the time of diagnosis being 59 years.[5,6,9]

PATHOLOGY

On the basis of the gross appearance, the tumors can be divided into two groups: polypoid and nonpolypoid infiltrating carcinosarcomas. The majority of them (80%) belong to the polypoid category. Their characteristic is the formation of a pedicle, most often is quite short, from which the tumor protrudes into the esophageal lumen. They may attain a quite large size.[1,2,4,6–10]

A small percentage (20%) belong to the infiltrating type. The tumors of this group expand into the wall of the esophagus in a manner similar to that of esophageal carcinomas.[5] The carcinomatous component is squamous cell carcinoma and occasionally adenocarcinoma or undifferentiated carcinoma. The sarcomatous part is commonly spindle-shaped sarcoma or more specifically a fibrosarcoma; however, there are several reports describing leiomyosarcomas, rhabdomyosarcomas, chondro-sarcomas, osteosarcomas, among others.[4,5,9,10]

CLINICAL

The presenting symptom is dysphagia. With the passage of time weakness, weight loss, and retrosternal discomfort appear. Cough, hemoptysis, and hematemesis are also among the expected clinical signs.[5,6] The interval between the onset of symptoms and the time of the diagnosis ranges between 6 and 12 months.[6]

Plain chest x-ray examination may reveal mediastinal widening as the large bulky tumors distend the esophagus unduly. On barium swallow, the pedunculated polypoid form projects as an intraluminal filling defect and renders smooth esophageal walls. Occasionally, the stalk may be identified, but usually it is not, because it is too short.[1,5] The infiltrative form produces esophageal constriction.[5]

In terms of location most of these tumors have occurred in the middle esophagus; however, cases have been described in the rest of the segments as well.[1]

The polypoid tumors grow and expand primarily locally, infiltrating the esophagus through the pedicle and thus extending in the later stages into the mediastinum. By this mechanism, extension into the bronchial tree may occur.[6]

Distant metastases or even regional lymph node metastases are not very common.[6,7]

TREATMENT AND RESULTS

Surgery offers the best possibility of cure, particularly for the pedunculated polypoid variety. However, against surgical success mitigates the fact that the nutritional status of practically all patients is very poor and this when combined with their advanced age makes them suboptimal operative candidates. For this reason, in more recent reports hyperalimentation prior to surgery has been recommended.[1] Among the 44 patients reviewed by McCort,[5] 24 were operated upon and, of these, 12 (50%) died in the immediate postoperative period. The aim of the operation is resection of the tumor with free margins above and below it. In spite of the difficulties there are several survivors reported in the literature following surgical resection.[3,6–8,10] There are no reports on the effects of chemotherapy in the management of these patients and radiation has been tried only on a very limited basis to this date.[5,8]

PROGNOSIS AND SURVIVAL

In the review by Calhoun et al.[1] among 45 cases of these rare neoplasms, only two patients had survived five years. Local persistent disease or recurrence was the main reason of failure. However, there have been several patients whose observation times were less than two years and a number of them were surviving without evidence of disease.[1,4] Should recurrence occur following definitive surgery, the average length of survival is approximately one year.[6]

REFERENCES

1. Calhoun, T., Ali, S.D., Muna, D., Kurtz, L.H., Simmonds, R.L., and Nash, E.C.: Carcinosarcoma of the esophagus. Case Report and review of the literature. *J Thorac Cardiovasc Surg* **66**:315, 1973.
2. Elton, S.E., and Joannides, M., Jr.: Carcinosarcoma of the esophagus. A review and case report. *Dis Chest* **41**:111, 1962.
3. Lichter, I., Smith, E.R., and Gwynne, J.F.: Carcinosarcoma of the esophagus. *Thorax* **23**:663, 1968.
4. Lin, M.H., Luna-Munoz, M.I., Kraft, J.R., and Marks, L.M.: Carcinosarcoma of the esophagus. *Am J Gastroenterol* **55**:249, 1971.
5. McCort, J.: Esophageal carcinosarcoma and pseudosarcoma. *Radiology* **102**:519, 1972.
6. Moore, T.C., Battersby, J.S., Vellios, F., and Loehr, W.M.: Carcinosarcoma of the esophagus. *J Thorac Cardiovasc Surg* **45**:281, 1963.
7. Palmer, J.A., and Mustard, R.A.: Carcinosarcoma of the cervical esophagus. *Can J Surg* **8**:56, 1965.
8. Stener, B., Kock, N.G., Petterson, S., and Zetterlund, B.: Carcinosarcoma of the esophagus. *J Thorac Cardiovasc Surg* **54**:746, 1967.
9. Stout, A.P., Humphreys, G.H., and Rottenberg, L.A.: A case of carcinosarcoma of the esophagus. *AJR* **61**:461, 1949.
10. Young, B., and Gardner, D.L.: Polypoidal carcinosarcoma of oesophagus. *Br J Surg* **51**:584, 1964.

66

Carcinosarcoma of the Stomach

MOST CASES WITH this tumor have been reported from Japan. It is a rare malignant neoplasm, many cases of which are seen in the region of the pylorus. The neoplasm could extend to involve the entire stomach as well.[1] Distant metastases are not common. It is estimated that they occur in approximately 30% of the cases. In spite of that, because of the local aggressiveness, the disease is uniformly fatal.

REFERENCES

1. Tanimura, H., and Futura, M.: Carcinosarcoma of the stomach. *Am J Surg* **113**:702, 1967.

67

Carcinosarcoma of the Kidney

TRANSITIONAL CELL carcinomas are known for the anaplasia they may exhibit; therefore renal pelvis carcinosarcomas should be viewed with this fact in mind.[4] However, there is evidence to suggest that true carcinosarcomas may be seen in the kidney.[2,3] Concomitant neoplasms, one mesenchymal and another epithelial in origin, have also been reported, arising independently in the same kidney.[1]

PATHOLOGY

The epithelial part may be a transitional cell carcinoma or clear cell adenocarcinoma. These are associated and intermingled with stromal sarcomas.[4]

CLINICAL

The patients are usually in their sixth decade of life or older. Hematuria is the commonest presenting symptom and this may be accompanied by flank pain and epigastric distress. The tumors infiltrate locally and metastasize widely.[3]

TREATMENT AND PROGNOSIS

Nephrectomy, if feasible, should be considered the treatment of choice. Renal pelvis carcinosarcomas may have a better prognosis than those arising in the parenchyma of the kidney.[2] Four patients reported by Fisher and Davis[3] and one reported by Hou and Willis[4] died of their disease in less than six months from the time of the diagnosis.

REFERENCES

1. De La Peña, A., Navarro, M., Pobil, J.L., Melicow, M.M., and Uson, A.C.: Concomitant unrelated neoplasms of the renal pelvis. *J Urol* **99**:21, 1968.
2. Fauci, F.A., Therhag, H.G., and Davis, J.E.: Carcinosarcoma of the renal pelvis. *J Urol* **85**:897, 1961.
3. Fisher, E.R., and Davis, E.R.: Carcinosarcoma of the kidney. *J Urol* **87**:109, 1962.
4. Hou, L.T., and Willis, R.A.: Renal carcinosarcoma, true and false. *J Pathol Bacteriol* **85**:139, 1963.

68

Carcinosarcoma of the Urinary Bladder

A REVIEW OF the literature up to 1970 by Brinton et al.[1] uncovered 28 cases, of which 20 were accepted as fulfilling the criteria of carcinosarcoma in this location. Until 1975 an additional 11 cases had been reported when the subject was again reviewed by Patterson and Dale.[3] As happens with carcinosarcomas of the lung and the esophagus, carcinosarcomas of the urinary bladder have a strong predilection (80%) for males.[3] The average age at the time of diagnosis is 64 years.

PATHOLOGY

The tumors are usually bulky and exophytic. They have been found to arise from the base and the walls of the urinary bladder. Histologically transitional cell carcinoma is the common epithelial element associated with spindle cell sarcoma or more well-defined leiomyosarcoma, chondrosarcoma, or osteosarcoma.[2,3] As with all carcinosarcomas, the question is raised whether or not they represent an oncological entity, or simultaneous "collision tumors," or whether the spindle cells are truly sarcomatous or just a manifestation of anaplastic carcinomas.[1]

CLINICAL

Hematuria is the presenting symptom and later on dysuria appears. Generally, these are slow-growing neoplasms that tend to extend locally and infiltrate the pelvis directly. There is no early propensity for metastasis and actually metastatic disease was found only in 25% of the autopsy patients, most commonly seen in the lungs and the liver. The cause of death is persistent pelvic disease frequently resulting in bladder perforation and peritonitis. The pelvic lymph nodes become involved and they have been shown to contain both epithelial and mesenchymal elements.[1,3]

TREATMENT AND RESULTS

The rarity of the disease has resulted in a variety of treatment programs. They range from fulguration and transurethral resection to cystectomy with urinary diversion. Radiotherapy has been used preoperatively or for palliative purposes in advanced tumors. As the disease tends to recur locally rather than to metastasize, total cystectomy with urinary diversion should be considered the proper therapy when feasible.[3]

PROGNOSIS AND SURVIVAL

A historical review reveals a poor prognosis, possibly because of failure in early diagnosis, possibly because of suboptimal therapy. The average survival has been 10–15 months from the time the diagnosis was made. The longest survival, 5 years, occurred in a patient treated by electrodesiccation by Powers et al.[4]

REFERENCES

1. Brinton, J.A., Ito, Y., and Olsen, B.S.: Carcinosarcoma of the urinary bladder. A case report and review of the literature. *Cancer* **25:**1183, 1970.
2. Holtz, F., Fox, J.E., and Abell, M.R.: Carcinosarcoma of the urinary bladder. *Cancer* **29:**294, 1972.
3. Patterson, T.H., and Dale, G.A.: Carcinosarcoma of the bladder: Case report and review of the literature. *J Urol* **115:**753, 1976.
4. Powers, J.H., Hawn, C., Van, Z., and Carter, R.D.: Osteogenic sarcoma and transitional cell carcinoma occurring simultaneously in the urinary bladder: Report of a case. *J Urol* **76:**263, 1956.

69

Carcinosarcoma of the Prostate

THIS IS AN entity with few documented cases.[1,2,4] The difficulty is in determining whether or not the lesion is a true carcinosarcoma or anaplastic carcinoma. Mostofi and Price[3] have stated that desmoplastic reaction of the stroma may occur secondary to estrogen administration. They consider true carcinosarcomas only those lesions whose mesenchymal component contains neoplastic cartilage or bone or definite stroma.

The tumors are not estrogen-dependent and they metastasize readily. Pulmonary nodules, liver metastases, spine, and viscera have been the recipient sites.[1,2,4]

REFERENCES

1. Haddad, J.R., and Reyes, E.: Carcinosarcoma of the prostate with metastasis of both elements: Case report. *J Urol* **103**:80, 1970.
2. Hamlin, W.B., and Lund, P.K.: Carcinosarcoma of the prostate: A case report. *J Urol* **97**:518, 1967.
3. Mostofi, F.K., and Price, E.B., Jr.: *Tumors of the Male Genital System.* Armed Forces Institute of Pathology, Washington, D.C., 1973.
4. Schmidt, J.D., and Welch, M.J., Jr.: Sarcoma of the prostate. *Cancer* **37**:1908, 1976.

70

Malignant Mixed Müllerian Tumors
of the Uterus
(Mixed Mesodermal Tumors of the Uterus)

MALIGNANT MIXED Müllerian tumors of the uterus (mixed mesodermal tumors) are a distinct group of uterine sarcomas. Characteristically, they represent an admixture of carcinomatous and sarcomatous elements, all of which arise in the uterus, an organ of Müllerian origin. Although the carcinomatous element is primarily adenocarcinoma in character and very occasionally squamous cell carcinoma, the sarcomatous counterpart has created several diagnostic problems and considerable confusion with regard to their classification, as witnessed in reviewing the literature.[4,10]

The histological patterns of the sarcomatous element reported have been great in number. In general the classification of uterine sarcomas presently used is that proposed by Ober and subsequently simplified by Kempson and Bari.[4] Thus, malignant mixed Müllerian tumors are subdivided into two broad categories: homologous type and heterologous type. In the former category are included those malignant mixed Müllerian tumors that are composed of carcinoma and whose sarcomatous element is leiomyosarcoma, stromal sarcoma, fibrosarcoma, or mixtures of these sarcomas. This group of tumors in earlier reports has been referred to as carcinosarcomas.[2,4,8,10] Heterologous

mixed mesodermal sarcomas are composed of carcinoma plus heterologous elements with or without homologous sarcoma. The basic heterologous elements to be encountered are rhabdomyosarcoma, chondrosarcoma, and osteosarcoma. These tumor components arise from striated muscle, cartilage, and bone elements, which are not part of the uterine anatomy under normal development from the Müllerian system.[10] This histological subclassification has some bearing, albeit not a great one, on prognosis and survival, as will be discussed later.

The relative incidence of mixed uterine sarcomas was 2% of all uterine malignancies in the series reported by Chuang et al.[2] In the series by Williamson and Christopherson[10] mixed Müllerian tumors composed 1.39%—34 cases of 2442-histologically verified malignant neoplasms of the uterus and the uterine cervix.

The majority of patients are postmenopausal. The average age at the time of the diagnosis was 67.3 years in the series by Chuang et al.,[2] 64.8 years in the series by Williamson and Christopherson,[10] and 63 years in the series by Schaepman-Van Geuns.[8] All these reports include both homologous and heterologous type of lesions. Norris and Taylor[7] reported on 31 carcinosarcomas of the uterus, the median age of the group being 62 years with a range from 48 to 76 years, and on 31 mixed mesodermal heterologous uterine neoplasms, the median age again being 62 years with a range from 45 to 91 years.[6,7]

PATHOLOGY

The gross appearance of the tumors in approximately 80% of the cases is that of a polypoid or pedunculated mass that is typically soft and contains areas of hemorrhage and necrosis. The mass fills and distends the uterine cavity, thus enlarging the uterus.[2,4,10] The average size of the tumor in its greatest diameter is 5–6 cm and in all cases there is involvement of the endometrium. Extension and invasion of the myometrium is also the rule.[6,7] Involvement of the cervix is uncommon.[6,7] Necrosis and hemorrhage are to be found in approximately 50% of the cases.[2]

Microscopically, the tumors exhibit a wide variation in histological patterns. The epithelial malignant element is adenocarcinoma in the majority of the cases. Squamous cell carcinoma, either alone or coexisting with areas of adenocarcinoma, is to be found in 25–30% of the cases.[10] The carcinomatous elements may be well differentiated in some areas and highly anaplastic in others. The main part of the histological picture, however, is that of a sarcomatous stroma into which the epithelial elements are intermingled. The sarcomatous stroma is composed of fusiform cells, usually highly anaplastic in character. In the homologous type the sarcomatous component is primarily formed of stromal sarcoma and to a lesser degree of leiomyosarcoma.[4,6,7] In the heterologous type in addition to the presence of stromal sarcoma and leiomyosarcoma they may contain rhabdomyosarcoma, chondrosarcoma, and osteosarcoma (Fig. 72.1). Obviously, not all tumors carry all histological patterns.[4,7,10]

The histogenesis of mixed Müllerian tumors during the previous century was attributed to embryonal rests, which were present but dormant within the uterus, potentially malignant in character and eventually giving life to this form of neoplasia. The modern view of development is different. Mixed mesodermal tumors are thought to develop from multipotent neoplastic cells and in particular stromal cells that have the capacity to differentiate into both epithelial and stromal components.[7]

Clement and Scully[3] reported on 10 mixed tumors of the uterus in which the stromal component was malignant but the epithelial element benign. These neoplasms the authors termed "Müllerian adenosarcoma."

CLINICAL

As with all uterine neoplasms, the commonest presenting symptom is that of abnormal vaginal bleeding. Less frequently pain and abdominal distention have been included in the symptomatology. Even less common are symptoms referable to the gastrointestinal and urinary tracts.[2,6,7,10] The duration of the symptoms prior to the time of diagnosis is in the range of 2.7–2.8 months.[6,10]

On physical examination, uterine enlargement was present in 69% of the cases in the series reported by Chuang et al.[2] Of them one-half had extension of the tumor beyond the uterus at the time of the diagnosis. In the series by Norris et al.[6] and Norris and Taylor[7] 50% of the patients with heterologous mixed mesodermal sarcoma and 25% of the patients with homologous mixed uterine sarcoma had extension of the disease beyond the uterus at the time of the diagnosis.

Dilatation and curettage usually leads to the diagnosis, but in a percentage of cases, although malignancy is found, the exact histology is not accurate. Protrusion of the tumor through the cervical os is common.[2,6]

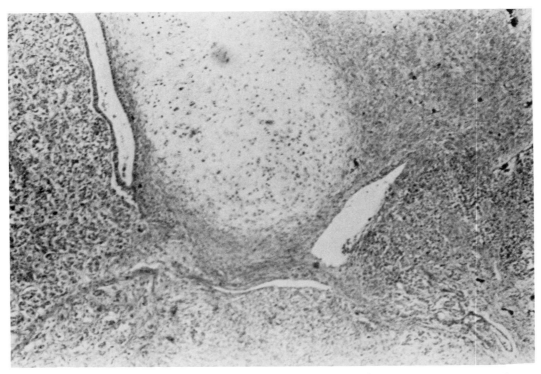

FIG. 70-1. Malignant mixed Müllerian tumor of the uterus. Irregular tubular structures, sarcomatous stroma, and a central area of cartilage are seen. Carcinosarcoma with heterologous element (cartilage).

It is significant and it should be noted that history of previous pelvic irradiation has been elicited and reported in the literature in a certain percentage of patients with mixed Müllerian uterine tumors. This percentage varies from author to author, ranging from 10 to 37%. In the usual case relatively high amounts of radiation have been delivered to the pelvis for a preexisting benign or malignant nonrelated disease. The interval between irradiation and the development of the mixed tumor has been long, in excess of 10 years.[2,6,10]

In the series by Williamson and Christopherson[10] of 48 patients with mixed Müllerian tumor, obesity was found in 20 patients (41.7%), hypertension in 15 (31.3%), and diabetes in 5 (10.4%).[10] In other series the incidence of these ailments has not been addressed and still others have found no increase of hyper-

tension, diabetes, and obesity among patients with uterine sarcomas compared to women having normal endometria.[1,8]

TREATMENT AND RESULTS

Total abdominal hysterectomy with bilateral salpingo-oophorectomy has been the most usual form of therapy. This has been combined in a certain number of patients with radiotherapy, either preoperatively in the form of radium placement or postoperatively in the form of external beam therapy, particularly for those with locally advanced disease. Radiation therapy alone has not been the primary treatment for early tumors that were deemed to be operable. It appears indeed that the radiosensitivity of mixed mesodermal uterine sarcomas is rather low, although occasional good responses have been noted.[4]

Norris and Taylor[7] encountered five

survivors among a group of 11 patients with homologous Müllerian sarcoma confined to the uterus treated by surgery alone. In the same series, of 10 patients with neoplasias confined to the uterus and treated with radiation combined with surgery, there were three survivors. On this basis, the authors express doubt about the effectiveness of radiotherapy. Norris *et al.*[6] found that radiotherapy was not capable of producing tumor sterilization in a series of 31 heterologous mixed tumors. Kempson and Bari,[4] on the other hand, as well as Badib *et al.*[1] and Vongtama *et al.*[9] favor the combined approach: before or after a total abdominal hysterectomy and bilateral salpingo-oophorectomy radiotherapy is applied. A critical review of their data, however, reveals a small number of cases and no substantial improvement of the survival rate when radiotherapy is added.[1,4,9] In our experience these neoplasms have been only modestly radiosensitive.

Reports on combination chemotherapy in the management of these tumors are not available at the present.

Cure can only be achieved for lesions at an early stage. Even those are considerably more difficult to control compared to adenocarcinoma of the endometrium. Autopsies of patients dying from their disease have shown pelvic recurrence or persistent disease being universally present (Fig. 70–2). In addition pelvic and periaortic lymph node involvement is a common finding, as well as extension of the tumor downward into the vagina. Distant organs commonly involved are the lungs and the liver.[6,7,10]

Prognosis and Survival

The extent of the disease at the time of the diagnosis greatly influences the prognosis. Actually it is the single most important criterion in determining the patient's survival. In the series reported by Chuang *et al.*[2] there were six survivors among 20

patients with intrauterine disease, whereas there were no five-year survivors among 22 patients whose tumor extended beyond the uterus. Norris and Taylor[7] found that among the cured patients with uterine carcinosarcomas, the median tumor diameter was 3.6 cm, compared to a median diameter of 7.0 cm observed among patients dying of their neoplasm. These authors reported on heterologous mixed mesodermal tumors and encountered similar findings. The cured patients as a group had smaller tumors, none exceeding 5.0 cm in diameter.[6] In the series by Kempson and Bari[4] patients with homologous tumors who survived had myometrial invasion no further than the proximal half. There were no survivors among 11 patients whose tumor extended beyond this point at the time of hysterectomy. Similarly, in the heterologous group the only survivors were patients with small superficial tumors.

The histological pattern regarding the presence or absence of chondrosarcoma and rhabdomyosarcoma in the heterologous group of tumors has been debated with regard to its prognostic value. More specifically, the presence of rhabdomyoblasts or osteoblasts is considered by some to affect the prognosis adversely.[4,6] The same authors feel that the chondrosarcoma elements represent a favorable sign. Others, however, do not agree with these assessments.[8]

The overall five-year survival was 32% in a series of 25 patients with mixed mesodermal tumors reported by Mortel *et al.*[5] For disease limited to the uterus, the five-year-survival rate was 60%. The five-year-survival rate in the series reported by Chuang *et al.*[2] on the basis of 49 cases of homologous and heterologous mixed mesodermal tumors was 30% among patients whose tumor was confined to the uterus and 0% when spread beyond the uterus had taken place. Norris and Taylor[7] pointed out that a difference in survival exists between patients

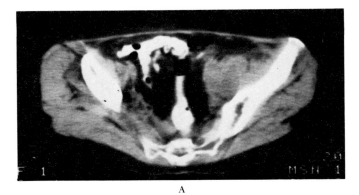

A

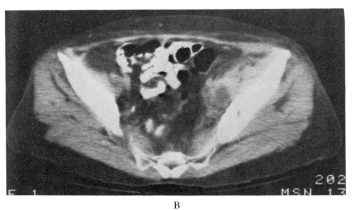

B

FIG. 70-2. Malignant mixed Müllerian tumor of the uterus in a 62-year-old female. Total abdominal hysterectomy and bilateral salpingo-oophorectomy performed two years earlier. The tumor invaded the middle third of the myometrium and was extending into the lymphatics. There was cartilage present. Computed tomography at the time of the recurrence reveals a mass lesion in the left posterior pelvis (A). Following palliative radiotherapy, there has been partial regression (B).

with homologous and heterologous tumors. In reviewing their data critically, indeed there appears to be a 10% difference in favor of carcinosarcomas. Thus, 6 of 31 patients with heterologous tumors (19.3%) survived at five years and so did 8 of 29 eligible patients (27%) with carcinosarcoma. In the series by Kempson and Bari[4] 32% of the patients with homologous type were alive at five years compared to 14% of those with heterologous type. The five-year-survival rate was 26.7% for patients with carcinosarcomas and 16.7% for patients with mixed mesodermal tumors in the series reported by Williamson and Christopherson.[10] The authors felt that the differences were not significant, however. Vongtama et al.[9] found the five-year-survival rate to be 31% for mixed mesodermal sarcomas and 41% for carcinosarcomas. The authors advocate the use of adjuvant pre- or postoperative irradiation, finding the five-year-survival rate in mixed mesodermal sarcomas to be 26% when surgery alone was used compared to 40% when surgery was combined with irradiation. So far as carcinosarcoma is concerned, the five-year-survival rate for surgery alone was 36%, reaching 57% for those patients receiving combined therapy.[9]

REFERENCES

1. Badib, A.O., Vongtama, V., Kurohara, S.S., and Webster, J.H.: Radiotherapy in the treatment of sarcomas of the corpus uteri. *Cancer* **24**:724, 1969.
2. Chuang, J.T., Van Velden, D.J.J., and Graham, J.B.: Carcinosarcoma and mixed mesodermal tumor of the uterine corpus. Review of 49 cases. *Obstet Gynecol* **35**:769, 1970.
3. Clement, P.B., and Scully, R.E.: Müllerian adenosarcoma of the uterus. A clinicopathologic analysis of ten cases of distinctive type of müllerian mixed tumor. *Cancer* **34**:1138, 1974.
4. Kempson, R.L., and Bari, W.: Uterine sarcomas. Classification, diagnosis, and prognosis. *Hum Pathol* **1**:331, 1970.
5. Mortel, R., Koss, L.G., Lewis, J.L., Jr., and D'Urso, J.R.: Mesodermal mixed tumors of the uterine corpus. *Obstet Gynecol* **43**:248, 1974.
6. Norris, J.H., Roth, E., and Taylor, H.B.: Mesenchymal tumors of the uterus. II. A clinical and pathologic study of 31 mixed mesodermal tumors. *Obstet Gynecol* **28**:57, 1966.
7. Norris, H.J., and Taylor, H.B.: Mesenchymal tumors of the uterus. III. A clinical and pathologic study of 31 carcinosarcomas. *Cancer* **19**:1459, 1966.
8. Schaepman-Van Geuns, E.J.: Mixed tumors and carcinosarcomas of the uterus evaluated five years after treatment. *Cancer* **25**:72, 1970.
9. Vongtama, V., Karlen, J.R., Piver, S.M., Tsukada, Y., and Moore, R.H.: Treatment, results and prognostic factors in Stage I and II sarcomas of the corpus uteri. *AJR* **126**:139, 1976.
10. Williamson, E.O., and Christopherson, W.M.: Malignant mixed müllerian tumors of the uterus. *Cancer* **29**:585, 1972.

71

Malignant Mixed Mullerian Tumors of the Ovary (Carcinosarcoma and Mixed Mesodermal Tumors of the Ovary)

THE INCIDENCE OF this malignancy among all malignant primary ovarian neoplasms was found to be 1.1% by Czernobilsky and LaBarre.[1] The patients are usually in their fifth or sixth decade.[1-3]

PATHOLOGY

The size of the primary ovarian neoplasms has varied from 3.0 to 30.0 cm. They are composed of cystic areas that are interspersed between soft to solid tissue. Microscopically the epithelial component is adenocarcinoma with glandular elements. This carcinoma takes the form of papillary well-differentiated carcinoma, medullary carcinoma, and endometrioid, squamous, or poorly differentiated carcinoma.[3] The stromal component, as far as the carcinosarcomas are concerned, presents nonspecific homologous sarcomatous elements, the cells being primarily spindle-shaped and in addition stellate-shaped cells and oval cells have been described.[1-3] In mixed mesodermal tumors heterologous tissues are present. Cartilage is seen in 57.0% of the cases; striated muscle, in 50.0%; and osteoid, in 21.0%. These heterologous foci are surrounded by nonspecific sarcomatous stroma.[2]

CLINICAL

The presenting symptoms are similar to those of carcinomas of the ovary. An abdominal mass associated with increasing girth and accompanied by abdominal pain and gastrointestinal complaints is the usual presentation.[1,2] The duration of the symptoms prior to diagnosis range from a few weeks to six months.[1] On pelvic examination, a mass can be found in 89.0% of the patients. During laparotomy 50.0–70.0% of the cases have metastases to the peritoneal surfaces and the omentum.[2] It follows that 50.0% or more are Stage III at the time of the diagnosis.[3] The tumors have a propensity for dissemination in the abdominal cavity, producing eventually peritoneal involvement with mass formations and ascites. Metastases occur to the liver and the lungs.[2,3] The periaortic lymph nodes are also involved, apparently with extension similar to that observed in carcinoma of the ovary. The sarcomatous elements tend to predominate histologically in the metastases.[3]

TREATMENT AND RESULTS

Exploratory laparotomy on the basis of the clinical findings and symptomatology is the usual course of events. According to the operative findings and on the basis of the extent of the disease and according to the criteria of the individual physician, hysterectomy and bilateral salpingo-oophorectomy, unilateral salpingo-oophorectomy, and bilateral salpingo-oophorectomy have been performed. Few advanced cases have been only biopsied. Postoperative radiotherapy has been administered to a considerable number of patients and chemotherapy has been used for recurrent disease.[1-3] We have participated in the management of one patient with carcinosarcoma of the ovary. At the time of the exploration, diffuse peritoneal involvement was noted. The year was 1970 and the patient was considered a candidate for abdominal irradiation. Prior to her starting radiotherapy, she developed intestinal obstruction and, following a downhill course, she died 2.5 months from the time of the diagnosis. An autopsy revealed tumor extension through the entire peritoneal surfaces with metastatic disease to the liver and periaortic lymph nodes. At the present time, we would recommend systemic chemotherapy rather than local radiotherapy postoperatively for the treatment of these patients.

PROGNOSIS AND SURVIVAL

The prognosis has been grim and actually there are, for practical purposes, no survivors and this even includes patients with Stage I lesions. The mean survival time from diagnosis to death has been six to eight months.[1,3] Dehner *et al.*[2] maintained that mixed mesodermal tumors, as happens in the uterus, have a better prognosis than carcinosarcomas. The median survival for both groups was six months; however, when considered individually, the mixed mesodermals had a median survival of 12 months and carcinosarcomas of two months.[2]

REFERENCES

1. Czernobilsky, B., and LaBarre, G.C.: Carcinosarcoma and mixed mesodermal tumor of the ovary. A clinicopathologic analysis of 9 cases. *Obstet Gynecol* **31:**21, 1968.
2. Dehner, L.P., Norris, H.J., and Taylor, H.B.: Carcinosarcomas and mixed mesodermal tumors of the ovary. *Cancer* **27:**207, 1971.
3. Fenn, M.H., and Abell, M.R.: Carcinosarcoma of the ovary. *Am J Obstet Gynecol* **110:**1066, 1971.

72

Malignant Mixed Müllerian Tumors of the Fallopian Tube

TWENTY-ONE CASES of carcinosarcomas and malignant mixed Müllerian tumors of the fallopian tube have been described. The average patient's age was 58 years and the presenting symptoms included abdominal pain and cramps, distention, and vaginal bleeding. The neoplasms grow as polypoid masses into the lumen. They metastasize readily by direct extension into the pelvis and the other parts of the genital tract and distantly to the liver, lungs, and bones.[1,2]

Surgery alone or surgery combined with postoperative radiotherapy, have been used in their management. The prognosis is serious; however, long-term survivors living for two years or more with or without signs of disease have been reported. The course of the disease can be slow. Most of the patients who die from it do so within the first 15 months.[1] However, the neoplasm has shown a slow progress in some instances. Manes and Taylor[1] reported two patients who survived more than four years before dying from their tumor.

REFERENCES

1. Manes, J.L., and Taylor, H.B.: Carcinosarcoma and mixed Müllerian tumors of the fallopian tube. Report of four cases. *Cancer* **38**:1687, 1976.
2. Wu, J.P., Tanner, W.S., and Fardal, P.M.: Malignant mixed Müllerian tumor of the uterine tube. *Obstet Gynecol* **41**:707, 1973.

73

Endometrial Stromal Tumors

INFILTRATING TUMORS of the uterus, composed of cells that resemble endometrial stroma, are rare. Koss *et al.*[7] found 10 such lesions in reviewing the records at Memorial Hospital between the years of 1939 and 1959, constituting only 0.2% of all uterine cancers seen during the same period. In the more recent publications on the subject these tumors have been subclassified on the basis of histology and natural history. Endolymphatic stromal myosis or endometrial stomatosis represents an infiltrating stromal tumor that may locally recur and occasionally metastasize; however, in general it pursues an indolent course and afford an excellent survival. Endometrial stromal sarcoma, on the other hand, infiltrates more widely the myometrium and is characterized by a high rate of local recurrence and distant metastases leading in the majority of the cases to the patient's death. A noninfiltrating variant appearing grossly as a well-circumscribed nodular tumor, solitary in character with pushing margins and lacking myometrial or endometrial infiltration is to be separated from the described groups as representing the most benign manifestation of endometrial stromal tumor.[4,6,8,10]

Due to the fact that the cells comprising circumscribed stromatosis, infiltrative stromatosis, and endometrial stromal sarcomas are similar in appearance, the lesions were described as a single entity in earlier reports.[3,5,7] Norris and Taylor[8] pointed out that infiltrating endometrial stromal tumors could be separated on the basis of their mitotic activity. It was on this basis that the present classification evolved. Subsequent reports have established its validity.[4,6,8,10]

The usual age of patients with endometrial stromal tumors is in the range of 42–47 years.[3,5,8] In general patients with endometrial stromatosis are about 10 years younger than those developing endometrial stromal sarcomas. Thus, the average age for the former is 40 years at the time of the diagnosis and for the latter, 50 or 51.[4,6,10]

PATHOLOGY

The gross appearance of the stromal neoplasms is that of a light yellow to gray-white tumor that typically produces bulging both outward toward the myometrium and inward toward the endometrial cavity. They result in uterine enlargement that is associated with nodular or diffuse expansion of the organ. The polypoid masses protruding into the endometrial cavity can be quite sizable, at times protruding through the cervical os. Within the tumor, areas of hemorrhage and necrosis are frequent.[3,4,6,7,10]

Histologically, both endometrial stromatosis and endometrial stromal sarcomas show a remarkably uniform cell pattern. The cells contain basophilic nuclei and indistinct cytoplasm. They are relatively small and they resemble hyperplastic endometrial stromal cells. Generally, they are very cellular neoplasms.[4,6,10] Epithelial glandlike arrangements and glands resembling those of the endometrium are seen in approximately 25% of the cases.[8] With regard to nuclear atypism, the cells of endometrial stromal sarcoma had larger nuclei and coarser irregularly distributed chromatin compared to those of endometrial stromatosis.[10] Norris and Taylor[8] divided the infiltrative tumors into two groups according to their mitotic activity: 1) neoplasms containing fewer than 10 mitotic figures per 10 high-power fields (HPF) and 2) those containing 10 or more mitotic figures per 10 HPF. It was the authors' observation that the former group had an actuarial survival of 100%, at 10 years, excluding nontumor-related deaths, as opposed to 26% six year actuarial survival for the latter group. Similar conclusions were reached later by Kempson and Bari[6] as well as by Yoonessi and Hart.[10]

In endometrial stromatosis, myometrial wall infiltration is the rule. Extension into the cervix may be noted. Typically there is growth of tumor within dilated veins and lymph vessels and it is on this basis that the term "endolymphatic stromal myosis" has been applied. In general there are few mitotic figures (one to five per 10 HPF).[4,6] The supportive elements of both variants is quite vascular.

According to recent publications, the frequency of endometrial stromatosis is similar to that of endometrial stromal sarcoma.[4,6,8,10]

CLINICAL

The most frequent and practically universal symptom in all patients is abnormal vaginal bleeding. For those who are premenopausal, it presents as cyclic menorrhagia or as intermenstrual bleeding and as postmenopausal bleeding in the remainder. This is associated at times with discharge and occasionally with abdominal pain and cramping.[3,7] Three of 35 patients presenting with vaginal bleeding in

the series reported by Norris and Taylor[8] had anemia ascribed to blood loss. Pelvic pain was present in 20% of the patients. The median duration of the symptoms prior to the diagnosis is approximately three to four months.[3,8] Occasionally, the patients will report the spontaneous passage of pieces of tumor.[10]

On physical examination, the uterus is found to be enlarged, at times irregularly, at times symmetrically. Due to the rarity of the tumor, however, preoperative diagnosis is rarely made.[7]

In approximately 20% of the patients there is an impression of extension of the tumor beyond the uterus into the pelvis.[8]

TREATMENT AND RESULTS

Dilatation and curettage, the initial steps of investigation of any uterine bleeding, will establish the diagnosis in the majority of the cases; however, cases do exist in which the diagnosis was not actually established until a hysterectomy was performed.[5,7]

In earlier reports, at a time when supracervical hysterectomy was an accepted procedure, several patients were managed by this method. As is evident from the same reports, this procedure is not adequate for managing either endometrial stromatosis or endometrial stromal sarcomas. Hunter et al.[5] comment on the fact that local recurrences may appear in the cervical stump, the vaginal walls, or the urinary bladder, particularly after subtotal hysterectomy. In the series by Koss et al.[7] five of seven patients had local recurrence following partial hysterectomy as their primary treatment. In the series by Norris and Taylor[8] patients with stromal sarcoma did better when treated by total abdominal hysterectomy and bilateral salpingo-oophorectomy. Patients with endometrial stromatosis (endolymphatic stromal myosis) treated initially by supracervical hysterectomy more often than not developed local recurrence. It is their view that supracervical hysterectomy does not appear to be an adequate therapy.

At the present, appropriate treatment for both entities is total abdominal hysterectomy as a minimum. Due to the fact that endometrial stromatosis tends to extend intravascularly into the parametrium and the broad ligament as well as into the adnexae, bilateral salpingo-oophorectomy should also be performed. In those particular cases in which the endometrial stromatosis presents as a solitary lesion—the stromal nodules of Norris and Taylor—removal of the tumor alone will be adequate treatment.[4,8] Histologically, the well-circumscribed nodular tumors can be distinguished from endometrial stromatosis and from endometrial stromal sarcoma by the fact that their margins are pushing rather than infiltrating the surrounding tissue and they are solitary in character. No myometrial or lymphatic infiltration is to be found for this particular group of lesions.[8] Endometrial stromal sarcomas carry a very serious prognosis regardless of the method of therapy.

After abdominal hysterectomy and bilateral salpingo-oophorectomy, and because of the dismal therapeutic results, radiation therapy and systemic chemotherapy are recommended as a supplement to the surgical procedure.[10] All six patients in the series by Yoonessi and Hart[10] who underwent total abdominal hysterectomy and bilateral salpingo-oophorectomy died of their disease with local recurrence, which eventually metastasized distally. The local recurrences included the vagina, the urinary bladder, the pelvis, and the abdomen. Distant metastases involved the lungs, the liver, the mesentery, the adrenals, abdominal lymph nodes, and peritoneum. Deaths occurred after intervals of 1–27 months from the time of the initial surgery. Of 10 patients with stromal sarcoma in the series by Norris and Taylor,[8] seven died of their disease during the ensuing six years. Seven of 10 patients with endometrial

stromal sarcoma reported by Kempson et al.[6] and treated by definitive surgery died from their disease during the subsequent months. So did the remaining three patients who were treated primarily by radiation.

The natural history and biological aggressiveness of endometrial stromatosis—endolymphatic stromal myosis—are different from that of endometrial stromal sarcomas. In spite of the fact that extension beyond the uterus is frequently present and involvement of the lymph vessels and the regional veins of the pelvis can be well demonstrated in several cases, these lesions tend to recur primarily locally, have a very long course in terms of years, and in the event of distant metastases resection of the metastatic focus results in a lengthy survival. Therefore it is important that they be approached aggressively from the surgical point of view. Once the histopathological diagnosis—on the basis of the low mitotic figures per 10 HPF—has been made, surgical resection to the maximum extent possible is recommended, even if that means cutting through tumor. There is evidence in the literature to support the belief that such resection when combined with postoperative radiotherapy has resulted in long-term survivals.[7] Several patients have been reported whose disease runs a span of several years with episodes of recurrences in between. Hunter et al.[5] reported seven such patients and reviewed the literature on the subject. The patients return typically with pelvic recurrences and if distant metastases are to be found they usually involve the lungs.[5]

Radiation therapy has been considered to be an effective means in the management of patients with endometrial stromal tumors. Because mitotic figure counts are lacking in earlier reports, the exact nature of these neoplasms treated by radiotherapy cannot now be determined. Be this as it may, Belgrad et al.[2] and Vongtama et al.[9] make a case for postoperative radiotherapy by showing an improved survival of patients receiving combined treatment over those having surgery alone. Tumor regression and objective responses to radiotherapy when applied to recurrent disease have been reported by Koss et al.,[7] Hunter et al.,[5] Hart and Yoonessi,[4] and others.

Of the chemotherapeutic agents available at this time Adriamycin and bleomycin appear to be the most active against endometrial stromal sarcoma.[1]

PROGNOSIS AND SURVIVAL

In considering the prognosis and the survival of endometrial stromal tumors it is necessary to assess them histologically and assign them according to the criteria established by Norris and Taylor[8] into two distinct groups on the basis of the number of mitotic figures per 10 HPF. The degree of mitotic activity provides an accurate estimate of their future behavior. According to the same authors in their own series, patients with fewer than 10 mitotic figures per 10 HPF have an actuarial survival of 100% at 10 years, after exclusion of deaths that were nontumor related. It is to be mentioned, however, that 31% of them were living with tumor activity at the time of last contact. In contrast, a group of 15 patients having stromal tumors with 10 or more mitotic figures per 10 HPF had much worse prognosis. Their five-year actuarial survival was 55% and at last contact only 26% were free of disease.

In the series by Kempson and Bari[6] there was 100% mortality for nine patients with stromal sarcoma. Their mean survival was four months. In the same series all seven patients with endolymphatic stromal myosis were alive and well for a mean observation period of six years.

Reports in earlier publications indicating reasonably favorable prognosis of endometrial stromal sarcomas compared to other sarcomas of the uterus are influenced by the fact that in their material both endometrial stromal sarcomas and endometrial stromatosis have been included.[2,9] It is now accepted that the clinical course of patients with stromatosis is considerably more favorable. Even in the face of recurrent disease, prolonged survivals or even cures can still be achieved by aggressive management. In contrast to these results patients with endometrial stromal sarcomas die of local or metastatic disease within months from the time of the diagnosis.[4,10]

REFERENCES

1. Barlow, J.J., Piver, M.S., Chuang, J.T., Cortes, E.P., Ohnuma, T., and Holland, J.F.: Adriamycin and bleomycin alone and in combination, in gynecologic cancers. *Cancer* 32:735, 1973.
2. Belgrad, R., Elbadawi, N., and Rubin, P.: Uterine sarcoma. *Radiology* 114:181, 1975.
3. Jensen, P.A., Dockerty, M.B., Symmonds, R.E., and Wilson, R.B.: Endometrioid sarcoma ("stromal endometriosis"). Report of 15 cases including 5 with metastases. *Am J Obstet Gynecol* 95:79, 1966.
4. Hart, W.R., and Yoonessi, M.: Endometrial stromatosis of the uterus. *Obstet Gynecol* 49:393, 1977.
5. Hunter, W.C., Nohlgren, J.E., and Lancefield, S.M.: Stromal endometriosis or endometrial sarcoma. A re-evaluation of old and new cases with especial reference to duration, recurrences, and metastases. *Am J Obstet Gynecol* 72:1072, 1956.
6. Kempson, R.L., and Bari, W.: Uterine sarcomas. Classification, diagnosis and prognosis. *Hum Pathol* 1:331, 1970.
7. Koss, L.G., Spiro, R.H., and Brunschwig, A.: Endometrial stromal sarcoma. *Surg Gynecol Obstet* 121:531, 1965.
8. Norris, H.J., and Taylor, H.B.: Mesenchymal tumors of the uterus. I. A clinical and pathological study of 53 endometrial stromal tumors. *Cancer* 19:755, 1966.
9. Vongtama, V., Karlen, J.R., Piver, S.M., Tsukada, Y., and Moore, R.H.: Treatment, results and prognostic factors in Stage I and II sarcomas of the corpus uteri. *AJR* 126:139, 1976.
10. Yoonessi, M., and Hart, W.R.: Endometrial stromal sarcomas. *Cancer* 40:898, 1977.

74

Angiosarcoma of the Skin and of the Head and Neck

CUTANEOUS ANGIOSARCOMAS tend to occur in older individuals but they may develop in the young. Although benign vascular tumors are rather common entities in the head and neck region, angiosarcomas are rare. Most of them are cutaneous in origin and infrequently described in other sites, such as the oral cavity and the upper respiratory passages.[3]

The age of patients with cutaneous angiosarcomas in the head and neck reported by Bardwil et al.[1] ranged from 45 to 72 years. Rosai et al.[5] in a clinical and fine structural study of 10 patients with cutaneous angiosarcoma encountered a median age of 66.1 years. Farr et al.[2] reported on 10 angiosarcomas of the head and neck region. Four of the patients were below the age of 30 years, four older than 60, and the remaining two were in their fourth and fifth decades. The youngest patient was 12 years and the oldest 74 years old. Girard et al.[4] in a series of 28 cases found the youngest patient to be 1 year old and the eldest 88. The authors state that hemangiosarcomas in children and young adults are usually of low-grade, having a slow progression, accelerating their growth after several years of stability. Males and females are affected equally.[4]

present.[2] The two cardinal histological features, according to Stout[6] are: the formation of atypical endothelial cells in numbers greater than those required for the lining of the vessels and the formation of vascular tubes with anastomosing lumens built within a framework of reticulin fibers. From this basic pattern variations are encountered according to the individual characteristics of the malignant endothelial cells. Silver reticulin stain readily outlines the tubular structures and thus defines the exact position of the abnormal proliferating endothelium.[6] A characteristic feature of this tumor which greatly affects treatment and prognosis is an apparent diffuse or even multicentric extension. This extension is far beyond the clinical boundaries of the lesion.[2] Rosai et al.[5] in their excellent histological description observed that vessels, at a distance from the tumor, appear normal when examined under low magnification, However, when seen under high power, they show a papillary arrangement of proliferating endothelium. This represents the earliest recognizable process of neoplastic transformation of the vascular endothelium. Commonly seen are normal capillaries intermingling with neoplastic ones.[5]

PATHOLOGY

During surgical removal and in the submitted specimen, no visible capsule is

CLINICAL

There is a definite preference for cutaneous hemangiosarcomas to develop in the skin of the head and the neck, especially in the scalp. Fourteen of the 28 patients (50%) reported by Girard et al.[4] had tumors originating in the head and the remainder in the trunk and extremities. All of the 10 lesions reported by Rosai et al.[5] were located in the head and actually all but one in the scalp. Other areas reported have been the lips, oral cavity, maxillary sinus, nasal cavity, orbit, and thyroid.[2,3,5,6]

The lesions have a subtle, inconspicuous beginning, being painless and flat. As they grow, they become papular or nodular and they have a red or purple color that bespeaks their origin. They are soft in consistency and commonly multiple. Satellite nodules were seen in 57% of all patients.[4] Their continuous growth leads to bleeding, either spontaneously or after a slight injury. Intratumoral small hemorrhages may take place.[5] Bardwil et al.[1] found the interval between the onset of symptoms and the diagnosis to range from 2 to 10 months. Four of seven cases reported by the authors had cervical lymph node metastases. Farr et al.[2] found lymph node involvement to occur in 30% of the patients during the course of the disease. Second in frequency as a metastatic site are the lungs.

In practically all cases in which metastatic disease develops, there has been previous local recurrence. The recurrences occur at the margins of previous resection or beyond the edges of previously irradiated regions because of the deceptive clinical appearance. As mentioned, the margins of the tumor do not correspond to the margins of the visible skin changes. Neoplastic endothelial changes continue for long distances into seemingly normal skin.

Seven of 28 patients reviewed by Girard et al.[4] developed recurrent ulcerating, fungating disease (25%). Rosai et al.[5] encountered five local recurrences among their 10 patients (50%). Of the seven patients reported by Bardwill et al.[1] local recurrence occurred in five and the remaining two had persistent local disease throughout their course.

Six of 10 patients reported by Farr et al.[2] developed local recurrence.

TREATMENT AND RESULTS

Surgical resection or excision has been the commonest form of therapy. This is the most appropriate approach, provided that the resection is adequate to encompass the involved area. All of 6 patients described by Stout,[6] 9 of 10 patients reported by Rosai et al.[5] five of seven primary cases seen by Farr et al.[2] six of seven patients reported by Bardwil et al.,[1] and 20 of 28 cases reviewed by Girard et al.[4] had surgery as their first modality of therapy. Unfortunately, the majority of the patients required further treatment because of locally recurrent or metastatic disease. Further therapy was in the form of additional surgery, radiotherapy, or chemotherapy.[1,2,4–6]

Local control is probable at relatively high-dose level of radiation; therefore 6000–7000 rad in six to seven weeks should be delivered and a wide margin should be kept. Rosai et al.[5] reported on three patients whose local recurrences were controlled by radiotherapy, one of them subsequently having a recurrence outside the irradiated field. Farr et al.[2] found the tumor to be responsive to radiation even at lower levels, with marginal recurrences being the cause of failure. Chemotherapeutic agents used for the management of angiosarcomas include vinblastine, vincristine, cyclophosphamide, actinomycin D, chlorambucil, and intraarterial infusion of methotrexate. With the exception of the methotrexate infusion, which produced a moderate short-lived tumor response, no appreciable change was brought about by the rest.[2] Currently, clinical chemotherapeutic trials are carried out under the auspices of Eastern Cooperative Oncology Group.

The possibility of regional lymph node involvement should be taken into consideration during the treatment planning.

We have participated in the palliative management of three patients with metastatic cutaneous angiosarcoma and in the definitive management of two patients both of which will be described briefly. The first is a 66-year-old female presenting with tumor in the right nasal vestibule whose chief complaint was one week of epistaxis. Upon inspection a sessile lesion was found in the apex of the right nostril. Following biopsy, radiographs of the region showed no osseous involvement. The proposed treatment was surgical resection, which she declined; therefore she was irradiated by means of a 6 MeV linear accelerator, receiving 6000 rad in 43 elapsed days. The treatment was delivered through a pair of oblique-wedged fields superiorly and inferiorly placed. The patient has survived for five years without signs of disease. The second patient is a 59-year-old female presenting with a cutaneous angiosarcoma of the scalp located in the right posterior parietal and occipital region. Bleeding to touch was the presenting symptom. The involved area was locally excised initially. The tumor recurred four months later, at which point a wide excision and skin graft was performed. However, at the same time a clinically suspicious posterior auricular lymph node was removed and proved to be involved with metastasis. Within two months, more nodes appeared in the right posterior cervical chain. The patient was treated by means of a 6 MeV linear accelerator, receiving 4000 rad in four weeks to the involved nodes. Following this a radium needle implant delivering 4000 rad

was performed because of clinically persistent disease. Two months from the completion of the course, recurrent disease reappeared in the scalp and simultaneously lung metastases developed. These were diffuse and eventually caused hemoptysis. The patient died one year after the diagnosis.

PROGNOSIS AND SURVIVAL

The best prognosis goes to small tumors diagnosed early and adequately resected.[2] Although local recurrence is a poor prognostic sign and it has signaled the beginning of dissemination in most patients, it should be treated vigorously because some patients have survived following successful treatment of these recurrences.

Compiling the data from the major publications on the subject we have found the five-year-survival rate to be approximately 40%.[1-3,5]

REFERENCES

1. Bardwil, J.M., Mocega, E.E., Butler, J.J., and Russin, D.J.: Angiosarcomas of the head and neck region. *Am J Surg* **116:**548, 1968.
2. Farr, H.W., Carandang, C.M., and Huvos, A.G.: Malignant vascular tumors of the head and neck. *Am J Surg* **120:**501, 1970.
3. Fu, Y.S., and Perzin, K.H.: Non-epithelial tumors of the nasal cavity, paranasal sinuses, and nasopharynx: A clinicopathologic study. I. General features and vascular tumors. *Cancer* **33:**1275, 1974.
4. Girard, C., Johnson, W.C., and Graham, J.H.: Cutaneous angiosarcoma. *Cancer* **26:**868, 1970.
5. Rosai, N.P., Sumner, H.W., Kostianovsky, M., and Perez-Mesa, C.: Angiosarcoma of the skin. A clinicopathologic and fine structural study. *Hum Pathol* **7:**83, 1976.
6. Stout, A.P.: Hemangio-endothelioma: A tumor of blood vessels featuring vascular endothelial cells. *Ann Surg* **118:**445, 1943.

75

Angiosarcoma of the Bone (Hemangioendothelioma)

MOST AUTHORS HAVE used the terms "hemangioendothelioma" and "angiosarcoma" when referring to bone tumors as being synonymous. This represents the basic vascular tumor described by Stout[7] in 1943 as hemangioendothelioma, whose primary cell originates from the endothelium of the vessels. Jaffe[4] considers all malignant vasoforming tumors of the bone as sarcomas and therefore has used the terms "angiosarcoma" and "hemangioendothelioma" as synonyms.

They are uncommon tumors; Unni *et al.*[9] in a review that included 4000 bone neoplasms from the Mayo Clinic found nine cases of hemangioendotheliomas among them. This represents an incidence of 0.2%.

They may occur at all ages, from the early months of infancy to persons in the seventh or eighth decades of life. The average age, however, is 30–35 years. The incidence is higher among males. Chow *et al.*[1] in their literature review found a male to female ratio of 3:1, with two-thirds of the patients being under the age of 50.

PATHOLOGY

Grossly, the lesions are soft and spongy in consistency and hemorrhagic bright red in color. They have irregular borders whose tendency is to erode the bone cortex locally and to extend and invade adja-cent soft tissues. Within the bone itself, the tumor extension is well beyond the area of destruction seen radiographically.[6,9]

Histologically, the basic criterion is the presence of neoplastic blood vessels lined by atypical endothelial cells and the production of anastomotic channels.[9] The individual cells are frequently large with large centrally placed nuclei and prominent nucleoli. Mitotic figures are not common and even in high-grade tumors, areas can be found where large blood-filled spaces are lined with atypical epithelium. The vascular channels are readily revealed by means of reticulin stains.[6] Reactive bone formation in the vicinity of the tumor is uniformly absent.[9]

CLINICAL

There is no definite site predilection. The skull, vertebral bodies, rib cage, clavicle, sternum, scapula, pelvis, and the extremities have all served as primary sites. The small bones of the hand and feet account for 20% of all tumor sites.[1,3,6,9] Another characteristic of osseous angiosarcomas is their multifocal presentation. In approximately 40% of the patients multiple adjacent bones were found to be involved at the time of the diagnosis.[3,6,9]

Pain in the region of the tumor is the commonest initial symptom and as the growth progresses this is followed by the presence of a local mass. The interval between the onset of symptoms and the time of the diagnosis has varied from 1 to 12 months, the average waiting period being five months.[6] On physical examination, if the mass can be palpated, it is soft in consistency.[1] Involvement of the vertebrae leads eventually to compression fractures.[5,8] Radiographically, these are purely lytic lesions without evidence of new bone formation. The undifferentiated ones have indistinct and irregular margins, whereas those of lower grade retain some trabeculae within the lytic process and they are better defined.[9]

TREATMENT AND RESULTS

Surgery, if feasible, is the therapy of choice. In contemplating manipulation of the tumor, awareness of its extreme vascularity is necessary, since there is a distinct possibility of severe hemorrhage.[1] There is evidence to support the fact that local excision alone is less successful than en bloc resection, particularly as far as the poorly differentiated tumors are concerned.[9] Otis et al.[6] found that each of the patients in their series who was alive and free of disease had been treated aggressively by means of amputation. This included the joint above the involved bone in four patients and a wide excision of a rib in a fifth. Before such a procedure, there is a need for metastatic work-up that should include a bone survey to rule out metastatic disease.

Tumors in areas not amenable to radical surgery are best treated by a combination of modalities, namely, surgery and radiation therapy. Radiation is effective when used at tumoricidal levels. Chow et al.[1] reported on a 21-year-old male whose skull angiosarcoma following biopsy was irradiated by means of a cobalt-60 modality, receiving 6000 rad in 34 treatments over a six week period. Six months later the area was resected to find only fibrosis

in the submitted specimen. Morgenstern and Westing[5] treated by radiotherapy a 40-year-old male with multifocal angiosarcoma involving the proximal and distal ends of the left clavicle as well as the acromion and the spine of the left scapula. The patient was irradiated by means of an orthovoltage modality, receiving approximately 5000 rad tumor dose over a four week period. The local pain and discomfort disappeared promptly and within one year the pronounced rarefied lesion was filling in with dense bone. The authors report a 14-year follow-up on the patient, during which time no local or distant recurrences developed. Glenn et al.[2] irradiated a multifocal malignant hemangioendothelioma of the first and second lumbar vertebrae. The patient, a 41-year-old man was treated by a cobalt-60 modality, receiving 3900 rad in three weeks to the involved region. During the following 24 months, he was virtually asymptomatic and radiographically a continuous improvement with recalcification was noted.

PROGNOSIS AND SURVIVAL

The most significant prognostic factor appears to be the degree of differentiation. Unni et al.[9] classified their material into low-grade tumors when there was abundant vasoformation, few mitotic figures present, and little atypia of the cells and their nuclei. High-grade tumors were those with less vasoformation, more mitotic figures, and more atypia. In what the authors considered Grade I, 13 patients were entered. Of these, nine were alive for periods ranging from 3 months to 12 years, two were dead of their disease, and two died of other causes. In Grade II four patients were entered, two dying of their disease and two surviving for 6 and 75 months. Those with the poorest histological features were allocated in Grade III. Included were five patients, all of whom died of their disease at intervals ranging from one month to two years, from the time of the diagnosis.

Multifocal disease need not necessarily have a poor prognosis. Actually, Otis *et al.*[9] are of the opinion that the outlook for these patients is better than the rest. Multifocal disease is not a metastatic situation and the authors urge that a vigorous and definitive treatment be applied. The degree of differentiation is the prognostically significant factor when multifocal disease is present.[9]

We have tabulated the results from four major publications on the subject. It appears that the two-year survival is 75%, and the survival at five years is 40%, approximately.[1,3,6,9]

REFERENCES

1. Chow, R.W., Wilson, C.B., and Olsen, E.R.: Angiosarcoma of the skull. Report of a case and review of the literature. *Cancer* **25**:902, 1970.

2. Glenn, J.N., Reckling, F.W., and Mantz, F.A.: Malignant hemangioendothelioma in a lumbar vertebra. A rare tumor in an unusual location. *J Bone Joint Surg* **56A**:1279, 1974.

3. Hartmann, W.H., and Stewart, F.W.: Hemangioendothelioma of bone. Unusual tumor characterized by indolent course. *Cancer* **15**:846, 1962.

4. Jaffe, H.L.: *Tumors and Tumorous Conditions of the Bones and Joints.* Lea & Febiger, Philadelphia, 1958.

5. Morgenstern, P., and Westing, S.W.: Malignant hemangioendothelioma of bone. Fourteen-year follow-up in a case treated with radiation alone. *Cancer* **23**:221, 1969.

6. Otis, J., Hutter, R.V.P., Foote, F.W., Jr., Marcove, R.C., and Stewart, F.W.: Hemangioendothelioma of bone. *Surg Gynecol Obstet* **127**:295, 1968.

7. Stout, A.P.: Hemangio-endothelioma: A tumor of blood vessels featuring vascular endothelial cells. *Ann Surg* **118**:445, 1943.

8. Sweterlitsch, P.R., Torg, J.S., and Watts, H.: Malignant hemangioendothelioma of the cervical spine. *J Bone Joint Surg* **52A**:805, 1970.

9. Unni, K.K., Ivins, J.C., Beabout, J.W., and Dahlin, D.C.: Hemangioma, hemangiopericytoma, and hemangioendothelioma (angiosarcoma of bone). *Cancer* **27**:1403, 1971.

76

Angiosarcoma of the Liver

SPONTANEOUS ANGIOSARCOMAS of the liver comprise 1% of all primary hepatic tumors. Better known and more numerous are those hepatic angiosarcomas that have resulted from a toxic pharmacological or industrial exposure.

Spontaneous hepatic angiosarcomas may occur in children—infantile form—or in adults. A high arteriovenous shunt is created in angiosarcomas of childhood, resulting in high-output failure. A failure to thrive and compression of the lungs and the gastrointestinal tract by the continuously enlarging liver are the usual causes of death. Spontaneous regression has been described in children and there are a few survivors following surgical resection.[1,6,11]

In adults the tumor has a progressive fatal course.

PATHOLOGY

The liver is grossly enlarged and most tumors measure in excess of 10 cm. They are composed of solid masses, among which cystic cavernous spaces containing blood are interspersed. Multiple tumor nodules, forming a congregation of masses, may be seen.[1,7]

Histologically, in the well-differentiated angiosarcomas, the vasoforming elements are promptly identified. In the more anaplastic tumors areas of spindle cell proliferation are seen, with numerous mitoses and giant cells present. An angiomatous pattern is seen and this can become more obvious with the use of the reticulin stain.[9]

Thomas et al.[10] distinguished three basic histological patterns in vinyl chloride-induced hepatic angiosarcomas. The sinusoidal pattern is characterized by dilated sinusoids lined by sarcomatous cells. The papillary pattern composed of larger vascular spaces has cords of sarcomatous cells projecting into them and the cavernous pattern, whose vascular spaces are even larger and filled by blood[10] (Fig. 76-1).

CLINICAL

The disease presents with epigastric or upper quadrant pain, which is accompanied by anorexia malaise and weight loss.[1,6] Jaundice ensues and an enlarged tender liver is found on palpation. Splenic enlargement occurs in 50% of the cases, mostly because of thrombosis of the portal vein, but tumor extension into the spleen has been seen. Hemorrhagic ascites is often present and hemoperitoneum from tumor rupture has been reported.[1]

The serum alkaline phosphatase, serum glutamic-oxaloacetic transaminase, and lactic dehydrogenase are elevated. Liver scans show filling defects. Arteriography demonstrates very large vascular tumors where great amount of contrast medium persists within large vascular pools. The opacification is more intense in the periphery than in the center.[5,12]

As the growth continues, the tumor lo-

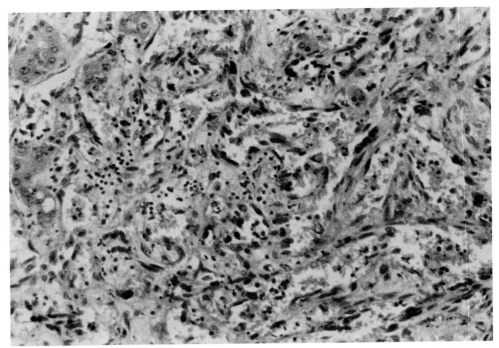

FIG. 76-1.   Angiosarcoma of liver. Sinusoidal pattern of blood vessels lined by bizarre endothelial cells infiltrating liver tissue, which can be seen in the left upper corner of the field.

cally extends to infiltrate the neighboring diaphragm, the abdominal wall, and the right kidney.[7] Metastatic spread takes place and it includes several organs. Deposits to the lungs, heart, bowel, skin, bones, and the lymph nodes have been reported.[6,7]

Thorium, in the purified form of thorium dioxide, was used as a radiographic contrast medium from 1930 through the 1950s. Under the trade name Thorotrast, it was the medium used for cerebral arteriography and in the colloidal form for the visualization of the spleen and liver, where the substance remained indefinitely due to phagocytosis. Thorium is a radioactive element emitting primarily alpha particles and has a half life of 400 years. An estimated 50,000 to 100,000 persons are at risk due to such radiographic exposures.[2] A total of 123 cases of liver sarcomas, including angiosarcomas, have been reported, for which thorium was considered the etiological factor.[5] The

interval between exposure and the appearance of the hepatic tumors has been, on the average, 20 years.

The latest group to develop hepatic angiosarcomas are industrial workers, who during the course of several years (10–20) have been exposed to gaseous vinyl chloride. Vinyl chloride, by polymerization, produces polyvinyl chloride, a commonly used plastic material.

Indeed, animal experiments have confirmed the genesis of hepatic angiosarcomas following exposure to vinyl chloride gas.[8] Creech and Johnson[4] reported the first clinical case and shortly thereafter Block[3] published on six similar patients. They were all male workers in their fourth and fifth decades of life who died of hepatic angiosarcomas following long-term exposure to vinyl chloride. Makk et al.[7] reported on 15 such patients. Their average age was 47.5 years and their exposure time averaged 17 years.

These findings led to a systematic

screening program of all those with a history of such exposure. Unfortunately, diagnosis at a preclinical level has not prevented the fatal outcome.[12]

PROGNOSIS AND SURVIVAL

The disease has had practically always a bad outcome. Theoretically, small lesions could be resected in their entirety, in reality, however, the growth is extensive and complete removal has been impossible. The average survival time, no matter what the etiological factor has been, was found to be seven months.[1,3,7]

Chemotherapy and radiotherapy have been used in an effort to decelerate the process. It is possible that life can be extended in this manner for three or four additional months.[7]

REFERENCES

1. Adam, Y.G., Huvos, A.G., and Hajdu, S.I.: Malignant vascular tumors of the liver. *Ann Surg* **175**:375, 1972.
2. Battifora, H.A.: Thorotrast and tumors of the liver. In *Hepatocellular Carcinoma*, Okuda, K., and Peters, R.L., Eds. John Wiley & Sons, New York, 1976.
3. Block, J.B.: Angiosarcoma of the liver following vinyl chloride exposure. *JAMA* **229**:53, 1974.
4. Creech, J.L., and Johnson, N.M.: Angiosarcoma of liver in the manufacture of polyvinyl chloride. *J Occup Med* **16**:150, 1974.
5. Curry, J.L., Johnson, W.G., Feinberg, D.H., and Updegrove, J.H.: Thorium induced hepatic hemangioendothelioma. *AJR* **125**:671, 1975.
6. Edmonson, H.A.: Differential diagnosis of tumors and tumor-like lesions of liver in infancy and childhood. *Am J Dis Child* **91**:168, 1956.
7. Makk, L., Delmore, F., Creech, J.L., Jr., Ogden, L.L., II, Fadell, E.H., Songster, C.L., Clanton, J., Johnson, M.N., and Christopherson, W.M.: Clinical and morphologic features of hepatic angiosarcoma in vinyl chloride workers. *Cancer* **37**:149, 1976.
8. Maltoni, C., and Lefemine, G.: Le potenzialita dei saggi sperimentali nella predizione dei rischi oncogeni ambientali: Un esempio: il clorruro di vinile. *Accad Nazion Linnei* **56**:1, 1974.
9. Stout, A.P.: Hemangio-endothelioma: A tumor of blood vessels featuring vascular endothelial cells. *Ann Surg* **118**:445, 1943.
10. Thomas, L.B., Popper, H., Berk, P.D., Selikoff, I., and Falk, H.: Vinyl-chloride-induced liver disease. From idiopathic portal hypertension (Banti's syndrome) to angiosarcomas. *N Engl J Med* **292**:17, 1975.
11. Videback, A.: Hemangioendothelioma of the liver. *Acta Paediat* **33**:129, 1946.
12. Whelan, J.C., Jr., Creech, J.L., and Tamburro, C.H.: Angiographic and radionuclide characteristics of hepatic angiosarcoma found in vinyl chloride workers. *Radiology* **118**:549, 1976.

77

Angiosarcoma of the Spleen

FEW CASES OF this very rare tumor have been reported. Angiosarcomas in the spleen are not related to toxic substances; they are spontaneous tumors.

Clinically, they present with splenomegaly associated with anemia, thrombocytopenia, reticulocytosis, and leukemoid reactions.[1-3] On physical examination, the patients appear chronically ill because of the anemia. They have pain in the left upper quadrant and the enlarged spleen is tender on palpation.

The disease has a rapid course with early metastases to the liver, the lymph nodes, and the bones. Another clinical development is splenic rupture. Stutz et al.[1] and Toghill et al.[2] have reported one case each of splenic rupture leading to death.

REFERENCES

1. Stutz, F.H., Tormey, D.C., and Blom, J.: Hemangiosarcoma and pathologic rupture of the spleen. *Cancer* **31**:1213, 1973.
2. Toghill, P.J., Rigby, C.C., and Hall, G.F.M.: Haemangiosarcoma of the spleen. *Br J Surg* **59**:406, 1972.
3. Wilkinson, H.A., III, Lucas, J.C., and Foote, F.W.: Primary splenic angiosarcoma. A case report. *Arch Pathol* **85**:213, 1968.

78

Angiosarcoma of the Heart

ANGIOSARCOMA, TOGETHER with rhab-domyosarcoma, represents the most common malignant cardiac tumor. Typically, it arises in the right atrium, where approximately 80% of all cardiac angiosarcomas are to be found. The rest arise in the pericardium (10%) and in the other chambers.

The average age of the patients at the time of the diagnosis has been 41 years. There is a male predominance, for 68% of the cases hitherto reported occurred in males and 32% in females.

A total of 58 cases have been published.[4,7,8]

PATHOLOGY

The most common finding is that of an intracavitary tumor that arises from the right atrium. It projects into the lumen producing obstruction. The presence of the tumor mechanically interferes with the blood flow into and from the right atrium, blocking the orifices of one or both the venae cavae or of the tricuspid valve. If the tumor is large enough, all these sites can be involved. Commonly, there is an outward extension and involvement of the epicardium. This eventually leads to the formation of hemopericardium, which is present in more than 50% of the cases.[3]

Histologically, the tumors are similar to hemangioendotheliomas in other locations.[2,8]

CLINICAL

There has been a remarkable uniformity in the clinical signs and symptoms. Chest pain, pericardial in origin, associated with temperatures higher than 100°F, cough, dyspnea, and weakness are the prominent clinical features. The composite of this symptomatology suggests viral pericarditis and this is a common initial diagnosis. Hemoptysis may occur and pleural effusions frequently develop. At this point, the clinical diagnosis of active pulmonary tuberculosis is often suggested.[8] Later, superior vena cava syndrome or inferior vena cava obstruction occurs in approximately 40% of the cases. Edema of the face and the upper extremities or hepatomegaly with peripheral edema are to be found clinically.[3]

Electrocardiographic changes are compatible primarily with pericarditis and are seen in most patients. Additional other nonspecific changes are frequently present.

Radiographically, there is cardiomegaly with prominence of the right cardiac border.

The disease follows a rapid downhill course, the average survival being six months.[4] During this short interval, however, metastases do develop, being encountered in 65% of the cases. Most commonly involved are the lungs (Fig. 78-1). Metastases also have been reported in the liver, the lymph nodes, and the bones.[4]

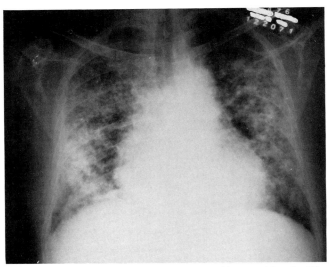

FIG. 78-1. Angiosarcoma of the heart in a 61-year-old male. The patient has angiosarcoma of the right atrium. At this time, chest x-ray demonstrates generalized cardiac enlargement and bilateral pulmonary metastases.

The usual cause of death is cardiac failure. This is due to mechanical obstruction of the blood flow into the right cardiac chambers. Hemopericardium, which eventually develops, adds to the difficulty of the cardiac flow.

TREATMENT AND RESULTS

In the majority of the reported cases the diagnosis was only of academic interest, often the extent and the exact nature of the disease being delineated during autopsy. In the recent years, however, with the advent of improved diagnostic and surgical techniques, a number of cases have been diagnosed early enough to allow application of therapeutic procedures. Hager et al.[5] resected a large left atrial tumor successfully. The patient was free of symptoms three years following the procedure. Hollingsworth and Sturgill[6] applied external beam radiotherapy following biopsy of a pericardial angiosarcoma. The patient received 5400 rad in 27 fractions and this therapy was followed by maintenance chemotherapy with cyclophosphamide and vincristine. At the time of the report, 10 months later, she remained symptom-free. Allaire et al.[1] demonstrated partial response of a cardiac angiosarcoma to combination therapy using radiation and cyclophosphamide. Rossi et al.[8] presented a case in which the exophytic tumor from the right atrium was completely resected. The patient had no further cardiac symptoms; however, he died of widespread metastases 4.5 months later. At the time of the autopsy no recurrent cardiac neoplasia was found.[8]

Surgery in combination with radiotherapy and chemotherapy have been effective, to a certain extent, in the management of angiosarcomas in other locations. As the limited experiences with cardiac angiosarcomas indicate, these modalities may be beneficial in cardiac angiosarcomas and they should be considered.

PROGNOSIS AND SURVIVAL

With few exceptions, the survival from the onset of the symptoms until death has been less than one year. Inability to control the disease locally and a high rate of distant metastases combined with the difficulties of an early diagnosis have been the major obstacles in containing the tumor.

REFERENCES

1. Allaire, F.J., Grimm, C.A., Taylor, L.M., and Pfaff, J.P.: Primary hemangioendothelioma of the heart. *Rocky Mt Med J* **61:**34, 1964.
2. Freeland, J.P., Sy, B.G., Ahluwalia, M.S., and Dunea, G.: Hemangiosarcoma of the heart. *Chest* **60:**222, 1971.
3. Glancy, D.L., Morales, J.B., and Roberts, W.C.: Angiosarcoma of the heart. *Am J Cardiol* **21:**413, 1968.
4. Gröntoff, O., and Hellquist, H.: Cardiac haemangio-endotheliosarcoma. *Acta Pathol Microbiol Scand [A]* **85:**33, 1977.
5. Hager, W., Kremer, K., and Miller, W.: Angiosarkom des Herzens. *Dtsch Med Wochr* **95:**680, 1970.
6. Hollingsworth, J.H., and Sturgill, B.C.: Treatment of primary angiosarcoma of the heart. *Am Heart J* **78:**254, 1969.
7. Robinson, D.S., and Machanic, P.B.: Hemangioendothelioma of the heart. *JAMA* **189:**1026, 1964.
8. Rossi, N.P., Koschos, J.M., Achenbrener, C.A., and Ehrenhaft, J.L.: Primary angiosarcoma of the heart. *Cancer* **37:**891, 1976.

79

Angiosarcoma of the Breast

THIS IS A rare neoplasm of which 48 cases had been recorded in the literature up to 1976.[1] The patients are females, commonly in their second or third decade of life.[1,2]

PATHOLOGY

The tumor size at the time of the diagnosis is 4.0–5.0 cm.[3] They arise in the breast parenchyma, having an ill-defined, spongy consistency due to the presence of dilated vascular compartments containing blood.[3] Histologically, intercommunicating irregular vascular channels are seen that are lined by endothelial cells exhibiting hyperchromic nuclei and great variations in terms of their appearance within different parts of the same tumor. The lining cells in certain areas proliferate into the lumen, producing papillary projections.[3] The growth actually extends in a fingerlike fashion into the breast parenchyma and involves areas far beyond those felt on clinical examination.[2]

CLINICAL

The common presentation is that of a mass in the breast that enlarges rather rapidly. In most patients it has been painless; however, painful tumors have also been reported.[2] Because of rapid enlargement, the duration prior to the diagnosis has been relatively short, in most patients only a few months. Metastases to the regional lymph nodes are rare. On the contrary, blood-borne metastases are common occurrences. They may be found in several organs and particularly in the skin, the bones, the lungs, the liver, the ovaries, and the gastrointestinal tract. Growing metastatic deposits to the liver and the gastrointestinal tract might cause hemorrhage and even death.[3]

TREATMENT AND RESULTS

In most patients, mastectomy has been performed. Steingaszner et al.[3] reviewed 10 cases of hemangiosarcoma of the breast from the files of the Armed Forces Institute of Pathology. Among the patients there were two long-term survivors, one for 14 years following radical mastectomy and another for seven years following local excision. There was a third patient alive and well 33 months after the original excision, which was followed by simple mastectomy for local recurrence. Dunegan et al.[1] had a four-year survivor without clinical evidence of disease in a patient who underwent radical mastectomy and a two-year disease-free survivor following simple mastectomy.

These results, however, are exceptional. The tumor has a poor prognosis and on the basis of the reported cases we found the two-year survival to be 37%. At five years only 5% of the patients were surviving.

REFERENCES

1. Dunegan, L.J., Tobon, H., and Watson, C.G.: Angiosarcoma of the breast: A report of two cases and a review of the literature. *Surgery* **79:**57, 1976.

2. Gulesserian, H.P., and Lawton, R.L.: Angiosarcoma of the breast. *Cancer* **24:**1021, 1969.

3. Steingaszner, L.C., Enzinger, F.M., and Taylor, H.B.: Hemangiosarcoma of the breast. *Cancer* **18:**352, 1965.

80

Hemangiopericytoma

STOUT AND MURRAY[14] in 1942 identified hemangiopericytoma as a separate entity among the group of vascular tumors. The cell of origin is the pericyte, originally described by Zimmerman, which normally is present around the capillary walls. The pericytes have contractile power and although they lack myofibrils it is assumed that they are related to the smooth muscle cells. Their function is to regulate the capillary lumen.[15,16]

On the basis of the reported series, it can be stated that the tumor may occur in any age group with slight preferential peak during the fourth and fifth decades.[1,3,10] It has been described at birth as the congenital form, in the early years of life as the infantile form, and in the very old.[8,15] Enzinger and Smith[3] are of the opinion that the congenital and infantile forms should be dealt with separately because of their uniformly benign course.

Both sexes are equally affected. This is well shown in a comprehensive literature review by Backwinkel and Diddams[1] who found the tumor occurring in 125 female and in 112 male patients.

PATHOLOGY

The tumors are well circumscribed in most instances and actually often they are well encapsulated. This is a gross appearance and does not necessarily imply benignity. Some may be firmly attached to the underlying structures and some are connected with a mesh of large vessels, being therefore prone to induce severe hemorrhage during their removal.[3] In general there is no skin redness or discoloration to be seen by which the vascular origin of the tumor could be suspected. This is because the proliferating pericytes compress upon the vascular spaces and obliterate their lumen.[2,15]

The size varies, but because the tumor growth is painless large masses are commonly encountered. Fisher,[5] reporting on 20 cases, encountered sizes ranging from 3.0 to 15.0 cm.

Histologically, this is a neoplasm of vascular origin that characteristically has vascular spaces surrounded by closely packed neoplastic pericytes (Fig. 80-1). These cells are spindle-shaped or oval-shaped, have no orientation, and their cytoplasm is ill-defined. The vessels are lined by thin endothelium and they are compressed by the neoplastic aggregates of pericytes. The size of the vessels varies from capillaries to large sinusoids.[15,16] Following his original description, Stout[16] wrote that no definite histological criteria could be found by which the metastasizing malignant form could be differentiated from the non-metastasizing benign variant. Enzinger and Smith,[3] analyzing 106 hemangiopericytomas from the files of the Armed Forces Institute of Pathology, found the following morphological features to be indicative of the malignant rather than the benign form: increased cellularity, prominent mitotic activity, and foci of necrosis or hemorrhage.

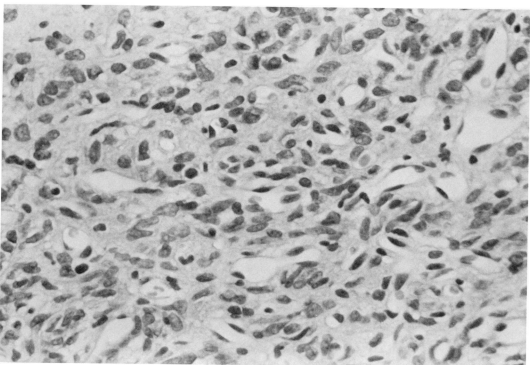

FIG. 80-1.   Hemangiopericytoma. Spindle-shaped cells arranged around vascular spaces lined by single layer of endothelium.

CLINICAL

Hemangiopericytomas arise from capillary vessels; therefore potentially they can be found anywhere in the body. In their review Backwinkel and Diddams[1] tabulated the following incidence by location: skin, muscles, and bones, 46.5%; intraabdominal, 17%; lungs and mediastinum, 9.5%; central nervous system, 6%; head and neck, 9.5%. The rest (11.5%) were unspecified in terms of origin and one arose in the thyroid gland. Stout[16] subdivided the tumors into those involving external tissues and those arising in internal organs and found the incidence of the two groups to be equal. Among the external sites, the lower extremities are affected the commonest. They are followed by the upper extremities and the external surfaces of the head and neck and the trunk.

Of the internal organs, the retroperitoneum leads, followed in incidence by the uterus, oral cavity and pharynx, the mediastinum, and the gastrointestinal tract.[16]

In the extremities and generally in the external tissues the clinical presentation is that of a painless growing mass. Pain occurs late and is produced only when nerve compression takes place. Hemangiopericytomas of the internal organs similarly create pressure phenomena and symptomatology, which depend on the site of origin. There is a great variation in the rate of tumor growth, but in most patients, the symptoms were present from six months to one year prior to the diagnosis.[5]

Radiographically, in the extremities, a soft tissue mass is demonstrated. Speckled calcifications may be present within it.[10,11]

Erosion of adjacent bone in long-standing soft tissue tumors or actual bone destruction produced by lesions originating in bone have been seen.[4] Pelvic or retroperitoneal hemangiopericytomas displace the normal structures and these changes can be detected by means of radiographic examinations of the colon and urinary tract.[3] Tumors in the region of the head and neck cast shadows like soft tissue masses and produce erosion of the adjacent bones.[9,13] Arteriography has shown hemangiopericytoma to be vascular, revealing a prominent regional arterial supply, dilated draining veins, and tumor blush.[7] Pulmonary metastases, should they occur, are commonly multiple; however, solitary lesions have been observed.[10]

Hemangiopericytomas show a great variation in biological behavior. Some grow rapidly with a fatal outcome, whereas others are quite benign in character, remaining unchanged for years.[11] Those with a malignant course tend to recur locally, following the original treatment. There is a 50% possibility for either a benign or a malignant behavior; therefore their overall management should reflect this.[1] Backwinkel and Diddams[1] found the rate of local and distant recurrences to be 52.2% among 224 cases reviewed.

Local recurrences are usually multiple, separated by intervals of several years. In most patients distal metastases have been preceded by local recurrences.[3] In the series by McMaster et al.[10] none of the 12 lesions with benign histological features metastasized, but 6 of 16 borderline and 25 of 32 malignant tumors developed distant metastases. The metastases are blood-borne and most commonly seen in the lungs and the bones.[10]

Treatment and Results

There is general agreement that surgical resection is the treatment of choice. In order to minimize the chance of local re-currence the resection should be wide of tumor. The operation is to be adapted to the location of the lesion. Lymphadenectomy is not required, since metastases to the regional nodes are uncommon. At times, for very large tumors of the extremities, amputation might be necessary in order to encompass the entire growth.

Hemangiopericytomas are only moderately radiosensitive, requiring relatively high dosages. Friedman and Egan[6] treated two patients with osseous hemangiopericytomas, delivering 8240 rad in 30 days and 9288 rad in 70 days. There were no signs of tumor activity during the follow-up periods, which were 3 and 2.5 years, respectively. Radiation has definite palliative effects at lower dosage.[4,11]

Chemotherapy has been used primarily when metastatic disease developed. The most common agents have been actinomycin D, cyclophosphamide, vincristine, and Adriamycin. Apparently the results were not satisfactory.[10]

We have participated in the management of four patients with hemangiopericytoma. A 3-year-old boy presented with a tumor in the left great toe. Following excision, recurrence occurred and amputation of the toe was performed six months later. The patient did well for an interval of nine years, when, at the age of 12, metastases in the lung and the pleura appeared. They continued to enlarge while the patient received Adriamycin. The second patient is a 31-year-old female with a hemangiopericytoma of the right buccal mucosa. Following resection, the area was locally implanted with radium needles and a tumor dose of 6000 rad was given. During a three-year follow-up no recurrent disease or metastasis has been identified.

In the third patient, a 64-year-old female, the tumor presented in the left anterior thigh. The treatment was surgical resection. Four years later local recurrence occurred and this was accompanied by lung metastases. She was placed on a combination chemotherapy program consisting of actinomycin D, cyclophosphamide, and Adriamycin, with partial response that lasted approximately nine months. Local regrowth of the mass in the thigh and hemoptysis with respiratory distress from the lung metastases necessitated the use of local radiotherapy to the right thigh and the largest of the lung lesions. At the 4000 rad level, moderate response was observed and the rate of growth was slowed down. The patient was subsequently placed on Razoxane. At this point she has been surviving with both local recurrence and distant metastasis for approximately three years. The last patient, a 73-year-old female had a tumor in the nasal cavity, left maxillary antrum, and the nasopharynx. It was surgically resected and controlled by this procedure for 12 years. At that point local recurrence developed, which again involved all the same sites. A Caldwell–Luc procedure was performed, nasal antrostomy, and excision of the tumor from the nasopharynx. She has been alive and well for three years following the second operation.

Prognosis and Survival

In addition to the histological features described earlier, the location of the tumor has a bearing on the prognosis. Tumors located in the central nervous system are apt to recur in approximately 80% of the cases. This is possibly due to incomplete resections because of their position. Tumors of the skin and the musculoskeletal system recur at a rate of 50% and the same rate of recurrence is observed for tumors of the lung and mediastinum.[1] It appears that hemangiopericytomas arising in the upper respiratory passages have a lower grade of malignancy compared to those arising in the extremities or the retroperitoneum.[2]

The difficulty in measuring survival rates is exemplified by the report of

O'Brien and Brasfield.[12] They reported on seven patients who achieved a five-year survival of 100%. Eventually, they lost four patients to the disease as years went by. It is important to remember that hemangiopericytomas have a long natural life and that local recurrence may occur several years after the original treatment. Enzinger and Smith[3] in plotting the survival rates against the mitotic activity found the relative 10-year survival to be 77% for patients whose tumors had from 0–3 mitotic figures per 10 high power fields versus 29% for those whose tumors had 4 mitotic figures or more. McMaster et al.[10] have reported similar findings. All their patients with histologically benign tumors survived free of disease and were followed for periods ranging from 3 to 16 years. Patients with borderline tumors or histologically malignant hemangiopericytomas had 20% disease-free survival for follow-up periods ranging from 3 to 22 years.[10] Hemangiopericytoma in children has a better prognosis.[8] The congenital and infantile form occurring during the first year of life have a benign course.[10]

References

1. Backwinkel, K.D., and Diddams, J.A.: Hemangiopericytoma. Report of a case and comprehensive review of the literature. Cancer 25:896, 1970.
2. Batsakis, J.G.: Tumors of the Head and Neck. Williams & Wilkins, Baltimore, 1974.
3. Enzinger, F.M., and Smith, B.H.: Hemangiopericytoma. An analysis of 106 cases. Hum Pathol 7:61, 1976.
4. Fink, H.E., and Oberman, H.A.: Hemangioendothelial cell sarcoma and hemangiopericytoma. Report of 9 cases. AJR 89:155, 1963.
5. Fisher, J.H.: Hemangiopericytoma: A review of twenty cases. Can Med Assoc J 83:1136, 1960.
6. Friedman, M., and Egan, J.W.: Irradiation of hemangiopericytoma of Stout. Radiology 74:721, 1960.
7. Jaffe, N.: Hemangiopericytoma: Angiographic findings. Br J Radiol 33:614, 1960.
8. Kauffman, S.L., and Stout, A.P.: Hemangiopericytoma in children. Cancer 13:695, 1960.
9. Lenczyk, M.J.: Nasal hemangiopericytoma. Arch Otolaryngol 87:536, 1968.

10. McMaster, M.J., Soule, E.H., and Ivins, J.C.: Hemangiopericytoma. A clinicopathologic study and long-term followup of 60 patients. *Cancer* **36**:2232, 1975.

11. Mujahed, Z., Vasilas, A., and Evans, J.A.: Hemangiopericytoma. A report of four cases with a review of the literature. *AJR* **82**:658, 1959.

12. O'Brien, P., and Brasfield, R.D.: Hemangiopericytoma. *Cancer* **18**:249, 1965.

13. Rhodes, R.E., Brown, H.A., and Harrison, E.G., Jr.: Hemangiopericytoma of the nasal cavity. Review of the literature and report of three cases. *Arch Otolaryngol* **79**:505, 1964.

14. Stout, A.P., and Murray, M.R.: Hemangiopericytoma; a vascular tumor featuring Zimmermann's pericytes. *Ann Surg* **116**:26, 1942.

15. Stout, A.P.: Hemangiopericytoma. A study of twenty-five new cases. *Cancer* **2**:1027, 1949.

16. Stout, A.P.: Tumors featuring pericytes. Glomus tumor and hemangiopericytoma. *Lab Invest* **5**:217, 1956.

81

Lymphangiosarcoma

STEWART AND TREVES[8] in 1948 described a previously unrecognized entity, lymphangiosarcoma, developing on a chronically edematous extremity. All six patients reported by the authors had a radical mastectomy for carcinoma many years earlier. Several publications on the subject followed as clinicians became aware of the entity.[4,7,9] Although the majority of the neoplasms have developed in the ipsilateral upper extremity of patients undergoing radical mastectomy for carcinoma of the breast, there is no doubt that a number of cases have arisen on a chronically lymphedematous extremity, whose lymphedema cause has been congenital, traumatic, or iatrogenic in character following multiple surgical procedures not cancer-related.[5,9] For this reason, lymphangiosarcomas arising in lymphedematous lower extremities and lymphangiosarcomas in males have been reported.[2,5]

The incidence in postmastectomy patients of complicating lymphedema of the upper extremity is estimated to be less than 1%, 0.45% according to one reviewer.[6] The average patient who presents with a lymphangiosarcoma in a postmastectomy lymphedematous extremity has been 62 years old. The age range extends from 41 to 84 years.[2] The average age of patients whose lymphangiosarcoma is not associated with mastectomy is lower. Mackenzie[5] in his literature review of this patient group found it to be 43 years.

PATHOLOGY

Grossly, the lesions appear as hemorrhagic skin nodules, discrete in the early stages, coalescing later into ulcerated fungoid masses. They are widespread, exhibiting a distinct tendency for multicentricity along the involved extremity.[9] This is a polymorphous lesion presenting as patchy ecchymoses, as frank nodules, or as bullae. Their color is pinkish or blue-purple. When advanced, they cover a large segment of the extremity.[2]

Histologically, a progressive change is to be found from the striking lymphangiomatosis that is composed of nonneoplastic endothelial-lined channels at the periphery of the lesion, to the frank malignant endothelial cells in the central part of the tumor. There, they form papillary intraluminal masses and they participate in the new vessel formation.[4]

Also, changes related to the chronic lymphedema are to be seen. Included are hyperkeratosis of the epidermis, increased pigmentation of the basal layers, mild lymphocytic infiltration of the upper part of the dermis, and associated thickening and edema of the interstitial tissues.[9]

According to Taswell *et al.*[9] a very striking papillary pattern with several islands and cords of connective tissue in the centers surrounded by several layers of malignant cells is the predominant histological picture. The cells are large, bizarre, and pleomorphic, with very large and hyper-

242

chromatic nuclei. In addition there may be areas composed only of solid sheets of anaplastic cells forming the so-called "medullary pattern." Areas of hemorrhage and necrosis are a constant feature within the neoplasm.[9] Stewart and Treves[8] as well as others described lymphoid cells arranged in folliclelike aggregates or scattered throughout the tumor. These folliclelike structures are particularly present near small arterioles and veins and it is thought that they represent lymphocytes extravasated from the lymphatic channel due to the lymph stasis.[4,8] The neoplasms even in their advanced form remain confined to the skin and subcutaneous tissues and the vessels, sparing in general the underlying muscles and bones.[8]

CLINICAL

The average time period from the mastectomy to the development of lymphangiosarcoma has been 10 years.[2,3] The shortest interval noted has been 1.5 years and the longest 24 years. The mastectomy has been radical in all patients. Following surgery, characteristically, the patients developed lymphedema of varying severity, a condition that has lasted throughout the postoperative period until the appearance of the new tumor. Radiation therapy in postoperative or preoperative adjuvant fashion was given in most but not all of the patients. It appears that the role radiation plays in their development is parallel to that of the surgical procedure. They both produce lymph stasis and lymphedema, a situation that is considered an essential predisposing factor. That radiation is not the direct cause of this tumor is further corroborated by the fact that it appears in areas usually not included in the field of treatment, such as the antecubital fossa, and by the fact that lymphangiosarcomas developing in the lower extremities or following trauma or congenital lymphedema is obviously nonradiation induced.[3,5]

The histological appearance of the breast cancer and the status of the axillary lymph nodes apparently have no bearing on the development of the tumor. Actually, it can be said that the majority of the patients have been stable in terms of their breast cancer, because long intervals of survival are required in order for the lymphangiosarcoma to appear.

The growth rate of the lymphangiosarcoma is rapid. The seemingly isolated nodule or nodules have considerable subcutaneous spread.

The tumors often appear in medial aspect of the upper arm near the axilla (68% of all cases) or in the region of the antecubital fossa, according to Herrmann,[3] who in 1965 published an excellent review on the subject. Unusual but occasional locations for initial presentation are the volar surface and the posterior aspect of the forearm. Eventually, as the disease progresses, extension into the chest wall takes place.

Due to the clinical appearance, as just described, differential diagnosis from Kaposi's sarcoma is often in order. The latter is a disease seen primarily in males and affecting the lower extremities. Both on clinical and histological grounds, differentiation is possible. The differential diagnosis should also include lymphangitic recurrence from the primary breast carcinoma, or a new carcinoma.

The development of the tumor nodules is accompanied or predated by progressive edema of the involved extremity. Tenderness or pain may also be present; however, this is not a universal symptom.[2]

Lymphangiosarcoma indeed is a lethal complication of chronic lymphedema because the neoplasm has a high tendency for distant metastases. Favorite metastatic sites are the lungs and the pleura.[3] Metastases, however, have been seen and described by various authors in several locations, including the dura, the bones, the thyroid, the peritoneal cavity, gastrointestinal tract, and the liver.

TREATMENT AND RESULTS

Local excision obviously is not a recommended approach for a tumor of this nature; however, the results with more radical procedures have been so poor that it is worth mentioning the existence of one long-term survivor whose only treatment was indeed local excision.[9]

The commonest definitive form of therapy has been forequarter amputation. In addition a number of patients have been treated by means of disarticulation. Eby et al.,[2] in their literature review, found four patients treated by definitive surgery surviving from 4 to 15 years postoperatively. In addition, two patients who received both surgery and radiotherapy were among the five-year survivors.[2] These six survivors were from a group of 34 patients definitively treated. Chemotherapy has been tried in the form of single drug treatment without success; however, it should be mentioned that recent data on this form of treatment are not available in the literature.[3]

The tumor appears to be moderately radiosensitive. Chu and Treves[1] obtained remissions with objective regression of the disease lasting five to eight months utilizing palliative radiotherapy in cases with advanced upper extremity disease. These responses were achieved with moderate doses in the range of 3000–4000 rad delivered by means of an orthovoltage apparatus.[1] Southwick and Slaughter[7] reported on a 41-year-old female with lymphangiosarcoma developing in postmastectomy lymphedema. The patient had a left radical mastectomy at the age of 41 for carcinoma of the breast. Multiple nodules were present, some of them becoming confluent in both of the upper and lower part of her extremity. Following biopsy, interscapulothoracic amputation was proposed; however, the patient refused and for this reason the entire extremity was irradiated. Four hundred rad were administered per treatment fraction in four fractions utilizing an orthovoltage modality.

The nodularity had disappeared six weeks after the completion of therapy and the patient was alive and well six years posttreatment. Eby et al.[2] reported only partial regression of the lesions following a course of radiotherapy by which 4500 rad were delivered to the tumorous extremity.[2] Taswell et al.[9] in their literature review found 3 of 12 patients who were treated solely by radiotherapy; two survived without recurrence for less than two years and one for 12 years. In addition two patients were living with recurrence after two years or less.[9] In view of the poor results encountered in the literature following radical surgery, we believe that radiotherapy should be considered in an adjuvant fashion pre- or postoperatively. It is also possible that irradiation at what we now consider to be a definitive level should be undertaken if distant metastases are not demonstrable at the time of the diagnosis.

PROGNOSIS AND SURVIVAL

This indeed is a lethal complication of the postmastectomy lymphedema. Data available in 65 treated patients collected from the literature indicate that only eight among them were long-term, five-year survivors. This represents a rate of 11.7%. The actual survival, however, is indeed much lower, for in several of the reported cases, which exceed at the present time 100, no follow-ups are given.[2] The mean survival time of patients who are known to have died of lymphangiosarcoma has been 19 months.[2]

REFERENCES

1. Chu, F.C.H., and Treves, N.: The value of radiation therapy in post-mastectomy lymphangiosarcoma. AJR 89:64, 1963.
2. Eby, C.S., Brennan, M.J., and Fine, G.: Lymphangiosarcoma: A lethal complication of chronic lymphedema. Report of two cases and review of the literature. Arch Surg 94:223, 1967.

3. Herrmann, J.B.: Lymphangiosarcoma of the chronically edematous extremity. *Surg Gynecol Obstet* **121**:1107, 1965.

4. Hilfinger, M.F., Jr., and Eberle, R.D.: Lymphangiosarcoma in postmastectomy lymphedema. *Cancer* **6**:1192, 1953.

5. MacKenzie, D.H.: Lymphangiosarcoma arising in chronic congenital and idiopathic lymphoedema. *J Clin Pathol* **24**:524, 1971.

6. Shirger, A.: Postoperative lymphedema: Etiologic and diagnostic factors. *Med Clin North Am* **46**:1045, 1962.

7. Southwick, H.W., and Slaughter, D.P.: Lymphangiosarcoma in postmastectomy lymphedema. Five-year survival with irradiation treatment. *Cancer* **8**:158, 1955.

8. Stewart, F.W., and Treves, N.: Lymphangiosarcoma in postmastectomy lymphedema. A report of six cases in elephantiasis chirurgica. *Cancer* **1**:64, 1948.

9. Taswell, H.F., Soule, E.H., and Coventry, M.B.: Lymphangiosarcoma arising in chronic lymphedematous extremities. Report of thirteen cases and review of literature. *J Bone Joint Surg* **44**:277, 1962.

82

Malignant Schwannoma

MALIGNANT SCHWANNOMAS are primary nerve tumors originating from the Schwann cells. Histologically, the individual neurons are completely engulfed by the myelin sheath, being the most intimate cover, followed by the sheath of Schwann. Electron microscopic studies have shown that the myelin sheath is a differentiated part of the Schwann cell and not a separate structure, as was earlier thought.[6,8]

A large number of synonyms exist relating to primary malignant nerve sheath tumors. Most often encountered are the terms "malignant neurinoma," "malignant neurilemoma," and "neurogenous sarcoma."[9]

On clinical grounds, malignant schwannomas can be divided into solitary tumors occurring spontaneously and into malignant schwannomas occurring in patients with neurofibromatosis (Recklinghausen's disease).

SOLITARY MALIGNANT SCHWANNOMAS

The tumors may appear in patients of all ages from the very young to the very old. Actually, 5% of them are younger than 10 years. The average age at the time of the diagnosis is 41–42 years. There is no definite sex predominance.[2,4,7]

Pathology

The main criterion in establishing the diagnosis is evidence of origin of the neoplasm within the nerve. Grossly, a fusiform or oval mass is encountered in the course of a nerve or a nerve trunk. This quite often is well circumscribed, white-grayish in appearance.

Microscopically, the tumor is composed of spindle-shaped cells that are arranged in bundles interlacing and wavy in character. The nuclei are ovoid and plump, the mitotic number varying from tumor to tumor. There is a distinct tendency for the malignant cells to extend and propagate along the nerve sheaths and it is believed that this is one of the mechanisms leading to local recurrence.[2,7,9]

It is the consensus at this time, that malignant schwannomas appear *de novo*, not arising from preexisting benign counterparts.[10]

Clinical

The commonest presenting symptom is that of a painless mass. In the series by Das Gupta and Brasfield[4] 73% of the patients had a painless tumor and the remaining had some form of pain or discomfort along the course of the peripheral nerves. Approximately 60% of the tumors are greater than 5.0 cm at the time of the diagnosis.[2,4,11]

In contrast to the benign schwannomas that are often found in the region of the head and neck, malignant schwannomas are uncommon in this area. The commonest involved regions are the extremities. Thus, 30–38% of all tumors are encountered in the lower extremities, 23–30% in the upper extremities, 15% in the trunk, and only 8–14% in the head and neck (Fig. 82-1). Malignant schwannomas can occur anywhere in the body and tumors have been described in such locations as the retroperitoneum, the mediastinum, and the pelvis[1,5,10] (Fig. 82-2).

Malignant schwannomas of the cranial nerves or the roots of the spinal nerves are uncommon. Regional lymph node metastases are rare or nonexistent.[4,7]

Large referral centers share a common experience, that of seeing a large proportion of patients with recurrent rather than with primary disease.

Treatment and Results

The commonest procedure is local surgical resection, which in the majority of the cases has led into local recurrence. In the series by White[12] of 15 patients who underwent surgical excision, only three were surviving, 2, 2.5, and 13 years postoperatively. D'Agostino et al.[2] reported local recurrences developing in 12 of 19 patients after simple or radical local excision.

In tabulating the rate of recurrence to the type of the operation Das Gupta and Brasfield[4] found it to be 73% following local excision and 21% following a wide soft tissue resection. Ghosh et al.,[7] however, demonstrated that for small tumors an adequate local excision with ample free margins surrounding the tumor may be sufficient therapy. As a rule, however, a major surgical resection should be undertaken. The inadequacy of local excision is most obvious in the head and neck area where there is a tendency to preserve the anatomy to the greatest extent. Conley and Janecka[1] reviewing 14 such patients found only two surviving free of disease for one and two years following surgery. The rest were either dead or were living with recurrent tumors.

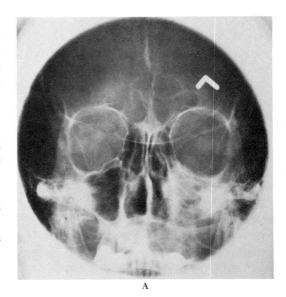

A

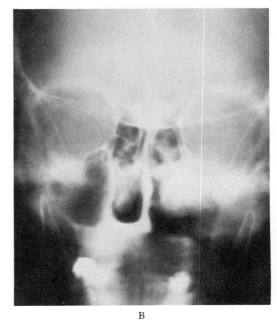

B

FIG. 82-1. Malignant schwannoma in a 63-year-old female. The tumor arose in the left maxillary antrum. The antrum is clouded and the inferior border is not well defined (A). Following surgical resection there was recurrence, especially in the superior aspect of the sinus. The tumor now extends medially to the nasal cavity and upward to the orbit and the ethmoids (B).

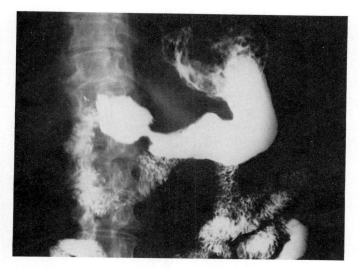

FIG. 82-2. Neurofibrosarcoma in a 73-year-old female. Upper gastrointestinal series demonstrates a large irregular filling defect in the fundus of the stomach.

The reluctance to proceed with an amputation for what appears to be a localized neoplasm combined with the characteristic propagation of tumor along the nerve trunks and with the fact that the individual experience of the practicing surgeons is limited when dealing with malignant schwannoma accounts for the high recurrence rates. It appears that the tumor is radioresistant, failing to regress even at definitive dose levels.

Prognosis and Survival

A major prognostic indicator is the tumor size. Among 58 patients whose tumor measured less than 5.0 cm, there was a 79.3% five-year survival, as reported by Ghosh et al.[7] In the same series for neoplasms infiltrating the surrounding muscles, a 54% five-year survival was found, whereas for large and recurrent neoplasms the five-year cure rate was 30%. These results are quite excellent, perhaps reflecting better understanding and better approach to this problem than reports published earlier. In the series by White[12] 9 of 15 patients died of their tumor within 20 months from the time of the diagnosis. In the series by Das Gupta and Brasfield[4] patients treated by local excision had a 29% five-year survival, whereas in those treated by radical surgical approach the survival rate at five years was 52%.

Local recurrence can be further managed and a considerable number of patients can be salvaged. Among 110 cases of locally recurrent tumor without distant metastases present, 40 showed no signs of disease following further surgery at five years.[4]

MALIGNANT SCHWANNOMAS ASSOCIATED WITH NEUROFIBROMATOSIS

The percentage of patients with multiple neurofibromatosis who develop malignant schwannoma has been variously reported between 5 and 15%. Generally, they are rather young in age, in the range of 28–30 years. There is no clear sex predilection[11] (Fig. 82-3).

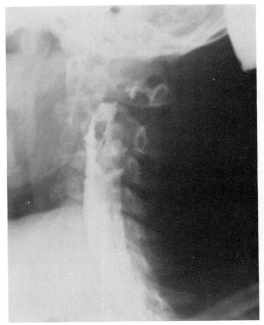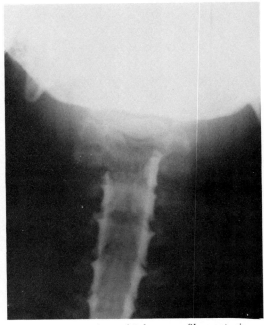

FIG. 82-3. Neurofibrosarcoma in a 15-year-old female. Patient with multiple neurofibromatosis. Myelogram in the posterioanterior and lateral projection demonstrates a filling defect that proved to be a neurofibrosarcoma arising in the region of the spinal cord.

Pathology

The neurofibromas of multiple neurofibromatosis have a distinct pattern, easily distinguishable from benign schwannomas. A malignant schwannoma, however, arising on a patient with multiple neurofibromatosis has a similar histological pattern as that of a solitary schwannoma [9,10] (Fig. 82-4).

Clinical

The common presentation is an enlargement rather fast and at times tender of a previously existing neurofibroma. The patient becomes aware that the growth rate is unusual and this combined with the local discomfort leads to further investigation. There is a predilection for the lower extremities; however, the upper extremities are also often involved.

Treatment and Results

These tumors have been treated primarily surgically. The procedures have varied from local excision to radical resection and amputation. As is the case in solitary malignant schwannomas, here, too, local excision has been followed by a high rate of recurrence and this in turn by a high rate of mortality.[3,12] For this reason, it is recommended by most authors that radical approach should be considered whenever feasible. In doing so, however, one must recognize that the patients have a systemic disease that is apt to produce similar malignant transformations in the years ahead.

The five-year-survival rate is inferior in this group as compared to patients with solitary malignant schwannomas. D'Agostino et al.[3] reported on 16 patients of 20 evaluable dying from their tumor. Ghosh et al.[7] encountered a 30% five-year survival.

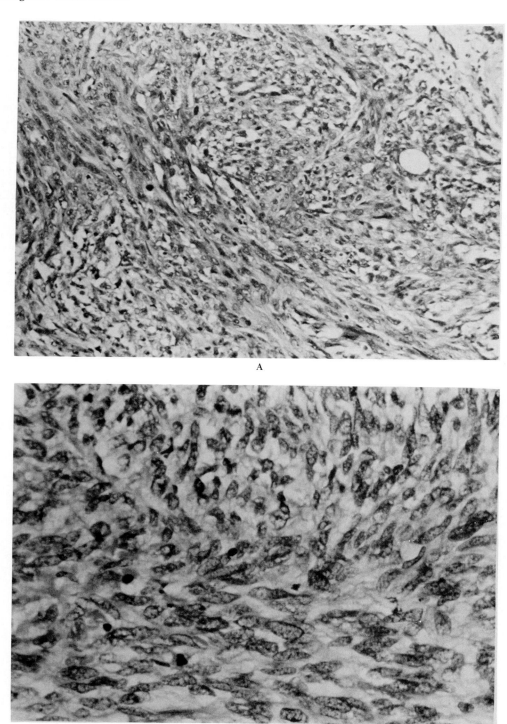

FIG. 82-4. Malignant schwannoma. (*A*): Spindle-shaped cells with oval nuclei forming multidirectional bundles. The tumor arose in the thigh of a 39-year-old male with Recklinghausen's disease. (*B*): Higher magnification shows a high mitotic rate.

REFERENCES

1. Conley, J., and Janecka, I.P.: Neurilemmoma of the head and neck. *Trans Am Acad Ophthalmol Otolaryngol* **80:**459, 1975.
2. D'Agostino, A.N., Soule, E.H., and Miller, R.H.: Primary malignant neoplasms of nerves (malignant neurilemomas) in patients without manifestations of multiple neurofibromatosis (von Recklinghausen's disease). *Cancer* **16:**1003, 1963.
3. D'Agostino, A.N., Soule, E.H., and Miller, R.H.: Sarcomas of the peripheral nerves and somatic soft tissues associated with multiple neurofibromatosis (von Recklinghausen's disease). *Cancer* **16:**1015, 1963.
4. Das Gupta, T.K., and Brasfield, R.D.: Solitary malignant schwannoma. *Ann Surg* **171:**419, 1970.
5. Eversole, L.R., Schwartz, W.D., and Sabes, W.R.: Central and peripheral fibrogenic and neurogenic sarcoma of the oral regions. *Oral Surg* **36:**49, 1973.
6. Fisher, E.R., and Vuzevski, V.D.: Cytogenesis of schwannoma (neurilemoma), neurofibroma, dermatofibroma and dermatofibrosarcoma as revealed by electron microscopy. *Am J Clin Pathol* **49:**141, 1968.
7. Ghosh, B.C., Ghosh, L., Huvos, A.G., and Fortner, J.G.: Malignant schwannoma. A clinicopathologic study. *Cancer* **31:**184, 1973.
8. Greep, R.O.: *Histology.* McGraw-Hill, New York, 1966.
9. Harkin, J.C., and Reed, R.J.: *Tumors of the Peripheral Nervous System.* Armed Forces Institute of Pathology, Washington, D.C., 1969.
10. Ingels, G.W., Campbell, D.C., Jr., Giampetro, A.M., Kozur, R.E., and Bentlage, C.H.: Malignant schwannomas of the mediastinum. Report of two cases and review of the literature. *Cancer* **27:**1190, 1971.
11. Vieta, J.O., and Pack, G.T.: Malignant neurilemomas of the peripheral nerves. *Am J Surg* **82:**416, 1951.
12. White, H.R., Jr.: Survival in malignant schwannoma. An 18-year study. *Cancer* **27:**720, 1971.

83

Malignant Granular Cell Myoblastoma

GRANULAR CELL myoblastoma was recognized as a separate entity and described first by Abrikossoff[1] in 1926. The tumor originated in the tongue and pursued a benign course.

In the following years several cases were reported. Most commonly, it was seen in the tongue, oral cavity, respiratory and digestive tracts, skin, and breast (Fig. 83-1). However, as many case reports indicate, it can actually be found anywhere in the body.

It was considered to be a uniformly benign neoplasm until 1945 when Ravich et al.[10] published the first unquestionably malignant case. This was a granular cell myoblastoma of the urinary bladder, which in spite of the benign histological appearance metastasized widely. The patient died 17 months after the diagnosis.

A comprehensive literature review by Cadotte[3] in 1974 revealed 22 cases of malignant granular cell myoblastomas among a total number of 600 cases. Thus, the incidence of the malignant variant is 3%.[3]

Two-thirds of the patients have been females. The average age at the time of the diagnosis was 45 years.

PATHOLOGY

Grossly, the tumors are circumscribed but not encapsulated. Thus, they are in intimate contact with the surrounding tissues.[2] The cells are polyhedral or polymorphic, having an abundant large granular eosinophilic protoplasm and a small central nucleus.[2] The malignant variant has no distinct histological or histochemical characteristics (Fig. 83-2). The appearance is similar to that of the benign form.[13] The granules are related to the Golgi apparatus and to the lysosomes of the cells.[12]

The presence of protein-bound lipids within the tumor cells, similar to those seen in myelin degeneration products, and the similarity between the granular cells and the Schwann cells of peripheral degenerating nerves raise the question of neural derivation.[2,4,5] The original proposal that the tumor was related to rhabdomyoblasts is no longer a consideration.

CLINICAL

Murphy et al.,[9] on the basis of 219 cases, estimated that 34% of granular cell myoblastomas occurred in the tongue. When considering the entire head and neck region, 52% of all tumors were encountered. Tumors of the skin and the subcutaneous tissues accounted for 16.6% and 7.9% occurred in the breast. A different distribution is to be found for tumors exhibiting a malignant course. Approximately 50% of them arose in the proximal extremities or in the area of the pelvis[3] (Fig. 83-3).

The commonest presenting symptom is that of a painless mass gradually enlarging and never ulcerating.[3,7,8,11] Also, symptoms specific to the tumor sites, such as hematuria or bowel obstruction, have

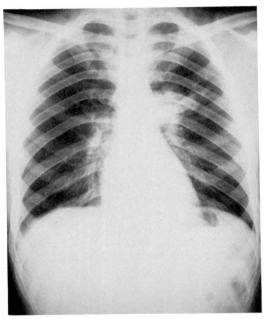

FIG. 83-1.   Granular cell myoblastoma of the lung in a 24-year-old male. There is a mass lesion in the hilar area of the left lung.

been noted.[6,10] At times, the tumor mass is tender.

Malignant granular cell myoblastomas metastasize via the lymphatics and the blood vessels. Regional lymph node metastasis is very common. The commonest distant sites are the lungs, liver, skeletal system, and the brain. In some patients metastatic disease occurred several years following the original diagnosis. More often, however, regional lymph node metastasis develops within the first two years.[3] Another frequent event is the local recurrence. This development has heralded the malignant course in a number of reported cases.[7,8,13]

TREATMENT AND RESULTS

Surgical resection is the proper therapy. Since the great majority of granular cell myoblastomas have a benign clinical course, this procedure is curative. Radical

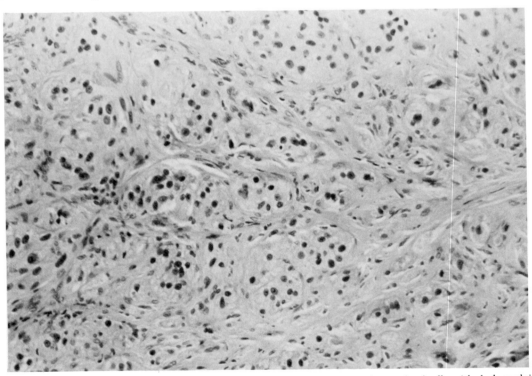

FIG. 83-2.   Malignant granular cell myoblastoma arising in bone. Organoid growth of cells with dark nuclei and large cytoplasm. A 38-year-old female.

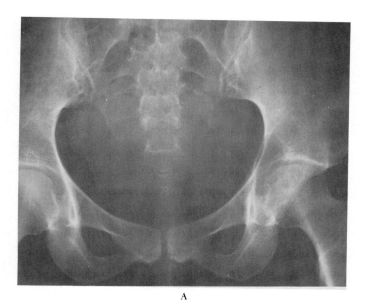

A

FIG. 83-3. Granular cell myoblastoma in a 39-year-old female. The tumor arose in the bones of the pelvis, presenting with left hip joint pain. There is a lytic lesion involving the roof and the medial aspect of the left acetabulum and extending toward the left iliac ring. Thought to be benign in character, it was twice locally excised and packed (A). Chest x-ray examination on the same patient 20 months later shows bilateral pulmonary metastases. The patient died of her disease (B).

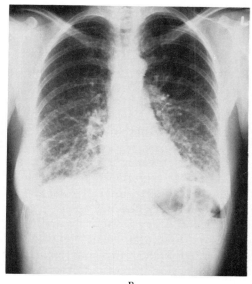

B

surgery should not be considered at this time. The benign histological appearance is another reason mitigating against a radical approach. It is the subsequent clinical behavior that determines the malignant or the benign nature of the disease. Unfortunately, by this time cure is impossible for the malignant form. With the exception of one patient who has been a long survivor following resection of a local recurrence, no other cures have been obtained.

There is a consensus that the tumor is radioresistant. Cadotte[3] reported on a patient who received 5500 rad for pulmonary metastatic lesions. There was no effect radiographically and actually the tumors increased during and following the course. MacKenzie[8] reported on a patient who received 5700 rad to a locally recurrent tumor in the lumbar region and to the regional metastatic lymph nodes. Six months following therapy, the tumor began regrowing. Ross *et al.*[11] reported failure of radiation to control recurrent skin nodules at a dosage of 2900 rad delivered in a period of eight days.

Data on the effects of chemotherapy are lacking in the literature at the present time.

We have participated in the management of a 38-year-old female whose tumor involved the ischium and the left ilium. The presenting symptom was pain and discomfort in the region of the left pelvis. Initial radiographs were interpreted as normal, later though, rarefaction in the region of the left acetabulum extending into the ischium and the adjacent ilium was identified. The area was biopsied and following consultations with several pathologists the diagnosis of granular cell myoblastoma was arrived at. The area was curetted and subsequently packed with graft bone. Four months later left inguinal adenopathy developed and biopsy revealed histology similar to that of the original lesion. Because of this development and because of further progression into the upper ilium, local radiotherapy was considered. At this point, the patient was requiring strong analgesics. A course of cobalt-60 teletherapy was planned and delivered to the region of the left pelvis. The patient received a total of 6500 rad as a calculated tumor dose via an arc technique in 48 elapsed days. There was only minimal and temporary pain relief. Radiographs of the chest two months following the completion of the radiotherapy indicated a suspicious interstitial infiltrate that was confirmed in subsequent films. Indeed, metastatic disease to the lungs developed in the form of a diffuse interstitial micronodular pattern, resulting eventually in severe shortness of breath. At this point, the patient had entered a program of systemic chemotherapy. Adriamycin, 80 mg intravenously and cyclophosphamide, 600 mg intravenously, were administered every four weeks. There was some occasional subjective improvement with regard to the pelvic pain and the dyspnea; however, radiographically, the disease progressed. The patient died two years from the time of the diagnosis.

PROGNOSIS AND SURVIVAL

The prognosis of the malignant granular cell myoblastoma is poor. One reason for this is the benign histology that makes an *a priori* diagnosis impossible. The malignant nature has been determined on clinical grounds, either because of local recurrence or because of distant metastases. Given the great propensity for lymphatic and hematogenous dissemination, it is questionable how much the survival would have been affected if early diagnosis were possible.

Review of the cases reported thus far indicates that the two-year survival for malignant granular cell myoblastoma has been 60%. The five-year-survival rate has been 25%, approximately.

REFERENCES

1. Abrikossoff, A.I.: Uber Myome ausgehend von der quergestreiften willkurlichen Muskulatur. *Virchow's Arch [Pathol Anat]* **206**:215, 1926.
2. Batsakis, J.G.: *Tumors of the Head and Neck.* Williams & Wilkins, Baltimore, 1974.
3. Cadotte, M.: Malignant granular-cell myoblastoma. *Cancer* **33**:1417, 1974.
4. Fisher, E.R., and Wechsler, H.: Granular cell myoblastoma—a misnomer. Electron microscopic and histochemical evidence concerning its Schwann cell deviation and nature. (Granular cell Schwannoma). *Cancer* **15**:936, 1962.
5. Garancis, J.C., Komorowski, R.A., and Kuzma, J.F.: Granular cell myoblastoma. *Cancer* **25**:542, 1970.
6. Hunter, T.D., Jr., and Dewar, J.P.: Malignant granular-cell myoblastoma: Report of a case and review of the literature. *Am Surg* **26**:554, 1960.
7. Krieg, A.F.: Malignant granular cell myoblastoma. A case report. *Arch Pathol* **74**:251, 1962.
8. MacKenzie, D.H.: Malignant granular cell myoblastoma. *J Clin. Pathol* **20**:739, 1967.
9. Murphy, G.H., Dockerty, M.B., and Broders, A.C.: Myoblastoma. *Am J Pathol* **25**:1157, 1949.
10. Ravich, A., Stout, A.P., and Ravich, R.A.: Malignant granular cell myoblastoma involving the urinary bladder. *Ann Surg* **121**:361, 1945.

11. Ross, R.C., Miller, T.R., and Foote, F.W., Jr.: Malignant granular-cell myoblastoma. *Cancer* **5:**112, 1952.

12. Sobel, H.J., Marquet, E., Avrin, E., and Schwarz, R.: Granular cell myoblastoma. An electron microscopic and cytochemical study illustrating the genesis of granules and aging of myoblastoma cells. *Am J Pathol* **65:**59, 1971.

13. Švejda, J., and Horn, V.A.: A disseminated granular-cell pseudotumor; so called metastasizing granular-cell myoblastoma. *J Pathol Bacteriol* **76:**343, 1958.

84

Clear-Cell Sarcoma of Tendons and Aponeuroses

ENZINGER[3] IN 1965 described a soft tissue sarcoma arising primarily from large tendons and aponeuroses of the extremities. The tumors lacked the biphasic pattern that characterizes the synovial sarcomas. Instead they were composed of uniform cells.[3] Twenty-one cases were reviewed in that original report and since that time several more have been reported.[1,2,4] The median age of the patients at the time of the diagnosis is 32 years. Obviously, this is a disease of the young, and there is equal distribution between the two sexes.[1]

PATHOLOGY

The gross appearance of the tumor is that of a firm rather spherical mass with a smooth or nodular surface. Characteristically, the overlying skin is not involved.[2,3] The average tumor size at the time of the diagnosis is 4–6 cm.[4] Microscopically, the tumors are composed of pale fusiform cells of epithelioid appearance which have round nuclei and prominent nucleoli. The clear appearance of the cytoplasm often is enhanced by the presence of minute vacuoles. The cells form compact nests and fascicles. A fine reticular stroma surrounding these formations is to be found (Fig. 84-1). There is generally a low mitotic figure count.[2,3]

CLINICAL

Literature review shows that the commonest presenting symptom is a mass or a swelling whose duration may vary from three months to 19 years.[2] The tumor is painless in the majority of the cases and in those patients who experience some discomfort it is only mild in character.[3]

They occur mainly in the extremities, especially the lower, where 80% of the total number are seen. More specifically, it is in the region of the foot and the ankle that 50% of all cases arise.[2]

TREATMENT AND RESULTS

In the majority of the patients the first treatment has been local excision of the tumor. The several reasons for this course of therapy include the peripheral location of the lesion, the lack of symptoms, the relative benign clinical appearance, and the reluctance of the patient to undergo major amputation once the diagnosis has been established.[1-4] The disease has a high tendency for both local recurrence and regional lymph node metastasis. Two-thirds of the cases reported in the literature developed, eventually, local recurrence. Distant metastases and lymph node involvement were seen in approximately 50% of the patients, the lungs being the commonest site. In addition

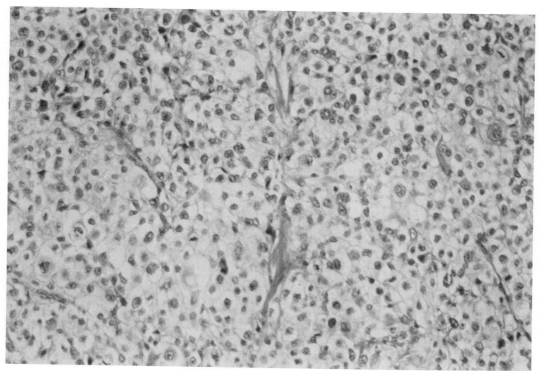

FIG. 84-1. Clear cell sarcoma of tendons and aponeuroses. Clusters and cords of cells with large clear cytoplasm and nuclei with prominent nucleoli. The clusters are separated by fine fibrous network.

metastasis to the bones, liver, heart, and adrenals have been reported.[1]

There is suggestive evidence derived from the literature that local excision when supplemented by definitive local radiotherapy provides a better control rate than excision alone.[1,3] The level of the radiation dose has been in the range of 6000 to 8000 rad. Amputation of the extremity, particularly in the early stages, yields good local control and provides reasonable expectations for cure. Of the seven patients who underwent amputation in the series by Tsuneyoshi *et al.*[4] four were alive and well at the time of the report without signs of recurrent disease and three were dead of their tumor. When radical surgery is performed, the regional lymph nodes should be considered as part of the procedure due to the high incidence of lymph node involvement.

In the original description by Enzinger[3] no mention was made regarding the presence or the absence of melanin within the tumor cells. Subsequently, however, several reports appeared in the literature describing tumors with the features of clear cell sarcoma that also contained melanosomes in their cytoplasm. This subgroup has been called melanotic type as opposed to the synovial type with the clear cells. It is presently believed that the melanotic type is indeed a malignant melanoma of the soft tissues and that it should be differentiated from the synovial clear cell sarcoma.[1,2,4]

The prognosis is worse for patients with the melanotic type, the five year survival being 29%.[3] The actuarial five year survival for the non-melanin containing tumors has been approximately 50%.[1]

REFERENCES

1. Alitalo, K., Paavolainen, P., Franssila, K., and Ritsilä, V.: Clear-cell sarcoma of tendons and aponeuroses. Report of two cases. *Acta Orthop Scand* **48:**241, 1977.

2. Boudreaux, D., and Waisman, J.: Clear cell sarcoma with melanogenesis. *Cancer* **41:**1387, 1978.

3. Enzinger, F.M.: Clear-cell sarcoma of tendons and aponeuroses. An analysis of 21 cases. *Cancer* **18:**1163, 1965.

4. Tsuneyoshi, M., Enjoji, M., and Kubo, T.: Clear cell sarcoma of tendons and aponeuroses. A comparative study of 13 cases with a provisional subgrouping into the melanotic and synovial types. *Cancer* **42:**243, 1978.

85

Epitheloid Sarcoma

EPITHELIOID SARCOMA is a soft tissue sarcoma related to the connective tissue parts of the extremities, primarily the tendons and the fascias. It was reported as a separate entity by Enzinger[1] in 1970, who presented the clinical and microscopic data on 62 tumors of this variety from the Armed Forces Institute of Pathology and reviewed previously reported cases with similar histology. Since that time, several new cases and series have been reported.[3-5] The exact cellular origin of epithelioid sarcoma remains speculative; however, most authors at the present time believe that it represents a variant of synovial sarcoma.[24]

Hajdu et al.,[2] reviewing 136 cases of tendosynovial sarcomas, found 12 among them with features of epithelioid sarcoma, an incidence of approximately 8.5%. This is primarily a disease of the young adult, with the average age at the time of the diagnosis being 23 years in the series by Enzinger[1] and 29 years in the series by Prat et al.[5] The peak is during the third decade of life.[5] There is a definite male predominance, the male to female ratio being in the range of 3:1.[2,5]

PATHOLOGY

The gross appearance of the lesions when present in the distal extremities is that of firm subcutaneous nodules. Their size ranges from 0.5 to 5.0 cm. They are associated with flexor tendons and with palmar aponeurosis. Larger tumors are to be found in the proximal extremities and in the region of the neck. These may attain sizes up to 10.0 cm.[1,5]

Histologically, the predominant cell is oval or polygonal in shape, containing densely eosinophilic cytoplasm. Enziger[1] states that the tumor has two characteristic features; a nodular arrangement of the cells and central necrosis within the nodule, hence the name "epithelioid." The overall pattern resembles that of a granuloma (Fig. 85-1). Occasionally areas of hemorrhage and fibrin deposits are associated with the lesions.

There is extension along fibrous structures, such as tendons, fascias, or periosteum, and proximal propagation along their planes. There is infiltration of the subcutaneous fat and of the overlying skin, which may eventually ulcerate.[1,5] Vascular invasion occurred in 5 of 22 cases reported by Prat et al.[5] This proved to be a grave prognostic sign.

CLINICAL

The onset of the disease is very gradual and very subdued. The patient presents with what he believes to be a "wart," a lump, or a "woody hard node," which in his estimate has grown slowly over some period of time. The duration of these lesions prior to the diagnosis is in the range of nine months to three years.[1,5]

The tumor favors the extremities and in particular the upper extremities. The commonest site of origin is the hand,

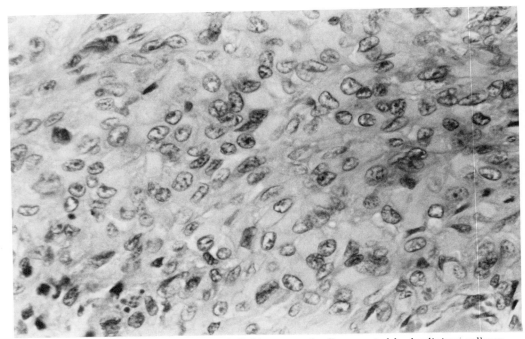

FIG. 85-1.   Epithelioid sarcoma. Primarily epithelioid pattern of cells separated by hyalinized collagen.

where 45% of the lesions are to be found. The tumors both in the hands and the feet involve the flexor surfaces.[1-5] The extensor surfaces of the forearms and the anterior tibial surfaces are also common sites.[1] When located in the hands, dysfunction due to tumor enlargement may be encountered. Pain is not a prominent feature of epithelioid sarcoma. Approximately 25% of the patients reported some pain or tenderness and this was usually mild in character.[1]

The reported incidence of regional lymph node metastasis has varied. This variation is due primarily to the length of the follow-up period. During the early stages of the disease, this occurrence is infrequent and therefore the percentage of lymph node involvement at this time is small. Eventually, particularly following local recurrences, the regional lymph nodes do get involved in approximately 40% of the cases.[5] During the early stages of the disease process, metastatic lymph node involvement is not a major factor.

TREATMENT AND RESULTS

Due to the deceptive clinical appearance resembling that of a benign condition, the overwhelming majority of the patients have had as their first therapy some form of local resection or excision. Following treatment of this type, local tumor recurrence is quite probable, seen in excess of 85% of the cases.[1] In many patients several local recurrences have taken place and treated with limited procedures as they appeared. Enzinger[1] in his review, found only 4% of the patients to have radical surgery—wide local excision or amputation—as the initial form of therapy. Due to the high local recurrence rate, however, 74% of the patients eventually underwent major surgery.[1] At the present time, it is obvious that in order to minimize the rate of local recurrence and avoid eventual involvement of the regional lymphatics, as well as the possibility of distant metastasis from active disease, the proper form of therapy is surgical amputation or an en bloc wide excision. The regional lymph nodes should be examined during the procedure; however, whether or not lymphadenectomy should be performed at this stage is questionable.[5] The neoplasm tends to infiltrate along tendons and fascias and therefore it can easily evade the therapeutic aspirations of a local excision.

Distant metastases occur primarily to the lungs and they may appear several years following the initial diagnosis. Practically all patients by that time have had local recurrence.

PROGNOSIS AND SURVIVAL

Histological evidence of vascular invasion was associated with death of all five patients who had it, according to Prat *et al.*[5] Similarly, lymph node involvement is a serious prognostic sign.

The survival rate at five years is 60%; however, disease-related deaths continue to occur up to the 10-year point and even beyond it.[5]

The best prognosis and the longest disease-free intervals go to patients whose original therapy was a major radical procedure in the form of amputation. Conversely, very few of those patients who had local excision are among the long-term survivors.[5]

REFERENCES

1. Enzinger, F.M.: Epithelioid sarcoma. A sarcoma simulating a granuloma or a carcinoma. *Cancer* **26:**1029, 1970.
2. Hajdu, S.I., Shiu, M.H., and Fortner, J.G.: Tendosynovial sarcoma. A clinicopathological study of 136 cases. *Cancer* **39:**1201, 1977.
3. Lo, H.H., Kalisher, L., and Faix, J.D.: Epithelioid sarcoma: Radiologic and pathologic manifestations. *AJR* **128:**1017, 1977.
4. Patchefsky, A.S., Soriano, R., and Kostianovsky, M.: Epithelioid sarcoma. Ultrastructural similarity to nodular synovitis. *Cancer* **39:**143, 1977.
5. Prat, J., Woodruff, J.M., and Marcove, R.C.: Epithelioid sarcoma. An analysis of 22 cases indicating the prognostic significance of vascular invasion and regional lymph node metastasis. *Cancer* **41:**1472, 1978.

86

Alveolar Soft Part Sarcoma

CHRISTOPHERSON et al.[5] in 1952 described 12 cases of a soft tissue tumor that had no histological similarity to any of the previously well-known and well-documented sarcomas. They attached to it the descriptive term "alveolar soft part sarcoma" because of the microscopic picture that gave the impression of an alveolus with cells arranged in a peripheral row around a central space devoid of organized structure.

At this time, approximately 70 cases have been reported in the English literature, most of the patients being young females. The average age of the female patients is 20 years and that of the males, 30 years.[9]

PATHOLOGY

Grossly, the tumors are moderately firm, for the most part seemingly well circumscribed and partially encapsulated.[5] Their size ranges from a few centimeters to more than 20.0 cm in diameter. A characteristic histological feature is the uniformity of morphology that is retained in the metastatic lesions as well. The cells are arranged in pseudoalveolar or organoid formations in relation to delicate, endothelial-lined vascular channels (Fig. 86-1). Septa separate the individual alveolar groups.[5] Electromicroscopic studies by Fisher and Reidbord[7] suggested that the tumor represents a variant of rhabdomyosarcoma, whereas Unni and Soule[14] following similar studies concluded that

alveolar soft part sarcomas are related to chemodectomas.

Review of the literature and in particular review of the clinical features and the natural history of the disease suggests that this is a specific entity quite different from any previously defined group of tumors, including those just mentioned.

CLINICAL

Basically, alveolar soft part sarcomas are associated with skeletal muscle. They occur primarily in the extremities, particularly in the proximal parts of the limbs. Lieberman et al.[9] noticed a definite laterality by which the tumors favored the right side of the body in almost a 2:1 ratio. A review of the individual case reports in the literature confirms this observation.[1,3,4,6,11,13]

Occasionally, the tumors have been seen in locations other than the extremities. One of Christopherson et al.'s[5] original patients presented with a lesion in the right abdominal wall; Olson and Perkins[11] reported on a patient with a tumor originating on the right side of the tongue; Balfour[3] reported on an alveolar soft part sarcoma in the area of the right masseter muscle; and Abrahams et al.[1] described an alveolar soft part sarcoma arising from the inferior rectus muscle of the right eye.

The presenting symptom is that of a painless, slowly growing mass that at times has been observed for considerably

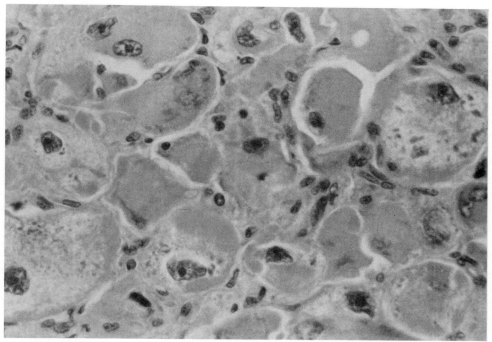

FIG. 86-1.   Alveolar soft part sarcoma. Large granular cells with abundant cytoplasm arranged in an organoid pattern.

long periods of time prior to seeking medical advice.[5] Metastasis to the lung has been reported as a first sign of the disease process.[5,10]

The disease usually progresses slowly, recurring locally and metastasizing distantly. However, particularly in older individuals, a rapid course may be seen. Metastasis may be seen a few months after the initial diagnosis or several years later.[3,4,8,12] Approximately 50% of the patients during the first five years following the diagnosis will develop metastases. The percentage increases to 70% at 15 years.[9] The commonest site (42%) is the lungs, followed by the skeletal system and the brain. Regional lymph nodes were involved only in 7% of the cases.[9] Local recurrence may take place more than once and it is seen in approximately 25% of the patients.[5,8,9]

Radiographically, the primary tumor usually does not extend to the underlying

bone. Arteriography reveals an extremely vascular lesion with arteriovenous shunting and dense tumor staining.[2,4] Rosenbaum et al.,[12] reviewing two patients with metastatic disease to the brain, reported similar hypervascularity. The lung nodules are usually round, well circumscribed, and the bone lesions are lytic in character.[2]

TREATMENT AND RESULTS

Conservative local excision was performed in 11 of the 12 original patients reported by Christopherson et al.[5] In the one case in which the tumor invaded the tibia and the fibula a low-thigh amputation was done. The tumor recurred locally in four patients, all of whom died with distant metastases. Five patients died with metastatic disease without prior local recurrence, and the remaining three were lost to follow-up.[5]

Lieberman et al.[9] in their series found no added value in radical surgery over local resection. The same authors state that on the basis of their results local radiotherapy administered postoperatively increased the mean survival time by 21 months.

The tumor basically is radioresistant; however, partial temporary responses or slowing of the growth have been observed. Furey et al.[8] reported on a 46-year-old female patient whose recurrent left buttock tumor was irradiated at 4500 rad level. This produced pain relief and provided a four-year interval of relative comfort. Local recurrence was reirradiated twice within a year, with poor response.

Rubenfeld[13] reported on the treatment of pulmonary metastasis by means of radiotherapy. The patient received 5500 rad in 37 elapsed days to the left upper lobe. Although no regression was observed, there was no progression either, as seen in radiographs one year following radiotherapy. Asvall et al.[2] reviewed four cases of alveolar soft part sarcoma, all treated by local resection and all recurring locally. Radiotherapy at the level of 4200 rad in 31 days given postoperatively in one patient did not prevent local recurrence three years later. The same authors reported beneficial response to Thiotepa in one of their cases. This was a 20-year-old female developing lung metastases one year postoperatively. Thiotepa was given for a total dose of 2 mg/kg over 16 days, producing disappearance of the lung lesion. The patient remained on the program for 2.5 years. Subsequent local recurrence some years later responded partially to Thiotepa.[2] Cyclophosphamide, actinomycin D, and vincristine resulted in temporary reduction of pain and diminution of trismus in a patient with alveolar soft part sarcoma of the right masseter muscle reported by Balfour.[3] Vincristine, Adriamycin, and cyclophosphamide were ineffective in treating pulmonary metas-

tases in two cases reported by Blumberg et al.[4]

PROGNOSIS AND SURVIVAL

The disease carries a serious prognosis, as lengthy follow-up examinations over several years have revealed. At the present time, the tumor is considered to be lethal. Because of the slow evolution, however, it may allow a long symptom-free survival before the development of metastases. In the series by Lieberman et al.[9] the mean survival time of patients undergoing surgical resection alone was 70 months, and those on whom postoperative radiotherapy was added had a mean survival time of 91 months. Young females under the age of 20 appeared to have a better prognosis than the rest. A cumulative two-year-survival rate from the same series was 82.8% with the 5- and 10-year rates being 59 and 47.1%, respectively.[9]

REFERENCES

1. Abrahams, I.W., Fenton, R.H., and Vidone, R.: Alveolar soft-part sarcoma of the orbit. Arch Ophthal 79:185, 1968.
2. Asvall, J.E., Hoeg, K., Kleppe, K., and Prydz, P.: Alveolar soft part sarcoma. Clin Radiol 20:426, 1971.
3. Balfour, R.S.: The alveolar soft-part sarcoma: Review of the literature and report of case. J Oral Surg 32:214, 1974.
4. Blumberg, M.B., and Chang, C.H.J.: Alveolar soft part sarcoma. South Med J 69:282, 1976.
5. Christopherson, W.M., Foote, F.W., and Stewart, F.W.: Alveolar soft-part sarcomas. Structurally characteristic tumors of uncertain histogenesis. Cancer 5:100, 1952.
6. Fisher, E.R.: Histochemical observations on an alveolar soft-part sarcoma with reference to histogenesis. Am J Pathol 32:721, 1956.
7. Fisher, E.R., and Reidbord, H.: Electron microscopic evidence suggesting the myogenous derivation of the so-called alveolar soft part sarcoma. Cancer 27:150, 1972.
8. Furey, J.G., Barrett, D.L., and Seibert, R.H.: Alveolar soft-part sarcoma. Report of a case presenting as a sacral bone tumor. J Bone Joint Surg 51A:185, 1969.

9. Lieberman, P.H., Foote, F.W., Stewart, F.W., and Berg, J.W.: Alveolar soft-part sarcoma. *JAMA* **198:**121, 1966.

10. McGlamory, J.C., and Harris, J.O.: Alveolar soft-part sarcoma. *Chest* **62:**762, 1972.

11. Olson, R.A.J., and Perkins, K.D.: Alveolar soft-part sarcoma in the oral cavity: Report of case. *J Oral Surg* **34:**73, 1976.

12. Rosenbaum, A.E., Gabrielsen, T.O., Harris, H., and Goldberg, S.: Cerebral manifestations of alveolar soft-part sarcoma. *Radiology* **99:**109, 1971.

13. Rubenfeld, S.: Radiation therapy in alveolar soft part sarcoma. *Cancer* **28:**577, 1971.

14. Unni, K.K., and Soule, H.H.: Alveolar soft part sarcoma. An electron microscopic study. *Mayo Clin Proc* **50:**591, 1975.

87

Malignant Fibroxanthoma
(Malignant Fibrous Histiocytoma)

THE TUMORS BELONG to the general group of fibrous lesions. The histological classification within this group has been often confusing due to a multitude of overlapping terms representing a multitude of clinical entities. These entities vary with regard to natural history, patient age, tumor location, and symptomatology.[5,7,8,10,14]

Ozzello et al.[11] were able to demonstrate that histiocytomas and fibroxanthomas have identical behavior in tissue cultures, thus presuming through their study a common origin. It is believed that the parent cell is the histiocyte, which can act not only as a phagocyte but also as a fibroblast—histiocytic facultative fibroblast—and thus it can form connective tissue fiber.[11]

The lesions derived from the histiocytic facultative fibroblast are numerous. Their clinical spectrum is very wide, ranging from the keloids to the undifferentiated fibrosarcoma.

O'Brien and Stout[10] reviewed a group of 1516 cases of fibrous lesions that at the time of their writing were considered to belong to the fibrous xanthomas group. Included were fibrous xanthomas, dermatofibrosarcoma protuberans, giant cell tumors, and villonodular synovitis of the soft tissues. Among the 1516 cases, they identified 15 tumors that behaved in an unquestionably malignant fashion and this group they called "malignant fibrous xanthomas." Thus, they represented 1% of the fibrous xanthomas group.[10]

The lesions have been seen in patients of all ages from the very young to the elderly and no definite age peak has been identified.[7,10,14] There is a clear male predominance. In the original series by O'Brien and Stout[10] 80% of the patients were males. In subsequent reviews the ratio of male to female has been 2:1.[8,10,14]

PATHOLOGY

Grossly, they are often associated with the skin, presenting as subcutaneous nodules or masses. Their color may vary from white-pink, gray-tan to yellow. The yellow color might be throughout the entire tumor or it might appear in the form of flecks or streaks.[7,10] Ulceration may eventually develop.[8] The lesions may be seated deeply below the skin, arising from the deep subcutaneous tissues. The extremities are common sites of involvement.[14] More recently malignant fibrous histiocytomas have often been reported in the head and neck region where they occur as masses involving soft tissues and bones.

Microscopically, a spectrum of histological presentations are to be encountered. They are histologically complex, and several cell types, including fibroblasts, histiocytes, and multinucleated giant cells participate in their histology (Fig. 87-1).

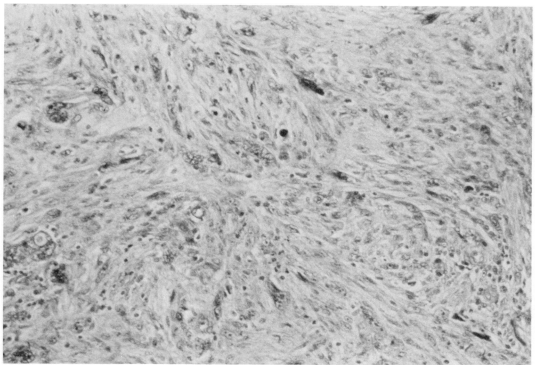

FIG. 87-1.   Malignant fibrous histiocytoma. Spindle cell stroma with bizarre multinucleated giant cells and foam cells.

Ozzello *et al.*[11] demonstrated conclusively through tissue culture studies that malignant histiocytomas and fibrous xanthomas derive from histiocytes, which are neoplastic in character and which can transform themselves into fibroblasts, giving rise to either histiocytomas or to fibrous xanthomas. It is now considered that dermatofibrosarcoma protuberans, malignant fibrous xanthomas (fibroxanthomas), atypical fibroxanthomas of the skin, fibrous xanthoma, histiocytoma, and malignant histiocytoma are all included under the same heading as tumors derived from histiocytes.

CLINICAL

The clinical presentation is that of a nodular lesion developing into a soft tissue mass, usually painless. Pain might accompany the tumor later on. At times,

rapid growth with bone involvement may occur (Fig. 87-2). Ulceration of the overlying skin is also a late event.[7] In many cases the patients stated that a mass was present for several years prior to the time of the diagnosis.[8,10,14]

There is a preference in terms of location, favoring the extremities and particularly the thigh. The tumors are to be found superficially or deep to the fascia within the extremities. They have been seen in the retroperitoneum, the chest wall, and the skin as well[5,8,10,12] (Fig. 87-3). There are several in the head and neck region. Malignant fibrous xanthomas have occurred in the larynx, maxilla, scalp, temporal bone, pharynx, mandible, and in the paranasal sinuses.[1-3,9,13,15,16]

Malignant fibroxanthomas have characteristically a high rate of local recurrence, which was reported to be 49% in the series by O'Brien and Stout.[10] In the series

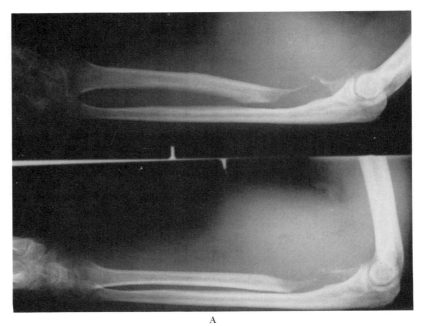

A

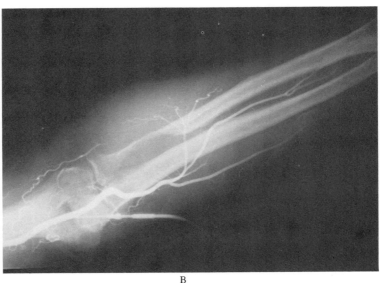

B

FIG. 87-2.   Malignant fibroxanthoma in a 76-year-old male. Tumor arising within the soft tissues of the forearm, recurring twice after local resection. Soft tissue view readily reveals the mass and the destruction of the proximal radius (*A*). Branchial arteriogram shows displacement of the branchial and radial arteries medially by the large tumor mass. The neoplasm is poorly vascularized, perfused by branches of the recurrent radial artery and of the radial collateral (*B*).

by Soule and Enriquez[14] the recurrence rate was 73%. They are multiple, occurring at frequent intervals despite wide local excisions.[14]

The incidence of distant metastases is also high. Approximately 25–30% of all tumors will metastasize to the regional lymph nodes and the lungs.[10,14]

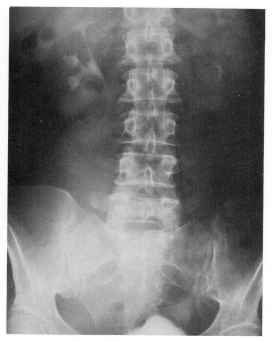

FIG. 87-3. Malignant fibrous histiocytoma in a 58-year-old female. There is a large retroperitoneal tumor seen as a soft tissue density producing stasis in the right pelvocaliceal system and compressing the superior aspect of the urinary bladder.

TREATMENT AND RESULTS

Surgical resection is the recommended treatment. It has been emphasized by all authors dealing with the subject that this should include a very adequate margin beyond the clinical boundaries of the tumor in order to prevent local recurrence. Of course, since the percentage of fibroxanthomas that pursue a malignant course is in the range of 1%, it is only through the clinical history and the behavior of the lesion that aggressive therapy will be dictated. Those that recur locally, invade underlying bone, ulcerate, or grow rapidly, as well as tumors large in size at the time of presentation, should be considered as locally aggressive and potentially lethal. The neoplasms tend to infiltrate along fascias and to extend deeper than clinically apparent, thus resulting in a high number of local recurrences.

By most accounts, radiation therapy appears to be incapable of containing the disease. Reports in the literature indicate that tumor dosages in the vicinity of 5500 to 6500 rad have failed locally to eradicate malignant fibrous xanthomas and malignant histiocytomas.[4,9,15,16] It is particularly important for tumors occurring in the head and neck region to keep in mind the radioresistance of this neoplasm. The treatment should rely solely on surgical resection and limited excisions planned in conjunction with radiation therapy will result in recurrence.

PROGNOSIS AND SURVIVAL

O'Brien and Stout[10] concluded that the histological differentiation between benign and malignant forms of fibrous histiocytomas may be difficult. Their mitotic rate counted in 50 high-power fields was an entirely unreliable index. The depth of tumor origin was likewise unreliable. Malignant behavior has been exhibited not only in tumors arising in the subcutaneous tissues but also in a number of those arising in the skin. On the other hand, the size, if in excess of 5–6 cm, is a good indicator of aggressiveness.[8,10]

In children the great majority of histiocytic tumors are benign in character, not exhibiting evidence of biological malignancy. Nevertheless, malignant forms have been reported and deaths have occurred from disseminated disease.[6] Therefore age is a limited prognostic criterion.

The survival rates are difficult to classify, since the aggressive behavior of the tumors even within the same histological subclassification varies from patient to patient. In the study by Soule and Enriquez,[14] the five-year survival for atypical fibrous histiocytomas was 90%, for malignant fibrous histiocytomas, 65%, and for malignant histiocytomas, 50%. The respective 10-year-survival rates were 82%, 38%, and 0%. The authors have reserved the designation of atypical fibroxanthoma only for skin lesions.[14]

Once metastasis develops, the prognosis is poor. O'Brien and Stout[10] had 15 patients with metastatic disease. Twelve of them died of their tumor within two years from the excision, one died of recurrent disease eight years later, and two were surviving with malignancy present.

REFERENCES

1. Barney, P.L.: Atypical fibrous histiocytoma (fibroxanthoma) of the temporal bone. *Trans Am Acad Ophthalmol Otolaryngol* **76**:1392, 1972.
2. Berschadsky, M., Gianetti, C.D., David, A., and LoVerme, S.R.: Atypical fibroxanthoma in the pharynx. Case report. *Plast Reconstr Surg* **52**:443, 1973.
3. Canalis, R.F., Green, M., Konard, H.R., Hirose, F.M., and Cooper, S.: Malignant fibrous xanthoma (xanthofibrosarcoma) of the larynx. *Arch Otolaryngol* **101**:135, 1975.
4. Jahrsdoerfer, R.A., Sweet, D.E., and Fitz-Hugh, G.S.: Malignant fibrous xanthoma with metastasis to cerebellopontine angle. *Arch Otolaryngol* **102**:117, 1976.
5. Kahn, L.B.: Retroperitoneal xanthogranuloma and xanthosarcoma (malignant fibrous xanthoma). *Cancer* **31**:411, 1973.
6. Kauffman, S.L., and Stout, A.P.: Histiocytic tumors (fibrous xanthoma and histiocytoma) in children. *Cancer* **14**:469, 1961.
7. Kempson, R.L., and Kyriakos, M.: Fibroxanthosarcoma of the soft tissues. A type of malignant fibrous histiocytoma. *Cancer* **29**:961, 1972.
8. Kempson, R.L., and McGavran, M.H.: Atypical fibroxanthomas of the skin. *Cancer* **17**:1463, 1964.
9. Norris, C.W.: Fibroxanthosarcoma of the neck. *Trans Am Acad Ophthalmol Otolaryngol* **80**:468, 1975.
10. O'Brien, J.E., and Stout, A.P.: Malignant fibrous xanthomas. *Cancer* **17**:1445, 1964.
11. Ozzello, L., Stout, A.P., and Murray, M.R.: Cultural characteristics of malignant histiocytomas and fibrous xanthomas. *Cancer* **16**:331, 1963.
12. Rosas-Uribe, A., Ring, A.M., and Rappaport, H.: Metastasizing retroperitoneal fibroxanthoma (malignant fibroxanthoma). *Cancer* **26**:827, 1970.
13. Solomon, M.P., and Sutton, A.L.: Malignant fibrous histiocytoma of the soft tissues of the mandible. *Oral Surg* **35**:653, 1973.
14. Soule, E.H., and Enriquez, P.: Atypical fibrous histiocytoma, malignant fibrous histiocytoma, malignant histiocytoma, and epithelioid sarcoma. A comparative study of 65 tumors. *Cancer* **30**:128, 1972.
15. Spector, G.J., and Ogura, J.H.: Malignant fibrous histiocytoma of the maxilla. A report of an unusual lesion. *Arch Otolaryngol* **99**:385, 1974.
16. Townsend, G.L., Neel, H.B., III, Weiland, L.H., Devine, K.D., and McBean, J.B.: Fibrous histiocytoma of the paranasal sinuses. Report of a case. *Arch Otolaryngol* **98**:51, 1973.

PART 3

UNCOMMON TUMORS SITE-SPECIFIC

88

Esthesioneuroblastoma

BERGER *et al.*[2] in 1924 were the first to describe a neoplasm in the nasal fossa containing olfactory neuroepithelial elements. They designated the tumor as olfactory esthesioneuroepithelioma. In subsequent reports the tumors were further subdivided into esthesioneuroepithelioma, esthesioneurocytoma, and esthesioneuroblastoma, on the basis of their microscopic appearance.[4] However, for practical purposes, all authors agree that the subdivisions represent various aspects of differentiation of the same tumor.[3,6]

The growth usually involves some area of the olfactory mucosa. The most plausible explanation with regard to the site of origin is the one advanced by Berger *et al.*,[2] who suggested the neuroepithelial cells of the olfactory membrane. This membrane contains neuroepithelial elements and tall epithelial olfactory cells.[9] Other possibilities of histogenetic derivation, according to Schall and Lineback,[11] include the olfactory placode, which is the primordium of the olfactory organ in the embryo, the organ of Jacobson, a vestigial organ in man located in some people in the lower anterior part of the nasal septum, and the sphenopalatine ganglion. The latter two sites, however, do not correspond well with the position where early small esthesioneuroblastomas have been found.[11] Sympathetic fibers of the nasal mucosa as well as ganglion cells from the nervus terminalis have been considered as potential sites.[1]

Herrold[5] has demonstrated the development of neuroepithelial tumors in Syrian hamsters by means of subcutaneous diethylnitrosamine injection. These tumors arise in the olfactory epithelium and are similar to the human esthesioneuroblastomas. This work raises the question of carcinogenic initiation of this tumor process in human beings.

The majority of tumors are to be found in young adults but esthesioneuroblastomas have been seen in all ages, from 3 to 79 years.[1,10] The peak incidence is, however, between 10 and 40 years, with 66% of the cases occurring within this age span.[1,10]

There is a slight male predominance.[1]

PATHOLOGY

The gross appearance is that of a polypoid red tumor, usually soft in consistency and quite vascular. Histologically, they share many features with the neuroblastomas. They are composed of nervous tissue. Neuroblasts and neurocytes are present and there may be a predominance of the one or the other cell type.[6] The neuroblasts resemble lymphocytes with a round or oval nucleus and scant cytoplasm (Fig. 88-1). The neurocytes have similarly round or oval nuclei, but in addition they have a distinct cytoplasm that is either tapered or presents as an elongated process. These processes are called neurofibrils and are helpful in making the diagnosis.[6]

Gerard-Marchant and Micheau[4] distin-

273

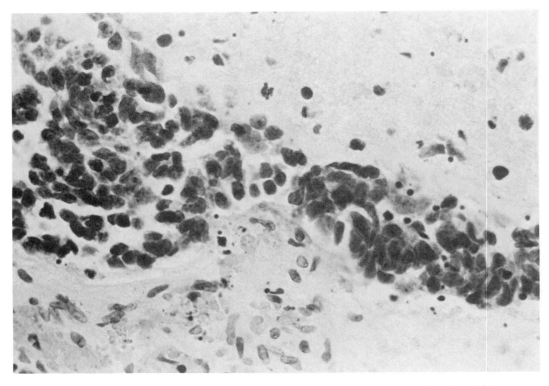

FIG. 88-1. Esthesioneuroblastoma. Clusters of small cells with hyperchromatic nuclei. The field contains areas of hemorrhage.

guish three histological types. 1) Olfactory esthesioneuroepithelioma, which has an epithelial component that serves as the supporting stroma and a nerve component that corresponds to the olfactory cells. Rosettes are the main features of this variety, being composed of epithelial elements. They consist of several rows of cells arranged around the central cavity, which is clearly outlined. The nerve cells resemble lymphocytes, as already described, with a hardly visible cytoplasm. 2) Olfactory esthesioneurocytoma, which has no epithelial supporting elements and may be confused with a lymphoma or an anaplastic carcinoma. The cells show a more or less regular diffuse distribution. 3) Finally, olfactory esthesioneuroblastoma contains many fibrils with which the central space of the rosette is filled; this is called pseudorosette.

Winestock et al.[15] suggest that the pres-

ence of chromaffin granules indicates a derivation from primitive neural crest cells. The adrenal medulla and the sympathetic paraganglia in the adult are of neural crest origin.

CLINICAL

The neoplasm is located in the nasal cavity. It arises from the olfactory epithelium in the roof of the nose and it grows downward into the nasal cavity, into the nasopharynx posteriorly, laterally into the ethmoids and the maxillary sinuses, and upward through the cribriform plate into the anterior fossa. It is a vascular tumor that bleeds easily, either spontaneously or on slight touch. For this reason, the commonest presenting symptom is unilateral nasal bleeding associated with nasal obstruction.[6,10,13] Other symptoms, as the tumor enlarges, include the presence of a tumor mass protruding through the nos-

trils, frontal headaches, and excessive lac-
rimation.[4] Anosmia is a less frequent
finding.[10] With progressing growth, erosion of the adjacent osseous structures
takes place and particularly of the medial
orbital wall, with the mass entering into
the retroorbital space and producing proptosis.[13]

On physical examination, the mass fills
the nasal fossa and the inferior aspect of it
is readily visible through the nostrils. Occasionally, a tumor component is found in
the nasopharynx. Radiographic examination of the sinuses in the early phase
shows clouding due to the presence of
tumor. The ethmoid sinuses, the maxillary
antrum, and the frontal sinuses are those
usually involved.[8] In more advanced cases
tomography will show bone destruction.
As stated, the ethmoids and in particular
the medial wall of the orbit are very vul-
nerable to this development. Arteriography discloses a vascular lesion that may
derive its blood supply from both the
internal and the external carotid arteries. It
is useful in demonstrating extensions,
particularly those occurring within the
cranium. More recently, computerized
transaxial tomography has been excellent
in outlining the tumor (Fig. 88-2).

Following extension within the
cranium, there is tumor propagation along
the meninges to the extent that it can be
found in the posterior fossa. These are
tumor implants, meningeal in character,
with the brain displaced rather than invaded. Distant metastases occur in
20–30% of the cases.

The most common sites involved have
been the cervical lymph nodes and the
lungs. Less commonly, the bones and
thoracic and abdominal lymph nodes have
been reported as showing metastatic deposits.[1,4,12]

TREATMENT AND RESULTS

By all indications, surgical therapy is
the treatment of choice. The question,
however, frequently posed is whether or

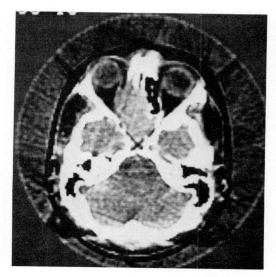

FIG. 88-2. Esthesioneuroblastoma in a 24-year-old
male. The tumor occupies the left nasal cavity, the
ethmoids bilaterally, the sphenoid sinus, and extends into the left medial orbit.

not surgery is feasible. In spite of the
marked radiosensitivity that has been
witnessed by practically all authors, this
neoplasm is not radiocurable. Apparently
residual disease is the rule following
radiotherapy, and from this recurrence
eventually develops. Because of the intri-
cate anatomy of the lesion, the extent of
resection is subject to limitations. It has
been suggested that a combined approach
of preoperative irradiation followed by
surgery might offer the best potential for
survival.

Lewis et al.[8] reviewed their experience
in terms of treatment and results at Memorial Hospital. The authors were pessimistic about the effectiveness of either modality. The recurrence rate was 100%,
regardless of whether surgery or
radiotherapy were used initially. The
five-year-survival rate was 50% and the
average life-span was six years.[8] Mendeloff[10] reported on six cases, all of whom
experienced recurrent or persistent disease. Three of the patients were treated to
what is considered adequate dose level, in
excess of 6400 rad.

Tingwald reported seven cases of olfactory tumors treated by combination therapy, mostly by surgery and postoperative radiotherapy. Chemotherapy was given for persistent tumors. There were five patients surviving for periods ranging from one to seven years without obvious disease and two patients living with tumor. These exceptionally good results raise some question about the accuracy of the histology.[13] Winestock et al.[15] preoperatively irradiated an 11-year-old male at 6000 rad in 25 treatment sessions. The treatments were given to the right antrum, ethmoid sinuses, orbit, and medial half of the nose. Subsequently, through a Caldwell–Luc approach, the area was cleared of the residual tumor, to the cribriform plate superiorly, sphenoid sinus posteriorly, and the eustachian tube laterally. A 16-year follow-up has been recurrence-free.[15]

Bailey and Barton[1] reported in 1975 on three cases of combined surgery and radiation therapy. The patients were surviving for three, five, and seven years, respectively, without signs of disease. Kadish et al.[7] expressed limited confidence that radiotherapy might control certain tumors. In their series of 17 patients, four were treated exclusively by irradiation. Of these one was surviving for 3.5 years without evidence of disease. The patient had an early lesion and received a total tumor dose of 5300 rad. In line with the rest of the reports the authors recommend a combined approach, using radiation therapy and surgery. They have proposed a system of staging, designating as a Group A, tumors limited to the nasal cavity; Group B, tumors localized to the nasal cavity and paranasal sinuses; and Group C, tumors extending beyond the nasal cavity and paranasal sinuses. For neoplasms of Group A and B, preoperative radiotherapy at a level of 5000 rad in 5–6 weeks to be followed by surgical resection is recommended. For Group C lesions, radiation at higher dosage levels (6000 to 7500 rad in seven weeks) is recommended, to be followed by resection of the residual disease if such a procedure is feasible.[7]

In our experience, in spite of the striking radiosensitivity, high radiation dosages failed to control the tumor in two recently treated patients. The first was a 24-year-old male with an extensive tumor involving the sphenoid and ethmoid sinuses, as well as the left maxillary antrum and left retroorbital space, and extending into the anterior fossa. He received 6500 rad to the tumor area by means of a 6 MeV linear accelerator. Following a complete clinical remission with actual radiographic restoration of the destroyed medial orbital wall, the patient developed recurrence eight months later. He was reirradiated, receiving 4000 rad in combination with intravenous cyclophosphamide and DTIC. He had a temporary response, which was followed by a series of recurrences and partial regressions to chemotherapy. The drugs were intravenous injections of cyclophosphamide in combination with DTC, and, later on, cyclophosphamide with Adriamycin. Eventually, he died from his tumor with intracranial extension two years after the initial diagnosis.

The second patient, a 20-year-old male presented with tumor in both nostrils and in the nasopharynx. He received 6480 rad as preoperative radiotherapy, which resulted in complete clinical remission. Following this, he underwent resection of the superior nasal turbinates and of the cribriform plate. Residual disease was indeed found in the apex of the nasal cavity. The patient has done well in the ensuing 2.5 years.

On the basis of this, it appears that a combined modality therapy with preoperative irradiation and surgical resection to follow offers the best chance of cure. It is to be said, however, that repeated courses of radiation as well as systemic chemotherapy may affectively prolong the life in patients with recurrent disease.

PROGNOSIS AND SURVIVAL

Whether or not the histological appearance is helpful in terms of prognosticating the outcome remains a point of conjecture. Gerard-Marchant and Micheau[4] suggest that olfactory esthesioepithelioma appears to be more malignant than the rest of the varieties and implicate the presence of rosettes in the malignant behavior. In their experience this variety showed the largest number of recurrences and the largest number of metastases. Lewis *et al.*[8] similarly noted that all their patients whose tumors contained rosettes died from their disease. Absence of rosettes or the presence of pseudorosettes was not necessarily associated with a good prognosis.[8]

Bailey and Barton,[2] reviewing 50 determinate cases from the literature, found the five-year cure rate without signs of recurrence in the interim to be 18%. The survey showed that an additional 10% of the patients were alive at five years with active disease present and 24% had succumbed to their illness beyond the five-year point. Actually, 38% of the patients died from their disease, having survived more than five years. On the basis of this collective review, the five-year-survival rate is approximately 50%; however, included are patients who have been cured from their tumor as well as those who are alive with disease. The same review showed that the best prospects were among patients who had been treated by a combination of surgery and radiation therapy. Their five-year-survival rate was 67%.[1]

Kadish *et al.*[7] obtained 100% three-year-survival for patients whose lesions were limited to the nasal cavity (Group A), 80% three-year survival for those whose tumors extended into the paranasal sinuses (Group B), and 40% three-year survival for tumors extending beyond these structures (Group C).

REFERENCES

1. Bailey, B.J., and Barton, S.: Olfactory neuroblastoma. *Arch Otolaryngol* **101**:1, 1975.
2. Berger, L., Luc, and Richard: L'esthésioneuroépithéliome olfactif. *Bull Assoc Franc Etude Cancer* **13**:410, 1924.
3. Castro, L., De La Pava, S., and Webster, J.H.: Esthesioneuroblastomas. A report of 7 cases. *AJR* **105**:7, 1969.
4. Gerard-Marchant, R., and Micheau, C.: Microscopical diagnosis of olfactory esthesioneuromas: General review and report of five cases. *J Nat Cancer Inst* **35**:75, 1965.
5. Herrold, K.M.: Induction of olfactory neuroepithelial tumors in Syrian hamsters by diethylnitrosamine. *Cancer* **17**:114, 1964.
6. Hutter, R.V.P., Lewis, J.S., Foote, F.W., Jr., and Tollefsen, H.R.: Esthesioneuroblastoma. A clinical and pathological study. *Am J Surg* **106**:748, 1963.
7. Kadish, S., Goodman, M., and Wang, C.C.: Olfactory neuroblastoma. A clinical analysis of 17 cases. *Cancer* **37**:1571, 1976.
8. Lewis, J.S., Hutter, R.V.P., Tollefsen, H.R., and Foote, F.W., Jr.: Nasal tumors of olfactory origin. *Arch Otolaryngol* **81**:169, 1965.
9. McCormack, L.J., and Harris, H.E.: Neurogenic tumors of nasal fossa. *JAMA* **157**:318, 1955.
10. Mendeloff, J.: The olfactory neuroepithelial tumors. A review of the literature and report of six additional cases. *Cancer* **10**:944, 1956.
11. Schall, L.A., and Lineback, M.: Primary intranasal neuroblastoma. Report of 3 cases. *Ann Otol Rhinol Laryngol* **60**:221, 1951.
12. Skolnik, E.M., Massari, F.S., and Tenta, L.T.: Olfactory neuroepithelioma. Review of the world literature and presentation of two cases. *Arch Otolaryngol* **84**:644, 1966.
13. Tingwald, F.R.: Olfactory placode tumors. *Laryngoscope* **76**:196, 1966.
14. Tyler, T.C., Chandler, J.R., Wetli, C., and Moffitt, B.M.: Olfactory neuroblastoma. *South Med J* **67**:640, 1974.
15. Winestock, D.P., Lansdown, E.L., Hammonic, M., and Meikle, A.L.: Esthesioneuroblastoma: A radiologic correlation. *J Assoc Can Radiol* **23**:38, 1972.

89

Chordoma

CHORDOMAS ORIGINATE from remnants of the embryonic notochord, which is the primitive skeleton of the vertebrates. They are rare neoplasms of low malignancy and they can be clinically separated into three groups on the basis of their location: cranial, sphenooccipital, or nasopharyngeal (36%); vertebral (15%); sacrococcygeal (49%).[5,8,9]

The notochord in the embryo extends from the sphenooccipital junction to the coccyx and as the development progresses during the fourth fetal week, mesodermal tissue surrounds it. In the sixth week cartilage forms the precursors of the vertebral bodies.[7] As the vertebral bodies and intervertebral discs are formed, the notochord disappears, the main remnant of it being the nucleus pulposus of the intervertebral disc. In addition, remnants of notochord may be found near the midline in the cephalic end of the notochord. These are located between the odontoid process of the axis and the occipital bone, in the clivus, in the dorsum sellae, and in the retropharyngeal region. There is accumulated evidence to suggest that from these remnants the cranial chordomas arise.[14] At the caudal end of the spinal axis, a coiling takes place by which the number of the distal vertebrae is reduced. During this time, detached masses of notochord can be found inside the coccygeal and sacral vertebral bodies and they are well seen in a 16-week-old embryo. It is probable that from these notochordal deposits chordomas originate later in life.[7,10]

The tumors have been reported in all age groups, from infancy to the very old.[2,5,9] In general, sphenooccipital chordomas are seen in younger patients than the sacrococcygeal ones. In the series by Dahlin and MacCarty[5] the average age was 38 years for the former and 53 years for the latter.[5,12] In the series by Higinbotham *et al.*[9] sphenooccipital chordomas were seen between the ages of 10 and 39, whereas most of the patients with sacral lesions were in the fifth and sixth decades. In yet another series by Windeyer[16] the average age of patients with tumors in the sacrococcygeal region was 49 years, as opposed to 36 years for the remainder. There is a sex predilection, the ratio of male to female patients being 2:1 in most series.[5,9,11]

PATHOLOGY

Grossly, the tumors are lobulated, fairly smooth, and mucoid in appearance, actually at times quite soft. Calcifications and hemorrhages may be present. The neoplasm destroys the bone of its origin; however, as far as the surrounding soft tissues are concerned, they are primarily displaced rather than invaded and infiltrated.[5]

Histologically, the tumor cells are arranged in cords. The cytoplasms often form a syncytium. There is abundant extracellular mucus in the background of these formations in most cases. In addition, there is intracellular mucus in the form of cytoplasmic vacuoles. These vac-

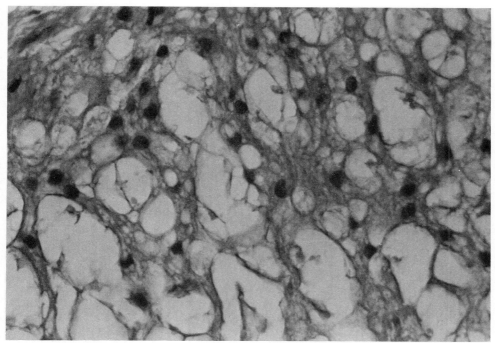

FIG. 89-1. Chordoma. Physaliphorous cells, in various degrees of development, containing mucus.

uoles vary in size from barely visible to very large, which actually are the characteristic physaliphorous cells of chordomas[1,5] (Fig. 89-1).

CLINICAL

Due to the slow growth, the tumors produce initially mild and intermittent symptoms and for this reason in the usual case there is a lengthy interval between the original presentation and the diagnosis. We will consider the symptomatology according to the anatomical location.

Cranial

Headache is a common sign for tumors with a nasopharyngeal presentation. This is mostly felt in the frontal and orbital areas, and visual disturbances, such as loss of acuity, diplopia, limitation of the visual fields, ptosis, and paralysis of the eye muscles, are common. Other cranial nerves involved are the trigeminal, the facial, and the acoustic. If there is an intracranial extension, hypophyseal and pontine symptoms appear. The diplopia is usually attributed to the oculomotor and the abducens nerves.[1,5,8] There is a clear tendency for the cranial nerve involvement to be unilateral. Epistaxis may occur in the case of nasopharyngeal chordomas. These tumors may be readily visible on examination in the postnasal space. In the cervical chordomas retropharyngeal or lateral neck masses develop.[11] There is a large variation of the time interval between the onset of symptoms and the diagnosis, which, according to the published reports, spans periods from a few weeks to 14 years. Usually, the interval has been between six months and three years.[8]

Radiographs of the skull reveal the osteolytic lesion occurring in various portions of the sphenoid bone, producing destruction of the clivus, the dorsum sellae, the posterior clinoid processes, and the sella floor (Fig. 89-2). Extension into the sphenoid sinus and the nasopharynx can also be noted. Calcifications within the mass have been stressed as a diagnostic feature by Heffelfinger et al.[8] and Wood and Himadi.[17] It has to be noted, however, that none of the five cases of nasopharyngeal chordomas described by Batsakis and Kittleson[1] contained calcium. Pneumoencephalograms have disclosed consistent abnormalities in the area of the third ventricle, cerebral aqueduct, and fourth ventricle. These structures have been displaced upward and posteriorly and filling defects are present in the basal cisterns. The dome of the mass can be seen posteriorly to the sella.[17]

Vertebral

Vertebral chordomas in the initial stage produce localized discomfort. As the tumors expand from the intervertebral discs into the vertebrae, bone destruction develops and compression fractures follow. Usually, one vertebral body is involved; however, the process may extend into a number of vertebrae.[6] Radiographically, the lesions are lytic and asymmetric and there is involvement of the intervertebral discs. Osteosclerosis may be seen frequently around the lytic areas. Associated with the bone destruction, soft tissue masses in the region of the compression may be seen (Fig. 89-3).

Sacrococcygeal

The earliest symptom is dull or intermittent pain that is felt in the region of the buttocks or in the rectum and the perineal area or it may follow the sciatic nerve distribution. Difficulty in walking can appear early. Similarly, due to nerve compression, difficulties from the bladder and the rectum may also appear. Later on, because of direct tumor extension and compression, urinary retention and constipation

occur.[7] Actually, constipation is the second commonest presenting symptom after pain.[5] Eventually, a lump in the pelvis is recognized, which on rectal examination is smoothly irregular, lobulated, fixed posteriorly, and usually large.[16] The duration of the symptoms is rather long. In the series by Dahlin and MacCarty[5] and MacCarty et al.[12] the average period was two years.

Radiographically, there are varying degrees of sacral destruction, which is associated with a simultaneous expansion of the bone, particularly in the anteroposterior diameter. In addition extraosseous tumor with areas of calcification can be seen in plain films of the pelvis. The commonest radiological findings to be seen are osteolysis and a soft tissue mass. Osteosclerosis and calcifications are seen in approximately 50% of the cases. Myelography reveals epidural defects or blocks and angiography has shown some tumor neovascularity, but primarily displacement of the normal vessels. Barium enema examination and intravenous pyelogram reveal extrinsic pressure defects upon the rectum and the bladder, best appreciated in the lateral projections[6] (Fig. 89-4).

Approximately 10% of the reported cases have been known to develop metastatic deposits. These occur late in the course of the illness, which, as we will be discussing, in most instances takes a long chronic course. The metastasizing tumors are to be found among the sacrococcygeal group. Vertebral chordomas only rarely metastasize and cranial chordomas probably never.[7] The common sites of metastatic deposits are the lungs and the liver.

TREATMENT AND RESULTS

The site of origin of these neoplasms is a very critical factor, which affects and limits the application of definitive surgery. For this reason and in spite of the fact that metastatic disease is very late and an infrequent development, surgical cures are

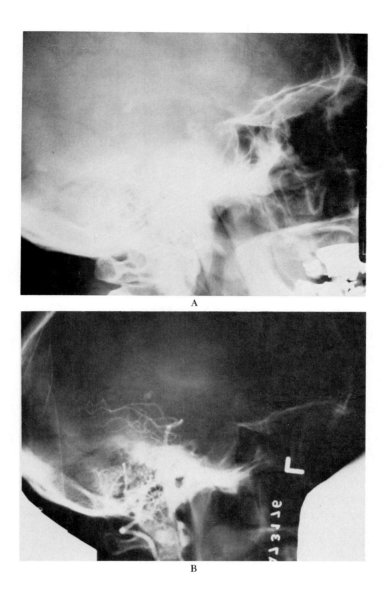

A

B

very uncommon. In all publications it is recognized that to devise a curative treatment is a difficult matter. Surgically, it is not possible to remove the base of the skull and it is not possible to remove the sacrum. Partial excision is excellent for palliation and many patients have been kept in good functional status for several years by this procedure.

Radiation therapy, although not curative, is quite effective in retarding the growth of the tumor and partially decreasing the size of it. In this way the useful life of the patient is considerably prolonged, in most cases for a number of years, and it also affords an overall lengthier survival.

The judicious combination of surgery and radiotherapy is essential for the optimal management of these patients.

In cranial tumors because of the location surgical intervention is indicated for biopsy, decompression, and shunting, to be followed by radiotherapy.[2,11] Ormerod[13] irradiated a nasopharyngeal

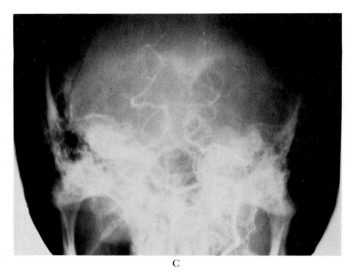

C

FIG. 89-2.   Chordoma of the clivus in a 44-year-old male. Lateral view of
the skull shows marked erosion of the posterior sella associated with
suprasellar calcifications (A). Left vertebral arteriogram shows marked
posterior displacement of the basilar artery by the tumor, especially
appreciated in the lateral view. (B) Asymmetry of the vessel is shown in
the anterioposterior projection (C).

chordoma at the level of 6157 rad. Two years later after local recurrence, an additional 3175 rad were delivered, which brought about the disappearance of the tumor. The patient was irradiated for a third time because of local recurrence, bringing the total dose of radiation to the nasopharynx to 13753 rad. The patient had a 13-year survival at the time of the report. A patient with clivus chordoma reported by Wood and Hamidi[17] was surviving for more than nine years following biopsy and external irradiation with a dose of 8000 rad to the tumor. The treatment had been given in eight series repeated at intervals over a total period of nine years. The same authors encountered a very sensitive nasopharyngeal chordoma in an 11-year-old boy which regressed completely following an estimated tumor dose of 2300 R with relief of the nasal obstruction and disappearance of the diplopia and the facial paresis. It is possible that in children chordomas are more radiosensitive.[17]

Boyle and Frank[3] reported on a 43-

year-old male with nasopharyngeal chordoma. The patient was irradiated by a cobalt therapy unit, receiving 6000 rad in 35 days. This was followed by partial tumor resection and the patient remained well until four years later, at which point the tumor recurred. A second course of radiation was given at the level of 5000 rad in 21 days. It was followed by one year's relief and a third local recurrence was managed by local radium placement. This resulted in regression of the mass. Eventually the patient died two years following his last treatment, surviving for a total of eight years. Richter et al.[15] reported on a 69-year-old man with a clivus chordoma and a large soft mass in the nasopharynx. The patient had impairment of several cranial nerves. Following biopsy, the nasopharynx was irradiated to 6630 rad. Initially, there was no obvious response; however, gradually the neurological symptoms disappeared and the patient was surviving without signs of recurrence 11 years later.[15]

Heffelfinger et al.[8] have drawn attention

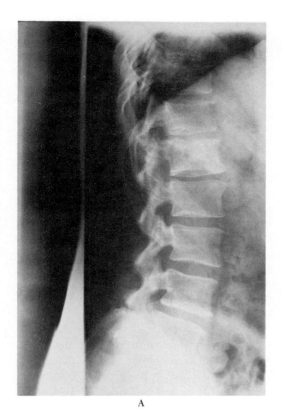

A

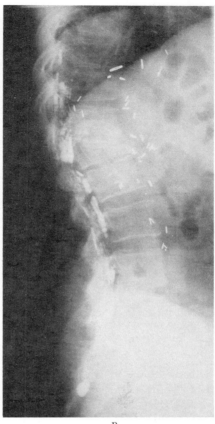

B

FIG. 89-3. Vertebral chordoma in a 59-year-old male. Lateral view of the lumbar spine demonstrates increased density of the L1 body associated with irregularity of the articular surfaces between L1 and T12 (*A*). Postoperative appearance. The lesion proved to be chordoma arising in the region of the T12-L1 vertebrae. The interspace now has disappeared and so has the inferior aspect of T12 and most of the superior anterior part of L1 following partial excision (*B*).

to a separate histological group of sphenooccipital chordomas that apparently exhibit a much better prognosis. The authors have designated a special group, the so-called "chondroid chordomas," which bear a histological similarity to chondromas or chondrosarcomas. They comprise approximately one-third of all chordomas and they have shown a greater curability by surgery and radiotherapy. For this reason, they also have a better prognosis.

Obviously there are many patients whose disease responds poorly and whose survival time is rather short.

For spinal, or vertebral, chordomas, partial resection and decompression laminectomy, if necessary, combined with external radiotherapy have been used.[11,14]

MacCarty *et al.*[12] reported on 18 patients with sacrococcygeal chordomas, who were evaluated and operated upon by a cooperative effort of neurosurgeons, general surgeons, and orthopedic surgeons. The coccyx was removed or posteriorly retracted and the rectum was freed from the coccyx and the sacrum. The tumor was identified during the surgical procedure and removed as completely as possible, preserving at the same time the nerves,

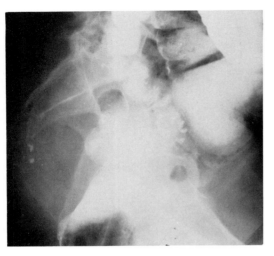

FIG. 89-4. Sacrococcygeal chordoma in a 56-year-old female. Lateral view during barium enema examination shows destruction with irregular margins of the inferior sacrum and of the coccyx. The rectum is markedly displaced anteriorly by a large soft tissue mass representing the neoplasm. Within it, characteristically, calcifications are seen.

especially the pudendal. The coccyx and the lower three sacral segments may be removed. Of the 18 patients, one died in the immediate postoperative period from a massive pulmonary embolus and another of coronary thrombosis 19 months following surgery. Four patients died because of their disease in 4, 4.5, 6, and 7 years after the original procedure. There were five patients alive with recurrent tumor and surviving five, six, seven, eight, and nine years, and there were seven patients alive without recurrent disease surviving 1, 2, 3, 4, 8, 9, and 12 years. Thus, among the long-term survivors, there are three patients surviving for 8, 9, and 12 years without evidence of recurrent tumor.[12]

Pearlman and Friedman[14] reviewed the radiation sensitivity of chordomas. This was accomplished by analyzing 81 cases from the literature plus 15 of their own. There was one patient surviving for 13 years following 8036 rad in 44 days deliv-ered for a sacral chordoma and an additional patient receiving similar amounts of radiation was surviving 10 years with disease present. In analyzing the tumor dosage necessary to produce a successful effect they concluded that 4000–6000 rad as a total tumor dose are more likely to fail than to succeed. On the contrary dosages from 6000–8000 rad have produced significant palliation or long intervals of apparent control.[14]

Partial excision is an excellent palliation and this in combination with sessions of radiation therapy to relatively high levels have provided most of the patients with a long-term survival and relatively useful life. The courses of radiation may be repeated and actually at times the second or third course appear to be more effective than the original.

We have participated in the management of six patients with chordoma. Two were cranial in location, one spinal at the L1–L2 level, and three were sacrococcygeal. Of the cranial, one patient died in the immediate postoperative period; the second was treated by radiation therapy, receiving 6000 rad in seven weeks. Stability was obtained for 14 months, at which time signs of recurrence developed. The patient with the vertebral chordoma underwent decompression laminectomy, during which the tumor was found extending from T12 to L2. Postoperative radiotherapy, 6000 rad in seven weeks, was administered. The patient has been active and well for two years. The treatment of the sacrococcygeal chordomas was a sequence of surgical and radiotherapeutic techniques. Two received definitive radiotherapy, 7000 rad in seven weeks and 8000 rad in eight weeks, whereas the third had multiple short radiation courses. All had surgical resection of their tumor. Their survival was 6, 7, and 10 years from the time of the diagnosis. They all died with active local disease; none had distant metastases.

PROGNOSIS AND SURVIVAL

Gray et al.[7] in a comprehensive literature review of 220 cases of sacrococcygeal
chordomas found the 10-year survival to
be approximately 15–20%. The average
life-span for those patients who succumbed to their tumor was 5.7 years.

As stated earlier, Heffelfinger et al.[8]
identified the good prognosis of the so-
called "chondroid chordoma" in the
sphenooccipital region; patients with this
particular histological type had a 60% 10-
year survival. Conversely, none of the patients with the typical form of chordoma
reached the 10-year mark. The average
survival time for the chondroid chordomas was 15.8 years, whereas the survival for the rest of the group was only 4.1
years.[8]

REFERENCES

1. Batsakis, J.G., and Kittleson, A.C.: Chordomas. *Arch Otolaryngol* **78**:168, 1963.
2. Becker, L.E., Yates, A.J., Hoffman, H.J., and Norman, M.G.: Intracranial chordoma in infancy. *J Neurosurg* **42**:349, 1975.
3. Boyle, T.M., and Frank, H.G.: The management of nasopharyngeal chordoma by repeated irradiation. *J Laryngol Otol* **80**:533, 1966.
4. Congdon, C.C.: Benign and malignant chordomas. A clinicoanatomical study of twenty-two cases. *Am J Pathol* **28**:793, 1952.
5. Dahlin, D.C., and MacCarty, C.S.: Chordoma. A study of fifty-nine cases. *Cancer* **5**:1170, 1952.
6. Firooznia, H., Pinto, R.S., Lin, J.P., Baruch, H.H., and Zausner, J.: Chordoma: Radiologic evaluation of 20 cases. *AJR* **127**:797, 1976.
7. Gray, S.W., Singhabhandhu, B., Smith, R.A., and Skandalakis, J.E.: Sacrococcygeal chordoma: Report of a case and review of the literature. *Surgery* **78**:573, 1975.
8. Heffelfinger, M.J., Dahlin, D.C., MacCarty, C.S., and Beabout, J.W.: Chordomas and cartilaginous tumors at the skull base. *Cancer* **32**:410, 1973.
9. Higinbotham, N.L., Phillips, R.F., Farr, H.W., and Hustu, H.O.: Chordoma. Thirty-five year study at Memorial Hospital. *Cancer* **20**:1841, 1967.
10. Horwitz, T.: Chordal ectopia and its possible relation to chordoma. *Arch Pathol* **31**:354, 1941.
11. Kamrin, R.P., Potanos, J.N., and Pool, J.L.: An evaluation of the diagnosis and treatment of chordoma. *J Neurol Neurosurg Psychiatry* **27**:157, 1964.
12. MacCarty, C.S., Waugh, J.M., Coventry, M.B., and O'Sullivan, D.C.: Sacrococcygeal chordomas. *Surg Gynecol Obstet* **113**:551, 1961.
13. Ormerod, R.: Case of chordoma presenting in nasopharynx. *J Laryngol Otol* **74**:245, 1960.
14. Pearlman, A.W., and Friedman, M.: Radical radiation therapy of chordoma. *AJR* **108**:333, 1970.
15. Richter, H.J., Batsakis, J.G., and Boles, R.: Chordomas: Nasopharyngeal presentation and atypical long survival. *Ann Otol Rhinol Laryngol* **84**:327, 1975.
16. Windeyer, B.W.: Chordoma. *Proc R Soc Med* **52**:1088, 1959.
17. Wood, E.H., and Himadi, G.M.: Chordomas: A roentgenologic study of sixteen cases previously unreported. *Radiology* **54**:706, 1950.
18. Wright, D.: Nasopharyngeal and cervical chordoma—some aspects in their development and treatment. *J Laryngol Otol* **81**:1337, 1967.

90

Chemodectoma of the Carotid Body

THE CAROTID BODIES are part of the chemoreceptor system and they function in parallel with the aortic bodies. These organs are stimulated by changes in the chemical composition of the arterial blood—Po_2, PCO_2, and H^+—reacting by reflex mechanism. Their reflexes are mediated through the vagus nerves affecting the blood pressure, the respiration, and the vascular resistance.

The normal carotid bodies are the largest collection of chemoreceptor cells, located in the posterior wall of the common carotid artery at the level of the bifurcation within the adventitia of the vessel. Their normal size is 5.0 by 5.0 mm and the neoplasia is the only known pathological condition that affects them.[8]

Carotid body tumors are the commonest chemodectomas, but even so only 500 cases have been reported in the literature since the original description of the tumor.[13]

Most chemodectomas are benign tumors, but a certain percentage pursue a malignant course. The incidence of malignancy among carotid body tumors has been in the range of 5–12%.[9,12] There is no striking sex predilection in the reported series.[4,8,9] Most patients at the time of the diagnosis are in their third or fourth decade.

PATHOLOGY

The carotid bodies, as is true of the rest of the chemoreceptor organs, are tissues of mural ectodermal origin. Macroscopically, the tumors of the carotid bodies are round in shape, encapsulated, and reddish in color. They attain sizes between 3 and 4 cm, classically located in the adventitia of the bifurcation of the common carotid artery, displacing away from each other the two branches and eventually encircling both the internal and the external carotid arteries. As the tumor enlarges at a later point, the vagus and the hypoglossal nerve may become involved.[5,8]

Histologically, they are composed of nests or clusters of epithelioid cells—"zellballen"—which are separated by a vascular and fibrous stroma. The vascularity varies within the tumor but it does represent a feature of this neoplasm. The individual cells are round, polygonal, or spindle-shaped, having a finely granular and faintly eosinophilic cytoplasm, a vesicular nucleus, and fairly prominent chromatin network and nucleolus (Fig. 90-1). The vascular spaces are lined by endothelial cells, although the principal tumor elements appear to be in direct contact with the blood.[3,8,9] Degenerative changes may be noted. There is no correlation between histology and future tumor behavior. Actually, infrequent mitotic figures were a feature of two metastasizing cases reported by Romanski.[11]

CLINICAL

The commonest presentation is that of a painless and otherwise asymptomatic

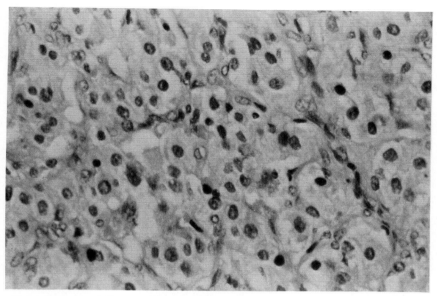

FIG. 90-1.   Chemodectoma of the carotid body. Organoid growth of cells separated by fine intervening stroma.

tumor mass that is felt in the neck just inferiorly to the angle of the mandible. Because the tumor is adherent to the carotid artery, the vertical mobility is restricted; however, it can be moved in a lateral direction. In most cases the patients admitted upon questioning that the mass had been present for many years, during which there has been a very slow and gradual growth.[5,8] Upon palpation, the mass is firm, and occasionally cystic or lobulated. In 5–10% of the cases extension into the parapharyngeal region produces a bulging that can be seen on oral examination.[8]

Blumenberg and Savlov,[2] in a retrospective review of the symptomatology of carotid body tumors, found that in approximately 10% of reported cases symptoms were present. Included were dysphagia, dyspnea, hoarseness of the voice, and the carotid sinus syndrome. All are related to direct extension into the adjacent structures and are the result of long-standing tumors.[10]

The slow growth has been pointed out by several authors. In a literature review by Monro[9] the average duration prior to the diagnosis was seven years.

Due to the rarity of the disease, correct diagnosis is made preoperatively in only 70% of the cases. The palpable neck mass at times exhibits a bruit. Evaluation of the oral cavity and the nasopharynx is necessary, since the tumor could conceivably represent metastatic lymphadenopathy. Roentgenograms of the sinuses and thyroid scans have been included in the work-up of these patients. Carotid arteriography will show in the typical case the internal carotid artery to be displaced laterally with a widening of the bifurcation. Carotid body tumors exhibit a vascular tumor stain[4,7] (Fig. 90-2).

There is no difference in presentation between benign and malignant chemodectomas. The main clinical manifestation of malignancy is local recurrence following local excision.[9] In most cases the tumor grows superiorly toward the base of the skull, but it may extend inferiorly toward the neck and the clavicle.[5]

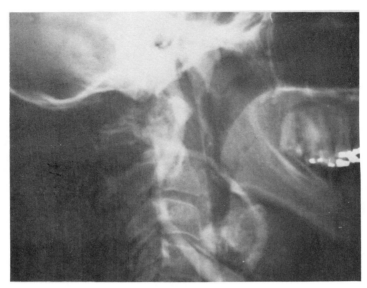

FIG. 90-2. Carotid body chemodectoma. Widening of the carotid bifurcation by a sizable tumor mass, which exhibits vascular blushing during arteriography.

Pathological bone fractures and compression of the spinal cord have resulted from metastatic deposits; however, it is also known that such deposits when occurring in the viscerae may be totally asymptomatic, being found only at autopsy.[10]

Fanning *et al.*[6] reported in 1963 a metastasizing carotid body tumor and reviewed previously published reports on an additional 25 such cases. About one-half of the metastases involved the regional lymph nodes and the remainder involved distant visceral sites, especially the lungs. The primary tumors, as a rule, had been present for several years before metastasizing.[6] The skeletal system, especially the vertebral bodies and the ribs have also been reported as metastatic sites[3] (Fig. 90-3).

In spite the rarity of metastases, a long follow-up is required, since patients have been reported developing such lesions for 7, 11, 14, and even 15 years following the tumor resection.[3,9]

Rapid growth, fixation of the tumor, local invasion into the surrounding tissues, and bony destruction are findings suggesting malignant behavior, regardless of the microscopic appearance, according to Conley.[5] In his review of 29 cases, the incidence of malignant carotid body tumors was less than 10%.

TREATMENT AND RESULTS

Surgical resection has traditionally been the treatment of choice. To be sure, chemodectomas are radioresistant tumors in the sense that they do not disappear after a course of definitive radiotherapy. However, as the experience in treating chemodectomas of the glomus jugulare has shown, arrest of the tumor growth and regression of the symptoms may be obtained.

Surgical removal, provided that operative complications are kept to a minimum, is a more definitive form of therapy. In recent years with the advent of angiography and vascular surgery, most carotid body tumors can be safely removed without interrupting the carotid circulation by a subadventitial approach.[4,13] The earlier

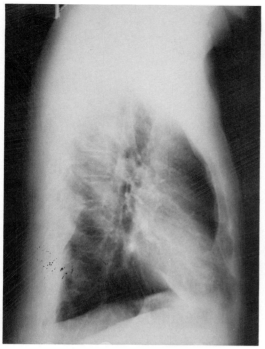 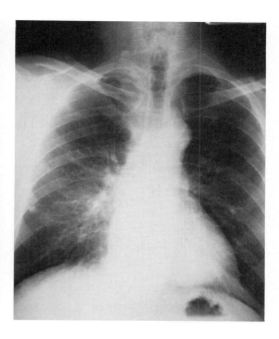

FIG. 90-3.   Chemodectoma of the right carotid body in a 65-year-old male. Partial resection of the right carotid body tumor nine years earlier. The patient returned with local recurrence, seen as a soft tissue swelling in the region of the right neck, and metastases to the cervical and thoracic epidural space, as well as to the posterior aspect of the right eighth rib.

practiced ligation of the internal carotid artery carried with it a 30% operative morbidity and mortality. Certainly, this is an unacceptable rate, far exceeding the risk from the tumor itself.[1] The mortality rate, when dissection is performed, is in the range of 6.5%.[9]

Chambers and Mahoney[4] reported a patient with an unresectable lesion who was treated by radiotherapy, receiving a total of 8000 R in intermittent dosages. The treatment afforded the patient a 20-year life-span. It is an observation that is in line with the results obtained by applying radiotherapy to tumors of the glomus jugulare.

Carotid body tumors are generally benign in character, the incidence of malignancy being 12%.[9] It is against this clinical background that judgment as to the applicable therapeutic modality should be made.

PROGNOSIS AND SURVIVAL

Death directly due to progressive growth of the tumor in patients for whom no therapy was attempted or whose therapy was inadequate occurred in 8% of such cases.[1]

Metastasizing tumors have afforded, generally, several years of survival. It seems that patients with metastatic disease more often than not have a lengthy and relatively symptom-free clinical course.[4,6,11]

REFERENCES

1. Batsakis, J.G.: *Tumors of the Head and Neck. Clinical and Pathological Considerations.* Williams & Wilkins, Baltimore, 1974.
2. Blumenberg, R.M., and Savlov, E.D.: Pain: An indication for carotid body tumor resection. *Arch Surg* **83**:205, 1961.
3. Brown, J.W., Burton, R.C., and Dahlin, D.C.:

Chemodectoma with skeletal metastasis: Report of two cases. *Mayo Clin Proc* **42:**551, 1967.

4. Chambers, R.G., and Mahoney, W.D.: Carotid body tumors. *Am J Surg* **116:**554, 1968.

5. Conley, J.J.: The carotid body tumor. A review of 29 cases. *Arch Otolaryngol* **81:**187, 1965.

6. Fanning, J.P., Woods, F.M., and Christian, H.J.: Metastatic carotid body tumor. Report of a case with review of literature. *JAMA* **185:**129, 1963.

7. Hewitt, R.L., Ichinose, H., Weichert, R.F., III, and Drapanas, T.: Chemodectomas. *Surgery* **71:**275, 1972.

8. McIlrath, D.C., and ReMine, W.H.: Carotid body tumors. *Surg Clin North Am* **43:**1135, 1963.

9. Monro, R.S.: The natural history of carotid body tumours and their diagnosis and treatment with a report of five cases. *Br J Surg* **37:**445, 1950.

10. Pinsker, K.L., Messinger, N., Hurwitz, P., and Becker, N.H.: Cervical chemodectoma with extensive pulmonary metastases. *Chest* **64:**116, 1973.

11. Romanski, R.: Chemodectoma (non-chromaffinic paraganglioma) of the carotid body with distant metastases with illustrative case. *Am J Pathol* **30:**1, 1954.

12. Rush, B.F.: Current concepts in the treatment of carotid body tumors. *Surgery* **52:**679, 1962.

13. Wilson, H.: Carotid body tumors: Surgical management. *Ann Surg* **159:**959, 1964.

91

Chemodectoma of the Glomus Jugulare

THE GLOMUS JUGULARE is composed of small clusters of paraganglionic cells that are located in the region of the temporal bone around the bulb of the jugular vein and extend along the tympanic branch of the glossopharyngeal nerve, the auricular branch of the vagus, and the jugular ganglion of the vagus. They all belong to the chemoreceptor system, but, unlike the carotid bodies, their exact function at this time is not well defined.[2,5,6] The structure was described as an anatomical entity by Guild[5] in 1941 and the first tumor in this location was reported by Rosenwasser[16] in 1945.

Glomus jugulare tumors occur less frequently than those of the carotid bodies.[15] There is a clear predominance of females, the ratio of female to male being 3.5:1.[1] Schermer et al.[17] found that the average age of the patients is 48.1 years, with a range from 23 to 78 years.

PATHOLOGY

The surgical specimen is usually composed of a small part of friable vascular tissue. Histologically, two main patterns are encountered. The alveolar pattern composed of cells exhibiting "zellballen" configuration occurs in approximately 70% of the cases. The angiomatous pattern is encountered in 17% of the patients and it is composed of dilated vascular spaces associated with the tumor. In the remaining patients there is a mixture of alveolar and angiomatous patterns.[4] The main cells are thought to be of neuroectodermal origin, being distinct from the cells that form the capillaries of the sinus vessels.[17]

The vascularity of the tumor is characteristic, and it is due to the fact that blood vessels are formed whose endothelial lining is a fine reticulum membrane. This rich vascular network of the tumor is the cause of profound bleedings during biopsy and surgery.[12]

CLINICAL

The commonest clinical symptom is tinnitus, commonly associated with a hearing loss. The tinnitus is of a pulsating nature and it is synchronous with the cardiac rhythm. The symptoms usually have been present for several years prior to the diagnosis.[4,14] In most patients no other neurological deficits are to be found except those from the eighth nerve. As the tumor enlarges, ipsilateral involvement of the seventh nerve brings about hearing loss and eventually the cranial nerves from 9 through 12 will be affected.[4,14]

With the passage of time, the patient becomes aware of a mass growing in the external ear, which characteristically has an extreme tendency to bleed following the slightest trauma. Local pain and otorrhea, as well as vertigo, may develop. The location of this growth may vary. Most commonly, it is encountered in the auditory canal but it may also develop behind the tympanic membrane (Fig. 91-1). Also it may extend toward the mastoid

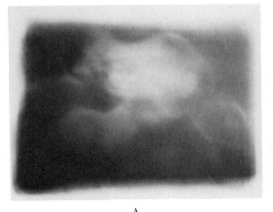

A

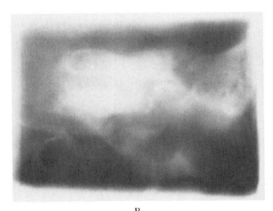

B

FIG. 91-1.   Chemodectoma of the glomus jugulare in a 60-year-old female. Polytomographic examination of the middle ears in the frontal projection reveals a normal right external auditory canal and normal middle and inner ear structures (A). On the left side, there is marked enlargement of the external auditory canal with extensive erosion of the inferior border, as well as a diffuse opacity in the region of the middle ear. On examination, the tumor could be seen within the external auditory canal (B).

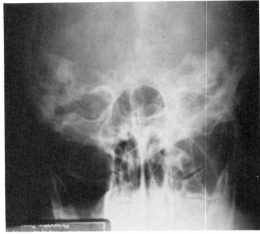

A

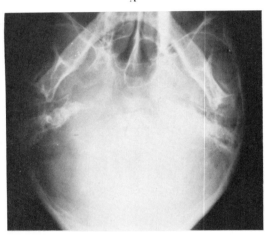

B

FIG. 91-2.   Chemodectoma of the glomus jugulare in a 71-year-old female. The tumor is located on the right side, producing considerable destruction of the medial aspect of the right petrous pyramid (A). In the base view of the skull there is a large lytic area at the tip of the petrous pyramid. The jugular foramen is destroyed (B).

process, producing radiographic images of clouded and sclerotic mastoids. Other radiographic findings include destruction or erosion of a portion of the petrous pyramid, as well as enlargement of the jugular foramen (Fig. 91-2). Arteriography demonstrates increased vascularity in the region of the tumor.[7,17] Occasionally, the mass has been found in the lateral part of the neck near the angle of the mandible or in the nasopharynx in the region of the eustachian tube.[4]

Examination reveals a tumor in the external auditory canal having a purplish color, being soft, polypoid, and friable in nature. Hemorrhage is easily produced on touch.[7]

In principle, this is a benign tumor; however, distant metastases have been described. Lattes and Waltner[12] reported a patient whose primary tumor invaded and extensively destroyed the temporal bone, entering the middle cranial fossa. Subsequently, liver metastases developed. The same authors reported on another patient with metastatic disease in the cervical lymph nodes. Other metastatic sites include the liver, lungs, spleen, and various bones. The incidence of distant metastases is in the range of 2–4%.[1,9]

Local recurrences do occur, especially among those patients who have been treated with surgery alone. They may, however, take 15 to 20 years before becoming obvious.[8]

TREATMENT AND RESULTS

When considering therapy for chemodectomas of the glomus jugulare, the long natural history of the tumor should be taken into consideration. Surgical resection when attempted in a radical fashion is accompanied by considerable difficulties. Weilen and Lane[19] presented the surgical problems involved. Included are hemorrhage during surgery, facial paralysis due to surgical injury, and recurrence of the tumor because of incomplete resection. Of those three, the major problem is profuse bleeding encountered during surgery. Capps[3] advocates surgery only for tumors arising within the tympanic cavity and not for those that affect the jugular bulb region. Due to the fact that the anatomical planes are difficult to define in this region, practically always following surgery the question arises as to whether or not a complete resection has taken place and eventually the outcome has been postoperative radiotherapy courses.[4,7,8] The actual surgical procedure performed is a radical mastoidectomy.[17]

There is considerable literature regarding the treatment of glomus jugulare tumors with radiation therapy. At this time, adequate clinical data are available, indicating that radiation in dosages ranging between 4000 and 5000 rad is capable of locally controlling the disease. This is delivered by means of a pair of wedged

fields that permit the tumor dose to be directed to the area of the tumor, sparing at the same time the brainstem.[11,14] Radiation brings about an arrest of the tumor growth rather than a disappearance of it. Maruyama et al.[13] reported on three patients, two of whom received 5000 rad tumor dose in five to six weeks and the third, 6000 rad in a six-week period. In all patients there was a clinical regression of the tumor and excellent clinical response in terms of alleviating most of their symptoms. Posttherapy arteriograms were performed two years after the completion of their treatment and surprisingly in spite of the clinical response there was very little if any change in the vascular character of the lesions. The authors explained the mechanism of the radiation action as based upon damage of small blood vessels whose caliber is below that of the arteriographic visibility.[13]

Following radiotherapy, the tumor response has generally been quite good. Radiation could be given either alone or in a postoperative fashion. Hatfield et al.[8] found that dosages in excess of 4000 rad were capable of locally controlling the disease for long periods of time. The average follow-up of patients treated in this manner in their series was 10 years. When less than 4000 rad were delivered, recurrences were seen but even these occurred more than 10 years posttherapy.

In contrast to these results, of 16 patients treated primarily by surgery, 8, or 50%, developed local recurrence in an average time of 4.3 years from the time of their therapy. Therefore radiation, when given in a definitive fashion, inhibits recurrent disease and affords a good survival.[8] Similarly, Grubb and Lampe[7] noted that five of nine patients treated primarily by surgery developed recurrent disease at five years or less. Within the same series, eight patients treated by radiation therapy either alone or in conjunction with surgery were surviving for an average period of six years without signs of recurrence.

The radioresistance of the tumors,

which was purported in the earlier reports by Rosenwasser,[16] was based on inadequate equipment and techniques. It is for this reason that he advocated surgery for those tumors deemed to be resectable. At the present time, however, the enthusiasm for surgery has dissipated and it appears that radiation is considered the main management.[14]

Prognosis and Survival

The disease even when recurrent or uncontrolled can afford a long survival. There are several patients who have died with their tumor rather than from it. Exceptions to this are neoplasms with extensive local destruction of the cranial fossa, which causes infection and bleeding, as well as those that have shown malignant tendencies, metastasizing to distal organs. The exceptions are, however, in the minority. The average survival of the patient with tumor of the glomus jugulare exceeds 10 years, according to the reported cases, and most probably it is much longer than that.[14]

It is important that the treatment be adequate so that recurrences do not occur. Uncontrolled recurrence over a period of several years will destroy vital adjacent structures and will lead to vascular and neurological complications, eventually threatening the life of the patient.[10]

Patients with metastatic disease have generally a poor prognosis with a fast downhill course. Their mean survival time is approximately five months from the time the metastases have been detected.[18]

References

1. Alford, B.R., and Guilford, F.R.: A comprehensive study of tumors of the glomus jugulare. *Laryngoscope* **72**:765, 1962.

2. Birrell, J.H.W.: The jugular body and its tumour. *Aust NZ J Surg* **24**:195, 1955.

3. Capps, F.C.W.: Tumors of the glomus jugulare or tympanic body. *J Fac Radiol* **7–8**:312, 1957.

4. Fuller, A.M., Brown, H.A., Harrison, E.G., Jr., and Siekert, R.G.: Chemodectomas of the glomus jugulare tumors. *Laryngoscope* **77**:218, 1967.

5. Guild, S.R.: A hitherto unrecognized structure, the glomus jugularis, in man. *Anat Rec (Suppl)* **79**:28, 1941.

6. Guild, S.R.: The glomus jugulare, a nonchromaffin paraganglion in man. *Ann Otol Rhinol Laryngol* **62**:1045, 1953.

7. Grubb, W.B., Jr., and Lampe, I.: The role of radiation therapy in the treatment of chemodectomas of the glomus jugulare. *Laryngoscope* **75**:1861, 1965.

8. Hatfield, P.M., James, A.E., and Schulz, M.D.: Chemodectomas of the glomus jugulare. *Cancer* **30**:1164, 1972.

9. Hawk, W.A., and McCormack, L.J.: Nonchromaffin paraganglioma of the glomus jugulare. *Cleve Clin Q* **26**:62, 1959.

10. Hoople, G.D., Bradley, W.H., Stoner, L.R., and Brewer, D.W.: Histologically malignant glomus jugulare tumor (Case report). *Laryngoscope* **68**:760, 1958.

11. Hudgins, P.T.: Radiotherapy for extensive glomus jugulare tumors. *Radiology* **103**:427, 1972.

12. Lattes, R., and Waltner, J.G.: Nonchromaffin paraganglioma of the middle ear. (Carotid-body-like tumor; glomus-jugulare tumor). *Cancer* **2**:447, 1949.

13. Maruyama, Y., Gold, L.H.A., and Kieffer, S.A.: Radioactive cobalt treatment of glomus jugulare tumors. Clinical and angiographic investigation. *Acta Radiol (Ther)* **10**:239, 1971.

14. Miller, J.D.R.: Results of treatment in glomus jugulare tumors with emphasis on radiotherapy. *Radiology* **79**:430, 1962.

15. Olson, J.R., and Abell, M.R.: Nonfunctional, nonchromaffin paragangliomas of the retroperitoneum. *Cancer* **23**:1358, 1969.

16. Rosenwasser, H.: Metastasis from glomus jugulare tumors. Discussion of nomenclature and therapy. *Arch Otolaryngol* **67**:197, 1958.

17. Schermer, K.L., Pontius, E.E., Dziabis, M.D., and McQuiston, R.J.: Tumors of the glomus jugulare and glomus tympanicum. *Cancer* **19**:1273, 1966.

18. Taylor, D.M., Alford, B.R., and Greenberg, S.D.: Metastases of glomus jugulare tumors. *Arch Otolaryngol* **82**:5, 1965.

19. Weile, F.L., and Lane, C.S., Jr.: Surgical problems involved in the removal of the glomus jugulare tumors. *Laryngoscope* **61**:448, 1951.

92

Chemodectoma of the Glomus Intravagale (Vagal Body Tumor)

WITHIN THE PERINEURIUM of the vagus nerve, just beneath the jugular foramen, a congregation of chemoreceptor cells is to be found in close proximity to the ganglium nodosum. No physiological function has been demonstrated, at this point, occurring within this structure. The original anatomical description was published by White[7] in 1935, and the first tumor in this location was reported by Stout[6] in 1935. Subsequently, tumors arising in this location were reported by other authors. Coldwater and Dirks[2] published the details about a patient whose tumor metastasized to the regional lymph nodes and Burman[1] reported on a patient with tumor extension into the occipital bone. The average age of the patients is 44–45 years at the time of the diagnosis and, as in tumors of the glomus jugulare, there is a female preponderance of approximately 2:1.[3]

PATHOLOGY

Usually at the time of the diagnosis, a sizable mass is present high in the neck and deep to the angle of the mandible. The average diameter has been 5.0 cm. The histological appearance is similar to that of the rest of the chemodectomas. Johnson *et al.*[3] found, in association with the tumor, nerve fibers and ganglion cells derived from the vagus nerve and the ganglion nodosum. Most authors agree that there is no distinct histological criterion to differentiate between metastasizing and non-metastasizing vagal body tumors.[3] It is possible that the glomus intravagale tumors as a group are more aggressive than carotid body tumors, because a greater percentage of them exhibit malignant characteristics in terms of both local invasion and distant metastases.[2]

CLINICAL

Practically all patients have as the presenting symptom a painless mass in the upper part of the neck. This is located behind the angle of the mandible and has been present for considerable length of time prior to the diagnosis. Other clinical symptoms include hoarseness and difficulty in swallowing, as well as nasal regurgitation and choking while swallowing, all difficulties associated with involvement with the vagus. Similarly manipulation of the tumor can produce reflex bradycardia and patients have been reported to have transitory episodes of unconsciousness for this reason. On physical examination, in addition to the mass, pulsation or bruit in the region of the tumor may be found.[2,3]

Malignant behavior manifesting itself in terms of metastatic disease and local invasion has definitely been noted in some of these tumors. Regional lymph node involvement has been reported by Coldwater and Dirks[2] as well as by Keener.[4]

TREATMENT AND RESULTS

Surgery in terms of total resection of the tumor has been the treatment in the reported cases. In all instances this has resulted in permanent damage of the ipsilateral vagus nerve. The tumor was found to extend upward into the region just beneath the jugular foramen. In a number of patients the hypoglossal nerve and the spinal accessory nerve were involved and therefore resected.[3] The interruption of the recurrent laryngeal nerve brings about fixation of the vocal cord, with hoarseness of the voice. Swallowing difficulty, particularly related to liquid intake, has also occurred. Damage to the hypoglossal nerve may lead to hemiatrophy of the tongue. Johnson *et al.*[3] stressed the importance of preserving the carotid circulation in order to keep the surgical mortality within acceptable limits.

Extension of the tumor into the base of the skull has been the mechanism of death for those patients who are inoperable at the time of the diagnosis. Deaths also have been reported as a result of postoperative cerebral complications following ligation of the common carotid artery.[2]

PROGNOSIS AND SURVIVAL

Nine of 10 patients with chemodectomas of the vagal body treated surgically at the Mayo Clinic and reported by Johnson *et al.* were surviving at the time of their report for intervals ranging from one month to five years. There was one death postoperatively following ligation of the common carotid artery. No patient from this group developed local recurrence or metastatic disease.[3] Lattes[5] has reported deaths occurring either from extension of inoperable tumors into the base of the skull or from surgical attempts to excise such tumors.

REFERENCES

1. Burman, S.O.: The chemoreceptor system and its tumor—the chemodectoma. *Int Abstr Surg* **102:**330, 1956.
2. Coldwater, K.B., and Dirks, K.R.: Chemodectoma of the glomus intravagale. Report of two cases: One with regional lymph node metastases. *Surgery* **40:**1069, 1956.
3. Johnson, W.S., Beahrs, O.H., and Harrison, E.G., Jr.: Chemodectoma of the glomus intravagale. (Vagal-body tumor). *Am J Surg* **104:**812, 1962.
4. Keener, E.B.: Chemodectomas of the vagal body. *Can Med Assoc J* **80:**173, 1959.
5. Lattes, R.: Nonchromaffin paraganglioma of ganglion nodosum, carotid body, and aortic arch bodies. *Cancer* **3:**667, 1950.
6. Stout, A.P.: Malignant tumors of peripheral nerves. *Am J Cancer* **25:**1, 1935.
7. White, E.G.: Die Struktur des Glomus caroticum seine Pathologie und seine Beziehung zum Nervensystem. *Beitr Pathol Anst Pathol* **96:**177, 1935.

93

Tumors of the Organ of Zuckerkandl

THESE TUMORS ARISE from a collection of paraganglia located around the origin of the inferior mesenteric artery. The structures were described originally by Zuckerkandl in 1901 and they are especially identifiable in fetuses. They develop earlier than the adrenal medulla and mature at a time when the medulla is still rudimentary. It is postulated that their function is to maintain the blood pressure of the fetus and the young infant. Gradually in the postnatal period degeneration takes place. Wrete identified the relationship between the chromaffin paraganglia of Zuckerkandl and the chromaffin tissue of the adrenal glands. Keene and Hewer published on the common embryological origin of the intraadrenal and extraadrenal chromaffin tissues from the sympathetic anlage.[3]

Approximately 10% of all pheochromocytomas have an extraadrenal origin, which in most cases is due to tumors of the organ of Zuckerkandl.[10] Glenn and Gray[3] in a literature review found 46 cases of such tumors reported up to 1976. Among them, the incidence of malignancy was 13%.

The average age of the patients at the time of the diagnosis is 33–38 years, with a rather wide range from 6 to 81 years. Possibly a slight male predominance exists.[1,3]

PATHOLOGY

The organs of Zuckerkandl are paired organs composed of chromaffin tissue around the origin of the inferior mesenteric artery. In the newborn infant they extended to the aortic bifurcation firmly attached to the surface of the aorta by the sympathetic plexus. In a small percentage of the cases they may extend above the orifice of the inferior mesenteric artery. The organs regress during childhood.[1,2] The cells are chromaffin positive and have been shown to contain epinephrine and norepinephrine.

The tumors grossly are lobulated light brown or reddish brown in color.[3] The histological pattern varies and two main cell types are to be found. One group has an appearance similar to that of non-chromaffin paragangliomas, such as carotid body tumors, while the other group of cells presents with histology similar to the pheochromocytomas. Commonly both elements are present.

The benign or the malignant behavior of the individual tumor cannot be assessed on the basis of histology. Literature review reveals seven such malignant tumors described.[1,3,5,7] The only reliable measure of malignancy has been the demonstration of metastatic disease or invasion of adjacent organs.

CLINICAL

The symptomatology is directly related to the catecholamine production by the chromaffin tumor cells. These catecholamines include dopamine, norepinephrine, and epinephrine. When norepinephrine is the dominant substance released, the common presenting symptoms are hypertension associated with headaches and tachycardia. When epinephrine dominates, metabolic changes, such as decreased gastrointestinal tract motility, sweating, and flushing, as well as diabetes, may be the presenting symptoms. Psychotic symptoms, hyperventilation with tachypnea, and weight loss accompany these. The picture may suggest thyrotoxicosis.[9]

The rarity of the disease requires a high index of suspicion and patients as a rule have often been misdiagnosed. Many patients notice that postural changes or pressure upon the abdomen will precipitate their symptomatology. The same effect may be achieved by palpation or pressure upon the tumor through the abdomen or while ingesting large quantities of food or during strenuous bowel movements.[3] Approximately 62% of patients present with the symptoms described. In the remaining the presenting symptom is that of a mass in the abdomen with discomfort and low back pain. Finally, the tumor may be totally asymptomatic and discovered at autopsy.[1]

Arteriography has been useful in identifying extraadrenal pheochromocytomas. In the past there has been reluctance to use arteriography because of the danger of hypertensive and cardiac crises. The radiologist should be prepared to treat such an occurrence, which may result when selective injection into the supplying vessel is performed. Preoperative localization of the tumor allows preplanned approach for surgical resection. It also helps in localizing multiple or bilateral tumors. The tumors have been reported to be quite vascular; however, they do not present the greatly intense vascularities seen with renal or adrenal neoplasms.[4,8]

Laboratory investigation reveals an elevated level of urinary catecholamines and elevated vanillylmandelic acid (VMA) levels as well.[3] Due to these diagnostic improvements provocative tests utilizing histamine or Regitine are no longer used, since they are dangerous and less specific. Diabetes may be among the presenting symptoms because of the inhibition the catecholamines exert on the uptake of glucose and on the production of insulin by the beta cells of the pancreas.[1]

TREATMENT AND RESULTS

Surgical resection is the basic form of therapy. It is important and necessary to prime the patient with alpha and beta adrenergic receptor blocking agents for days or even weeks prior to operation in order to prevent cardiovascular mishaps during anesthesia and surgery. Their use prevents the precipitous fall of the blood pressure due to the extensive increase of the vascular space following release of the spasm brought about by the catecholamine secretion. Prior to surgery, identification of the relationship between the tumor and the surrounding structures, namely, adrenals, kidneys, and ureters, as well as identification of the vascular branches that supply the tumor, is necessary. The vascular supply is primarily from vessels directly arising from the aorta and the venous return is to the inferior vena cava. More than one vessel is involved usually in this process.[1,3] Ventricular arrhythmias or hypertensive crises may develop during the actual procedure, therefore lidocaine hydrochloride should be available in the operating room. During the operation, there should be intraarterial monitoring of the blood pressure.[9]

Malignant tumors that appear to be unresectable due to their local extension or that have metastasized distantly can be palliatively irradiated with good prospects of control. Holsti[5] reported on two patients treated with external beam therapy receiving 5000 and 5500 rad as a calculated tumor dose. A drop in the blood pressure and a decrease in the urinary catecholamines associated with radiographic improvement in terms of diminution of the pathological vessels was found in one patient who remained asymptomatic two years following his therapy. In the second patient local recurrence occurred two years following the treatment. Joseph[7] reported successful symptomatic relief and reduction of the blood pressure following therapy of metastatic disease to the left clavicle. Radiographically sclerotic healing changes were noted.

PROGNOSIS AND SURVIVAL

There is considerable lack of follow-up information in most of the reported cases. It appears that for those patients in whom the tumors are removed completely and timely there is no obvious effect on the survival.[3] In long-standing and neglected cases hypertensive disease produces generalized arteriosclerosis associated with left ventricular hypertrophy. Hypertension also produces hyalinization of the glomeruli and marked sclerosis of the arterioles in the kidneys with areas of fibrinoid necrosis. Sustained high blood pressure leads to heart failure and cerebral episodes.[6] Patients with malignant disease have developed generalized metastases involving the liver, lungs, bone, and regional lymph nodes.[5,7]

REFERENCES

1. Brantigan, C.O., and Katase, R.Y.: Clinical and pathologic features of paragangliomas of the organ of Zuckerkandl. *Surgery* **65:**898, 1969.
2. Coupland, R.E.: Post-natal fate of the abdominal para-aortic bodies in man. *J Anat* **88:**455, 1954.
3. Glenn, F., and Gray, G.F.: Functional tumors of the organ of Zuckerkandl. *Ann Surg* **183:**578, 1976.
4. Hahn, L.C., and Nadel, N.S.: Angiographic localization of a pheochromocytoma of the organs of Zuckerkandl. *J Urol* **111:**553, 1974.
5. Holsti, L.R.: Malignant extra-adrenal phaeochromocytoma. *Br J Radiol* **37:**944, 1964.
6. Isaacson, C., Rosenzweig, D., and Seftel, H.C.: Malignant pheochromocytoma of the organs of Zuckerkandl. *Arch Pathol* **70:**725, 1960.
7. Joseph, L.: Malignant phaeochromocytoma of the organ of Zuckerkandl with functioning metastases. *Br J Urol* **39:**221, 1967.
8. Kinkhabwala, M.N., and Conradi, H.: Angiography of extra-adrenal pheochromocytomas. *J Urol* **108:**666, 1972.
9. Lulu, D.J.: Pheochromocytoma of the organs of Zuckerkandl. *Arch Surg* **99:**641, 1969.
10. Watkins, D.B.: Pheochromocytoma: A review of the literature. *J Chron Dis* **6:**510, 1957.

94

Paragangliomas in Other Locations

THE TERM "paraganglia" was introduced by Kohn in 1903. As such, he designated anatomical formations that arise from neural crest cells and that are related to the ganglia of the sympathetic and parasympathetic nervous system. The paraganglia migrate with the autonomous nervous system elements and therefore are to be found in more or less the same anatomical locations.[6,7,14]

Among the prominent paraganglia, the carotid bodies and the glomus jugulare formations are nonchromaffin-staining structures whose main function is that of a chemoreceptor. On the other hand, the adrenal medulla and the paraaortic ganglia, which form the organ of Zuckerkandl, are related to the sympathetic system. They are catecholamine secreting and the majority of them are chromaffin positive.

Because the migration of the neural crest cells takes place early in life and because they lack differentiation, paraganglian cells can be found in several organs. It is from these cells that functioning or usually nonfunctioning paragangliomas have been reported in such organs as the lung, prostate, gallbladder, and pancreas.[2,5,7,14]

Spitzer et al.[8] presented a case of functioning paraganglioma of the urinary bladder. A review of the literature reveals approximately 25 such cases reported.[1,8] The patients may present with hematuria or with symptoms related to paroxysmal or sustained hypertension, which includes headaches, profuse sweating, and pallor. Often the symptoms appear when micturition takes place because the pressure on the tumor increases. Radiograpically, they are quite vascular neoplasms, producing prolonged tumor stain, just as the pheochromocytomas do. Certainly, their vascularity is much more distinct than that of a carcinoma of the urinary bladder.[4,7]

Westbrook et al.[13] reported a malignant nonchromaffin paraganglioma of the stomach. The tumor arose in the fundus and was initially treated by a wedge resection. The patient did well for three years, when she developed metastasis with collapse and fracture of the second lumbar vertebral body. This was proved histologically. Further therapy was refused and she died one year later. In a review of the literature the authors uncovered 11 cases on nonchromaffin paragangliomas involving the intestinal tract, all of them located in the duodenum. All the tumors were located in the submucosa and none of them metastasized.[9,12,13]

Paragangliomas may be found in the superior mediastinum, presumably arising from the aortic bodies.[14] Enquist et al.[3] reported such a lesion with malignant characteristics in a 20-year-old man. The clinical presentation was that of a pathological fracture of the left humerus and the chest roentgenogram showed a superior mediastinal mass with osseous metastases to several ribs. A bone survey revealed extensive involvement. Some of the lesions were irradiated to a total dose of 5000 rad over 35 days. There was no change noted in the radiographic appearance.[3]

In the lung solitary paraganglia have been described; however, more commonly seen is the so-called "pulmonary chemodectomatosis." In this condition multiple minute paragangliomas are found in both lungs, lacking any functional or clinical features. This is simply a proliferation of glomic tissue and is estimated to occur in 0.3% of the population.[5,14]

In the thyroid region, as well as in the larynx and the trachea, paragangliomas have been described occasionally. The vast majority of them have been benign in character.[6,11]

In the orbit, in the retrobulbar area, a chemodectoma was reported by Thacker and Duckworth.[10] The tumor surrounded the optic nerve and extended into the apex of the orbit.

Chemodectomas may be encountered in every organ and tissue. Indeed, some investigators think that they are more common than the literature indicates.

REFERENCES

1. Albores-Saavedra, J., Maldonado, M.E., Ibarra, J., and Rodriguez, H.A.: Pheochromocytoma of the urinary bladder. *Cancer* **23**:1110, 1969.
2. Cope, C., Greenberg, S.H., Vidal, J.J., and Co-hen, E.A.: Nonfunctioning nonchromaffin paraganglioma of the pancreas. *Arch Surg* **109**:440, 1974.
3. Enquist, R.W., Tormey, D.C., Jenis, E.H., and Warkel, R.L.: Malignant chemodectoma of the superior mediastinum with elevated urinary homovanillic acid. *Chest* **66**:209, 1974.
4. Glucksman, M.A., and Persinger, C.P.: Malignant non-chromaffin paraganglioma of the bladder. *J Urol* **89**:822, 1963.
5. Goodman, M.L., and Laforet, E.G.: Solitary primary chemodectomas of the lung. *Chest* **61**:48, 1972.
6. Kay, S., Montague, J.W., and Dodd, R.W.: Nonchromaffin paraganglioma (chemodectoma) of thyroid region. *Cancer* **36**:582, 1975.
7. Olson, J.R., and Abell, M.R.: Nonfunctional nonchromaffin paragangliomas of the retroperitoneum. *Cancer* **23**:1358, 1969.
8. Spitzer, R., Borrison, R., and Castellino, R.A.: Functioning nonchromaffin paraganglioma (chemodectoma) of the urinary bladder. *Radiology* **98**:577, 1971.
9. Taylor, H.B., and Helwig, E.B.: Benign nonchromaffin paragangliomas of the duodenum. *Virchows Arch [Pathol Anat]* **335**:356, 1962.
10. Thacker, W.C., and Duckworth, J.K.: Chemodectoma of the orbit. *Cancer* **23**:1233, 1969.
11. Tobin, H.A., and Harris, H.H.: Non-chromaffin paraganglioma of the larynx—case report and review of the literature. *Arch Otolaryngol* **96**:154, 1972.
12. Weitzner, M.D.: Benign nonchromaffin paraganglioma of the duodenum. *Am J Gastroentol* **53**:365, 1970.
13. Westbrook, K.C., Bridger, W.M., and Williams, G.D.: Malignant nonchromaffin paraganglioma of the stomach. *Am J Surg* **124**:407, 1972.
14. Zak, F.G., and Chabes, A.: Pulmonary chemodectomatosis. *JAMA* **183**:887.

95

Acinic Cell Carcinoma

THIS IS AN uncommon tumor involving primarily the parotid gland. Its existence has been known since 1892 at which point Nasse described the first case.[11] Until 1953, it was considered a benign tumor. Godwin et al.[9] called attention to the fact that some of these lesions are malignant, but in order to demonstrate their malignant nature a very long follow-up is required. In subsequent series the histological and clinical characteristics of the disease were better delineated.[1,4-6,8,9]

Of 2102 parotid tumors reviewed by Eneroth et al.[4] 63 (3%) were found to have histological features characteristic of acinic cell carcinoma. Grage et al.[8] in reviewing 272 tumors of the major salivary glands found 11 acinic cell carcinomas, an incidence of 4%. Among all primary malignant tumors of the parotid gland in the same series, acinic cell carcinoma was found to constitute 16.9%.

Seventeen of the 27 patients from the series by Godwin et al.[9] were women. A ratio of 2:1 between female and male patients has been observed by other authors. Eneroth et al.[4] encountered 42 women and 21 men and in the series by Grage et al.[8] there were 7 women and 4 men. The age range has been rather wide, from the early teens to the late decades of life. It appears that the peak incidence is in the fourth and fifth decades.[3,4]

PATHOLOGY

The majority of acinic cell carcinomas arise in the parotid gland. Abrams et al.,[1] reviewing 77 cases examined at the Armed Forces Institute of Pathology, found 71 to have originated in the parotid gland, an incidence of 92%. Rarely, they have occurred in the submandibular gland and single case reports of acinic cell carcinoma involving the base of the tongue, the lung, the paranasal sinuses, the palate, and the lip have been published in the recent years.[1,7,10,12,13,14,15]

The tumor size varies from 1.0 to 10.0 cm or more. In most patients it measures about 3 cm.

Grossly, they are usually sharply circumscribed masses varying in consistency from soft to hard, depending on the number of cystic areas present. The impression was entertained that the lesion produces a capsule; however, Eneroth et al.[4] pointed out that this apparent capsule actually represents a compression of the surrounding tissue produced by the tumor. Occasionally neoplastic cells are to be found within this condensed fibrous tissue and thus the false impression of infiltrative growth may be generated.[4,9]

The commonest histological appearance is that of granulated cells that are much larger than the normal acinic cells (Fig. 95-1). Their granules are identical histologically and histochemically to the granules of the normal acinic cells. The membranes of the cells are distinct and the nuclei uniform, small, and dark in color. Occasionally the cells are clear. In such tumors, the cells are similar to those seen in the intercalated ducts, or those present at the junction of the acinous and the in-

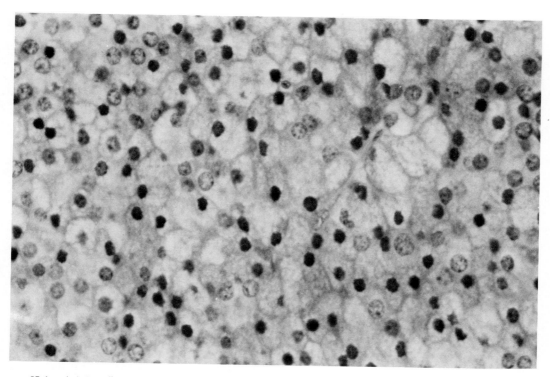

FIG. 95-1.   Acinic cell carcinoma of the salivary gland. Trabecular formations of polyhedral cells with large clear-to-granular cytoplasm.

tercalated ducts.[9] Erlandson and Tandler[5] examined by electron microscopy acinic cell carcinomas and they identified indeed two basic cell types: serouslike cells with numerous secretory granules and smaller cuboidal cells without granules.[5] A more detailed analysis of the cellular pattern was provided by Abrams et al.[1] who further subdivided the two major cell groups. Most frequently, the cells were arranged in a solid parenchymatous mass and occasionally microcystic configurations as well as papillary or follicular growth patterns were encountered in the material review by the same authors.

Because the tumors are composed of well-differentiated cells, the pathologist is faced with the problem of attaching the term "carcinoma" to such a lesion. This is even more disquieting when many of these patients have tumors that behave in a benign fashion. For this reason, some

authors advocate the noncommittal term "acinic cell tumor," which might be more appropriate because the histology does not convey information relative to the natural history of the disease.[2,5]

CLINICAL

The commonest clinical presentation is slowly progressive unilateral swelling of the face, which is due to a mass developing in the parotid gland. The lesion is painless and it is only in advanced stages where hearing defects, dysphagia, or pain may occur along with paralysis of the facial nerve. All these events are extremely rare. The duration of the symptoms varies from 3 months to 20 years and on the average the tumor has been known to be present 5.5 years prior to the time of the diagnosis.[1,3,8,12]

On physical examination, the mass is mobile in most cases; however, in about one-third they are fixed. They are firm but not hard and the overlying skin is not adherent to them.[1]

Metastasis to the regional lymph nodes is uncommon but has been reported. This takes place to the contiguous lymph nodes.[4,9] Characteristically, the tumor shows a tendency for local recurrence and also characteristically several years are required to elapse before distant disease becomes obvious. In the series by Godwin et al.[9] local recurrence was seen in 50% of the patients. Many of these patients had several recurrences at various intervals over long periods of time. In a literature review Abrams et al.[1] found local recurrence in 64 patients of a total of 161 reported.[1] Distant metastases, hematogenous in character, occurred primarily to the lung. Even with the development of metastasis, the prospects of long-term survival remain good.[8]

TREATMENT AND RESULTS

Surgical resection is the recommended treatment by all reviewers of the subject. In the earlier report by Godwin et al.[9] excision of the tumor with a margin of parotid gland was considered to be an adequate method of therapy. Subsequent authors, armed with the benefit of long-term follow-up observation, do not consider simple excision as the proper from of therapy. In most cases a parotidectomy with sacrifice of all or part of the facial nerve is required for an adequate removal of this neoplasm and only in the occasional case superficial parotidectomy may be sufficient, based on the anatomical orientation of the tumor.[1,8,9] Chong et al.[3] in retrospective analysis evaluated the treatment program of 73 patients with acinic cell carcinoma seen at the Mayo Clinic. Patients whose primary tumors were treated by local excision or by enucleation had been followed for a mean period of 11.8 years. Among them, 66.7%

developed local recurrences and 22.2% died as a result of their disease. Patients treated primarily by total parotidectomy were followed for a shorter period of time (mean follow-up period of 5.2 years), since this treatment program had been applied to the most recent cases. Within this group, local recurrence occurred in 9.5% of the patients and there were no deaths related to the disease.[3]

Indeed, local recurrence is the main difficulty in managing acinic cell carcinoma and this, as is evident from the results of all reviewers, is related to the mode of therapy. Eneroth et al.[4] advocate lymph node dissection in addition to the radical surgery. This is based on their experience with 63 patients, among whom six developed regional lymph node metastases. It is not clear, however, whether or not the same patients had local recurrence of their disease.[4] In the experience of most authors lymph node metastasis at the time of the diagnosis is a rare event and lymphadenectomy is not recommended.[3]

The effectiveness of radiotherapy is questionable. Four patients treated for recurrent tumors with radiotherapy in the series by Grage et al.[8] failed in terms of local control.

PROGNOSIS AND SURVIVAL

The disease has an indolent course and several years are required in order to determine patient survival. In the series by Godwin et al.,[9] of 27 patients, three patients were dead at the time of the report because of their disease. There were three additional patients living with recurrence. In the series by Abrams et al.[1] 84.7% of the 72 patients included have had neither recurrence locally nor distant metastasis. Local recurrence alone was seen in 8.3% and metastasis developed in 6.9% of the patients. The lungs, the spine, pelvis, skull, and femurs are favorite sites of dissemination. Eneroth et al.[4] compiled the survival rates from their material and determined that a fall in survival occurs with the passage of time. The survival rate at five years was 90%, dropping to 50% at 25 years.

It is important to remember in determining survival that the majority of the patients had disease present several years prior to the time of the diagnosis. Therefore the actual survival rates, if they were to be measured from the onset of the disease, would be considerably longer.

REFERENCES

1. Abrams, A.M., Cornyn, J., Scofield, H.H., and Hansen, L.S.: Acinic cell adenocarcinoma of the major salivary glands. A clinicopathologic study of 77 cases. *Cancer* **18**:1145, 1965.
2. Batsakis, J.G.: *Tumors of the Head and Neck. Clinical and Pathological Considerations.* Williams & Wilkins, Baltimore, 1974.
3. Chong, G.C., Beahrs, O.H., and Woolner, L.B.: Surgical management of acinic cell carcinoma of the parotid gland. *Surg Gynecol Obstet* **138**:65, 1974.
4. Eneroth, C.M., Hamberger, C.A., and Jakobsson, P.A.: Malignancy of acinic cell carcinoma. *Ann Otol Rhinol Laryngol* **75**:780, 1966.
5. Erlandson, R.A., and Tandler, B.: Ultrastructure of acinic cell carcinoma of the parotid gland. *Arch Pathol* **93**:130, 1972.
6. Evans, R.W., and Cruickshank, A.H.: *Epithelial Tumors of the Salivary Glands.* W.B. Saunders, Philadelphia, 1970.
7. Fechner, R.E., Bentinck, B.R., and Askew, J.B., Jr.: Acinic cell tumor of the lung. A histologic and ultrastructural study. *Cancer* **29**:501, 1972.
8. Grage, T.B., Lober, P.H., and Arhelger, S.W.: Acinic cell carcinoma of the parotid gland. A clinicopathologic review of eleven cases. *Am J Surg* **102**:765, 1961.
9. Godwin, J.T., Foote, F.W., Jr., and Frazell, E.L.: Acinic cell adenocarcinoma of the parotid gland. Report of twenty-seven cases. *Am J Pathol* **30**:465, 1954.
10. Manace, E.D., and Goldman, J.L.: Acinic cell carcinoma of the paranasal sinuses. *Laryngoscope* **81**:1074, 1971.
11. Nasse, D.: Die Geschwülste der Speicheldrüsen und verwandte Tumoren des Kopfes. *Arch Klin Chir* **44**:233, 1892.
12. Rivlin, R.S.: Acinic cell adenocarcinoma of the parotid gland. *Am J Surg* **100**:639, 1960.
13. Trodahl, J.N.: Case for diagnosis. *Milit Med* **137**:234, 1972.
14. Walker, W.E., Rosenfeld, L., and Hartmann, W.H.: Salivary gland carcinoma of the palate. *J Oral Surg* **33**:936, 1975.
15. Wendling, D.: Acinic cell adenocarcinoma of the base of the tongue. *Laryngoscope* **78**:64, 1968.

96

Pulmonary Blastoma

THIS IS A rare, perhaps the rarest, pulmonary neoplasm. A literature review in 1976 by Peacock and Whitwell[7] revealed 30 cases reported. The tumor was first described by Barnard in 1952,[1] occurring in the right lung of a 40-year-old female. Histologically, it consisted of tubules lined with epithelium and surrounded by connective tissue. The overall pattern was reminiscent of a Wilms' tumor of the kidney. It also resembled the arrangement observed in the developing lungs of an embryo when bronchial buds grow into adjacent undifferentiated mesoderm.[1]

Contrary to the Wilms' tumors, pulmonary blastomas have occurred primarily in adults and occasionally in children. The ages have ranged from 2 months to 77 years, the mean average age for the male patients being 45 years and for the females, 36. Males have outnumbered females by a ratio of 3:1.[7]

PATHOLOGY

Spencer[8] in 1961 reported three cases similar in histology to the case of Barnard. He introduced the term "pulmonary blastoma" as an analogue to the nephroblastoma of the kidney.

Their gross appearance has been rather uniform. All are well circumscribed, arising in the periphery of the lung, often being subpleural in location, without bronchial connections. They expand and compress the surrounding lung parenchyma, which creates a form of capsule around the tumor. Grossly, they are soft with a shiny cut surface containing areas of hemorrhage and occasional necrosis.[1,5,6]

The basic histological features are a sarcomatous component, either undifferentiated or forming fibrous, muscle, or cartilage elements and epithelium-lined tubes and tubules, which are interspersed in the stroma[1,5] (Fig. 96-1). The currently accepted origin of pulmonary blastomas is based on the embryogenesis of the lung, as advanced by Waddell.[9] According to this theory, the distal lung—alveoli—develops from mesenchymal tissue, whereas the bronchi and the bronchioles are formed by the central laryngotracheal bud. Later, fusion between the peripheral and central parts takes place and with the process of canalization continuity of the respiratory system is established.[9] It is believed that pulmonary blastomas arise from the peripheral bipotential part of the embryonic lung, that mesenchymal part that gives genesis to the alveoli. The mechanism of origin of pulmonary blastomas explains the absence of epidermoid elements and their peripheral location. It also explains their histological similarity to nephroblastomas (Wilms' tumors).[1,2]

Pulmonary blastomas are to be differentiated from pulmonary carcinosarcomas. The latter are a mixture of epidermoid and mesenchymal elements originating in the bronchi, having an age distribution similar to that observed in carcinoma of the lung, and much poorer prognosis.

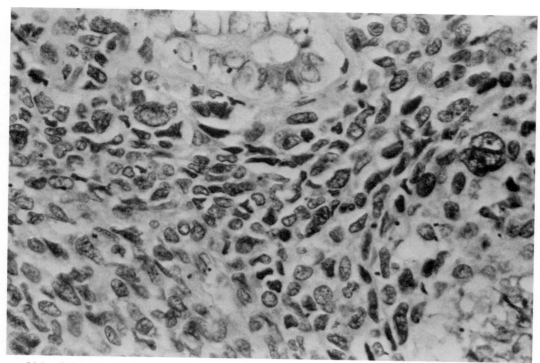

FIG. 96-1. Pulmonary blastoma. Abnormal glandular formation against a background of sarcomatous stroma.

CLINICAL

Chest discomfort, pain, and shortness of breath are the earliest elicited symptoms. As they progress, cough, persistent in character, and hemoptysis develop. Because of the insidious onset, frequently the diagnosis of "flu" or "cold" is made prior to the development of hemoptysis.[3-5] At times, the lesion is completely asymptomatic the diagnosis is made unexpectedly on a "routine" chest x-ray examination.[6]

Most of the tumors are quite large by the time of the radiographic diagnosis. They are unilateral, well-circumscribed masses, somewhat lobulated, occasionally cavitating, and generally located peripherally.[5,6] Reportedly, the left lung is favored over the right as a site of origin.[2]

Sputum cytology and bronchoscopy have occasionally indicated the diagnosis of malignancy; however, the percentage of failure of both of these methods is considerable, since there is no bronchial connection.[7] Metastasis to the hilar nodes is not a common occurrence, seen in approximately 20% of the cases.[5] Hematogenous dissemination has been seen to take place in several organs, including the opposite lung, brain, liver, and skeletal system.

TREATMENT AND RESULTS

Surgery has been the primary method of therapy. In their literature summary, Peacock and Whitwell,[7] found that of the total of 30 patients, 10 underwent pneumonectomy, 11 had lobectomy, and 3 had lesser surgical resections. Radiation therapy, chemotherapy, or no treatment at all were applied to the remaining six patients, all of whom had far-advanced disease. The longest survivor among them lived for seven months. Of the 24 patients operated on, 10 were known dead as a result of their tumor, and three were surviving with recurrent local, or distant disease.[7]

The effectiveness of radiotherapy is unclear. Parker et al.[6] stated, in one of their case reports, that irradiation dissolved completely several metastatic nodules in the lung. Ghaffar et al.[3] reported on a 9-year-old boy whose primary therapy had been left pneumonectomy. Because of residual mediastinal disease, postoperative radiotherapy to the left hemithorax and mediastinum, 3500 rad, was given. This was followed by several courses of methotrexate and bleomycin. In spite of that, the patient died with a large locally recurrent tumor mass, as well as with widespread metastases, nine months following radiotherapy.

Data on the effectiveness of chemotherapy are lacking at the present time.

PROGNOSIS AND SURVIVAL

The most important prognostic factor is the local extent of the disease at the time of the surgery. Patients with hilar lymph node involvement or other intrathoracic extensions have not survived, in general, beyond the first year. It is among patients with localized disease that long survivors may be found.[3,4,7] In the review by Peacock and Whitwell,[7] of 30 patients reported, the authors found 10 living without evidence of disease. Of the remaining, 17 were dead because of their tumor, and three had active disease present.

It is to be noted that among the long-term survivors, the patient originally described by Barnard is included. Reportedly, she was alive and well 15 years postoperatively.[5]

REFERENCES

1. Barnard, W.G.: "Embryoma of lung." *Thorax* 7:299, 1952.
2. Cox, J.L., Fuson, R.L., and Daly, J.T.: Pulmonary blastoma. A case report and review of the literature. *Ann Thorac Surg* 9:364, 1970.
3. Ghaffer, A., Vaidynathan, S.V., Elguezabal, A., and Levowitz, B.S.: Pulmonary blastoma. Report of two cases. *Chest* 67:600, 1975.
4. Iverson, R.E., and Straehley, C.J.: Pulmonary blastoma; Long term survival of juvenile patient. *Chest* 63:436, 1973.
5. Karcioglu, Z.A., and Someren, A.O.: Pulmonary blastoma. A case report and review of the literature. *Am J Clin Pathol* 61:287, 1974.
6. Parker, J.C., Payne, W.S., and Woolner, L.B.: Pulmonary blastoma (embryoma). Report of two cases. *J Thorac Cardiovasc Surg* 51:694, 1966.
7. Peacock, M.J., and Whitwell, F.: Pulmonary blastoma. *Thorax* 31:197, 1976.
8. Spencer, H.: Pulmonary blastomas. *J Pathol Bacteriol* 82:161, 1961.
9. Waddell, W.R.: Organoid differentiation of the fetal lung: A histologic study of the differentiation of mammalian fetal lung in utero and in transplants. *Arch Pathol* 47:227, 1949.

97

Myxoma of the Heart

MYXOMA OF THE heart is the most common intracavitary cardiac tumor. Seventy-five percent of them occur in the left atrium at the fossa ovalis. Other locations include the right atrium, both atria, or the ventricles. It may occur in any age from early infancy up to the late decades of life, seemingly with a slight female predominance.

PATHOLOGY

For several years the prevailing notion was that cardiac myxomas represent organized thrombi. More recently, histological, histochemical, and electron microscopy studies have shown that cardiac myxomas are composed of neoplastic cells (myxoma cells), which exhibit a wide range of differentiation. Actually, the observed cells were endothelial, fibroblastlike cells, macrophages, and mature and immature smooth muscle cells. In addition stellate-shaped cells and variously differentiated vascular structures are present. It is thought that cardiac myxomas arise from multipotential mesenchymal cells.[1] Symbas et al.,[4] proceeding with similar methods, suggested that the myxoma cells are active cells of endothelial origin[4] (Fig. 97-1).

Cardiac myxomas are basically benign tumors. However, the potentiality of a left atrial myxoma in behaving as a malignant neoplasm by local recurrence or embolization metastases requires awareness and aggressive management. Histologically,

on electron microscopy the features of recurrent tumors are identical to those of nonmetastasizing myxoma. The future behavior cannot be predicted accurately from the microscopic appearance of the primary tumor.[3] Murphy et al.[2] have reported on a myxosarcoma arising in the left atrium. The tumor was composed by poorly differentiated stellate and spindle cells lying in a myxoid stroma. Numerous mitotic figures were present and there was marked nuclear pleomorphism.

CLINICAL

Because of the consistent tumor location in the right atrium, the symptoms are relatively typical of those of tricuspid stenosis with pulmonary hypertension (Fig. 97-2). Systemic embolization at times has been a part of the clinical picture. The presentation may also include a constellation of systemic symptoms, such as fever, weight loss, anemia, hematological changes, and cyanosis.[4] The diagnosis can be established by means of echocardiography and especially by angiocardiography.

TREATMENT AND RESULTS

Cardiac myxomas are treated by surgery under direct vision and under total cardiopulmonary bypass. After excision of the tumor, the valves should be inspected and both atria should be examined for multicentric myxomas.[4]

The patient described by Murphy et al.[2]

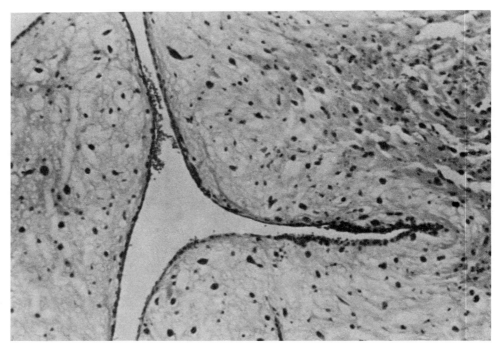

FIG. 97-1.   Myxoma of the heart. Polypoid growth of myxomatous stroma containing bizarre nuclei.

was a 16-year-old girl whose left atrial tumor was removed under total cardiopulmonary bypass. She remained well during the first seven postoperative

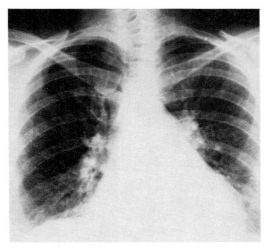

FIG. 97-2.   Myxoma of the right atrium in a 48-year-old female. There is cardiac enlargement associated with congestive heart failure.

months. Subsequently, there was gradual appetite loss accompanied by cough, fever, and finger clubbing. A holosystolic murmur was heard. Work-up led to a second thoracotomy, at which point she was found to have recurrent tumor involving the major portion of the atrial septum. This was biopsied and the patient underwent a course of postoperative radiotherapy, receiving 5000 rad to the heart in 30 days. She survived four years following the first operation, developing at that time metastasis to the left hip. This was histologically identical to the cardiac myxosarcoma and was treated with vincristine and actinomyxin B. The patient died five years following the original diagnosis.

Read *et al.*[3] reported on three patients whose left atrial tumors following the initial resection either recurred locally or metastasized distally. The authors reviewed the literature and found 10 similar patients who had undergone open heart surgery for locally recurrent left atrial myxomas. The authors advocate that, in order to avoid residual disease, all cardiac chambers should be inspected by means of a biatrial approach. Frequent and closer follow-up visits are also recommended. Due to the improvement of the surgical techniques, an increasing number of patients with cardiac myxomas are surviving now, following cardiac surgery, thus providing a chance for the tumor to better manifest its nature and biological behavior.[3]

REFERENCES

1. Ferrans, V.J., and Roberts, W.C.: Structural features of cardiac myxomas. Histology, histochemistry, and electron microscopy. *Hum Pathol* **4:**111, 1973.
2. Murphy, W.R.C., Carter, J.B., Lucas, R.V., Moller, J.H., Edwards, J.E., and Castaneda, A.R.: Recurrent myxosarcoma of left atrium. *Chest* **67:**733, 1975.
3. Read, R.C., White, H.J., Murphy, M.L., Williams, D., Sun, C.N., and Flanagan, W.H.: The malignant potentiality of left atrial myxoma. *J Thorac Cardiovasc Surg* **68:**857, 1974.
4. Symbas, P.N., Hatcher, C.R., Jr., and Gravanis, M.B.: Myxoma of the heart: Clinical and experimental observations. *Ann Surg* **183:**470, 1976.

98

Tumors of the Aorta

NEOPLASIA OF THE aorta is a rare entity. Until 1977, 15 documented cases existed in the English literature. The tumors occurred primarily during the fifth and sixth decades, the median age being 56 years. With the exception of one case in which the patient was a 3.5-month-old infant the rest of the patients have all been adults.[5-7] In spite of the small number of cases, it appears that males are more prone to develop aortic neoplasms, with 11 males and 4 females encountered thus far.

PATHOLOGY

The primary sites of the reported aortic tumors were as follows: thoracic aorta, two; abdominal aorta, seven; and thoracoabdominal aorta, six.

On the basis of the gross appearance, the neoplasms can be classified as[2]:

1. Polypoidal, which form long intraluminal projections attached to the arterial wall by a stalk or small base. This type is prone to produce tumor emboli resulting in multiple kidney and spleen infarcts.
2. Infiltrating tumors that progress by extension along the aortic surface in the form of plaques.
3. Finally, the adventitial type, which unlike the previous two, does not produce obstruction of the lumen extending and growing away from the vessel.

Histologically, these tumors are basically sarcomas. Several authors have stressed the presence of multinucleated giant cells. Some of them have a marked myxomatous appearance, which is reminiscent of the endocardial myxomas. The majority could be classified as fibromyxosarcomas. One patient with leiomyosarcoma has been described and three were found to have endothelial sarcomas.[2,4-6]

CLINICAL

The clinical diagnosis is extremely difficult. The symptoms are vague and the original diagnosis has been incorrect in practically all patients. Renal colic, hypertension, peripheral vascular disease, and herniated disc are among the initial diagnoses. Of the 15 reported cases, only two were diagnosed antemortem.[1,6]

All the symptoms are derived from and related to the vascular obstruction. They include migraine, intermittent claudication, intestinal colic, hypertension, low-back pain extending to the lower extremities, and embolic episodes with varied manifestations from various organs. General symptoms included nausea, vomiting, fever, and cachexia.[2-4,6] Hypertension in the upper extremities, frequently considered "malignant hypertension," combined with diminished femoral pulses has been the main clinical manifestation in four patients.[1,4,5]

Tumors of the aorta may give rise to

metastatic pulmonary neoplasm, idiopathic pulmonary hypertenson, aortic stenosis, and psychosomatic disorder.

With the exception of the lung, metastases to other organs have been infrequent. In the lungs it extends in the form of emboli. In reviewing the autopsy material, peripheral tumor emboli were found in 66% of the cases. Sarcomatous metastases to the hilar and mediastinal nodes were seen in 16%.[8]

TREATMENT AND RESULTS

Very few patients have been treated surgically for this tumor. Killebrew and Gerbode[6] reported on a 62-year-old man with a leiomyosarcoma involving the posterior wall of the pulmonary artery, extending from a location just distal to the pulmonary valve into the left pulmonary artery. The main pulmonary artery and the left pulmonary artery were replaced by a Dacron prosthetic composite graft. The patient died on the 12th postoperative day of right ventricular failure.

DiGilio et al.[2] reported on a 45-year-old man presenting with syncopal attacks. Cardiac catheterization and right ventricular angiocardiograms showed a filling defect in the main pulmonary artery and in the left pulmonary artery. The tumor was resected and in spite of its benign arrearance it proved to be a myxosarcoma. Six months later the lesion recurred and repeated ventricular angiocardiogram showed a large mass arising from the pulmonary valve and occupying most of the main pulmonary artery. A second operation was performed and the main pulmonary artery, the pulmonary valve, and adjacent portion of the anterior surface of the right ventricle were resected. The right ventricular outflow tract was reconstructed, utilizing a Dacron tube containing a porcine xenograph valve. The patient was surviving several months following surgery.

Schmookler et al.[8] reported on a 34-year-old woman whose presentation was a sudden severe substernal chest pain associated with dyspnea and fainting. Following catheterization studies, angiography was performed, which disclosed large filling defects in the pulmonary tract and both the right and the left main pulmonary arteries with lack of filling of the arteries to the lower lobe of the left lung and diminution of the filling of the arteries to the upper lobe of the same lung. At operation, a large tumor completely occupying the pulmonary tract extending into the right and the left main pulmonary arteries was found. The entire tumor was excised intact. The patient recovered uneventfully and she was placed on Adriamycin. Six months later, the systolic murmur returned and repeat right ventricular angiogram revealed a round filling defect in the anterior wall of the pulmonary trunk. Thoracotomy was again performed and a tumor mass was removed from the previous suture line. Histologically, this was an undifferentiated sarcoma.

With the exception of the cases just mentioned, in the great majority of patients (25 of 37) the diagnosis was made postmortem. The effectiveness of modern chemotherapy or radiotherapy on these neoplasms has not been determined. Haythorn et al.[5] used radiation in the management of a patient with primary fibromyxosarcoma of the pulmonary artery without success; however, the tumor dosage was inadequate.

PROGNOSIS AND SURVIVAL

Obviously, the prognosis is extremely poor, the average survival being 12 months. The duration of the disease, from the onset of the symptoms until the patient's death, has ranged from 1 to 39 months.[8]

REFERENCES

1. Ali, M.Y., and Lee, G.S.: Sarcoma of the pulmonary artery. *Cancer* 17:1220, 1964.

2. DiGilio, M.M., Tatooles, C.J., Rosen, K.M., and Rahimtoola, S.H.: Myxosarcoma of the pulmonary valve. *Chest* **62:**639, 1972.

3. Friedman, H.M., and Smith, C.K.: Leiomyosarcoma of the pulmonary artery. *JAMA* **203:**809, 1968.

4. Goldstein, B., and Joubert, E.J.: Solid pulmonary artery. *Thorax* **19:**322, 1964.

5. Haythorn, S.R., Ray, W.B., and Wolff, R.A.: Primary fibromyxosarcomas of the heart and pulmonary artery. *Am J Pathol* **17:**261, 1941.

6. Killebrew, E., and Gerbode, F.: Leiomyosarcoma of the pulmonary artery diagnosed preoperatively by angiocardiography. Replacement with composite graft. *J Thorac Cardiovasc Surg* **71:**469, 1976.

7. Rao, N.G., Krishnaswami, S., Cherian, G., and Krishnaswami, H.: Sarcoma of the pulmonary artery with metastases to pancreas and adrenal glands. *Chest* **66:**459, 1974.

8. Shmookler, B.M., Marsh, H.B., and Roberts, W.C.: Primary sarcoma of the pulmonary trunk and/or right or left main pulmonary artery—a rare cause of obstruction to right ventricular outflow. Report on two patients and analysis of 35 previously described patients. *Am J Med* **63:**263, 1977.

9. Wackers, F.J.T., Van Der Schoot, J.B., and Hampe, J.F.: Sarcoma of the pulmonary trunk associated with hemorrhagic tendency. A case report and review of the literature. *Cancer* **23:**339, 1969.

100

Tumors of the Superior and Inferior Vena Cava

PRIMARY TUMORS OF the venous system are rare. Light *et al.*[11] in a literature review found 22 malignant tumors involving the veins. Of these, nine arose in the inferior vena cava.

Bailey *et al.*[3] in 1976 encountered 35 cases of leiomyosarcoma involving the inferior vena cava reported in the literature, to which they added one of their own. In the same year Davis *et al.*[5] reported on a case of leiomyosarcoma involving the superior vena cava. This was the second such malignant case involving the superior vena cava reported.

Among 14,000 autopsies performed at the University of Michigan, Abell[1] was able to find only two cases of leiomyosarcoma of the inferior vena cava. Indeed, all cases reported in the English literature of tumors involving the venae cavae were leiomyosarcomas.

There is an overwhelming preference for females. Tabulating data from the literature, we found that 39 of the reported cases involved females and only seven were males. The average age at the time of the diagnosis has been 60 years. Nevertheless, the tumor can be seen in younger patients below the age of 40. Eight such patients have been reported.

PATHOLOGY

Staley *et al.*[12] for purposes of clinicoanatomical correlation divided the inferior vena cava into three segments: 1) a lower segment, extending from the junction of the right and left common iliac veins to an arbitrary point slightly below the renal veins, 2) a middle segment that continues up to the entrance of the hepatic veins, and 3) a superior segment that extends from the region of the hepatic veins to the right atrium. There is more or less an even distribution of tumors along those segments and in addition 37% of all reported cases had involvement of more than one segment.[3]

Neoplasms that arise in the wall of the middle and superior segment exhibit primarily an intraluminal growth. This is due to the presence of the liver and to the confinement by the surrounding structures. Leiomyosarcomas of the lower segment may extend intraluminally but occasionally the entire growth has been extraluminal in character.[12]

The tumors are slowly growing, not readily diagnosed, and therefore they usually attain a large size. In most patients the greatest diameter was in excess of 10.0 cm. Direct invasion of adjacent organs and extension into venous tributaries is often present.

The gross appearance is that of a nodular, lobulated, and firm mass. The color is gray-white or reddish-brown. Central necrosis has been recorded.[10,12]

They originate from the smooth muscles of either the media or from the adventitial vasa vasorum.[12] They are composed of cells that are spindle shaped or round in bizarre giant forms. Usually a combination of these groups is present. An increased number of mitotic figures is a prominent feature.[11]

They are generally of low-grade malignancy and metastases usually develop late.[1] The histological diagnosis of leiomyosarcomas involving the vena cava has not been a diagnostic problem.[12]

CLINICAL

The clinical signs and symptoms depend on the location of the lesion.

The patient reported by Davis *et al.*[5] with leiomyosarcoma involving the superior vena cava presented with malaise and discomfort of the chest. X-ray examination revealed the presence of a right paramediastinal mass.

Growths involving the inferior vena cava below the entrance of the renal veins present with edema of the lower extremities. This, however, may be minimal in character, particularly when the tumor is slow in growth, thus giving the opportunity for collaterals to develop.[12] For patients of this kind, the main finding many times is a palpable abdominal mass. Symptoms from adjacent organs of the gastrointestinal and urinary tract, as well as back pain, may predominate.[10]

Tumors of the middle segment produce renal vein thrombosis. When the renal vein is occluded, nephrotic syndrome and renal failure follow. When the hepatic vein is invaded and occluded by tumor, there is as a result hepatomegaly, ascites, and jaundice, actually a Budd-Chiari syndrome develops. Many times the hepatic failure is more dramatic than the syndrome itself.[8-10]

The leiomyosarcomas of the inferior vena cava may propagate upward and reach the right atrium. Such cases have been reported in the literature. The diagnosis was made at autopsy.[6,7]

Distant metastases occur late, primarily to the liver (17%) and to the lung (15%). In several patients, particularly those seen in earlier years, the diagnosis was made only during autopsy. However, during the last decades, practically in every case, exploratory laparotomy and an attempt at resection has been made.

TREATMENT AND RESULTS

Inferior venocavography and improvement in surgical techniques have resulted in attempts of surgical resection in practically all patients with tumors of the vena cava at this time. Cope and Hunt[4] were the first to report a long-term survivor following surgical resection of a tumor located in the middle and lower part of the inferior vena cava. The vein was resected from a point below the renal veins to the iliac veins and postoperative radiotherapy was delivered. Recurrence developed 16 months later involving the right renal vein. A right nephrectomy was performed in association with removal of the vein of the right kidney, to be followed one year later by a new recurrence involving the second lumbar vertebral body. Palliative radiotherapy was employed. Stuart and Baker[13] reported on a 58-year-old female with leiomyosarcoma involving the middle segment and liver metastases. Palliative resection resulted in a 14-month-survival period.

In general there are technical problems involved with a surgical procedure. Local recurrences have occurred in 36% of all operated patients. Obviously, there is concern of thrombotic episodes and involvement of the renal veins represents another technical problem. Human venous grafts and synthetic materials have been employed.[3,8,10,12]

Radiation therapy can be used palliatively for pain relief. Such a case has been reported by Allen *et al.*[2] Similarly, Davis *et al.*[5] employed cobalt radiotherapy postoperatively following the removal of a leiomyosarcoma of the superior vena cava. The patient received 5500 rad and was surviving without recurrence of metastases four years later.

Prognosis and Survival

Both the prognosis and the survival rate have changed within the last 15 years. This is due to the fact that the diagnosis is more accurate and the surgical treatment greatly improved. Of 21 patients who underwent tumor resection, 13 were surviving for more than one year following surgery. There were nine patients surviving for two years or longer.[3] As usually is the case, the smaller the tumor the better the prognosis.

References

1. Abell, M.R.: Leiomyosarcoma of the inferior vena cava. Review of the literature and report of two cases. *Am J Clin Pathol* **28**:272, 1957.
2. Allan, J., Burnett, W., and Lee, F.D.: Leiomyosarcoma of the inferior vena cava. *Scott Med J* **9**:352, 1964.
3. Bailey, R.V., Stribling, J., Weitzner, S., and Hardy, J.D.: Leiomyosarcoma of the inferior vena cava: Report of a case and review of the literature. *Ann Surg* **184**:169, 1976.
4. Cope, J.S., and Hunt, C.J.: Leiomyosarcoma of inferior vena cava. *Arch Surg* **68**:752, 1954.
5. Davis, G.L., Bergmann, M., and O'Kane, H.: Leiomyosarcoma of the superior vena cava. A first case with resection. *J Thorac Cardiovasc Surg* **72**:408, 1976.
6. Dmoulin, J.C., Sambon, Y., Baudinet, B., Beaujean, M., Jeukens, J.M., and Delvigne, J.: Leiomyosarcoma of the inferior vena cava; An unusual cause of pulmonary embolism. *Chest* **66**:597, 1974.
7. Deutsch, V., Fraenkel, O., Frand, U., and Hulu, N.: Leiomyosarcoma of the inferior vena cava propagating into the right atrium. *Br Heart J* **30**:571, 1968.
8. Dube, V.E., and Carlquist, J.H.: Surgical treatment of leiomyosarcoma of the inferior vena cava: Report of a case. *Am Surg* **37**:87, 1971.
9. Hallock, P., Watson, C.J., and Berman, L.: Primary tumor of inferior vena cava with clinical features suggestive Chiari's disease. *Arch Intern Med* **66**:5a, 1940.
10. Johansen, J.K., and Nielsen, R.: Leiomyosarcoma of the inferior vena cava. Report of a case. *Acta Chir Scand* **137**:181, 1971.
11. Light, H.G., Peskin, G.W., and Ravdin, I.S.: Primary tumors of the venous system. *Cancer* **13**:818, 1960.
12. Staley, C.J., Valaitis, J., Trippel, O.H., and Franzblau, S.A.: Leiomyosarcoma of the inferior vena cava. *Am J Surg* **113**:211, 1967.
13. Stuart, F.P., and Baker, W.H.: Palliative surgery for leiomyosarcoma of the inferior vena cava. *Ann Surg* **177**:237, 1973.

101

Insulinoma

THE FIRST CASE of carcinoma arising in the islands of the pancreas and producing hyperinsulinism and hypoglycemia was described by Wilder et al.[24] in 1927. Howland et al.[10] in 1929 reported the first patient with a solitary hyperfunctioning islet cell adenoma. Insulinomas are islet cell tumors arising from the beta cells of the pancreas. They belong to the APUD system of tumors and they can be seen alone or they may be part of a syndrome of multiple endocrine adenopathies.[16,22] The three cardinal symptoms of insulinoma were described by Whipple.[23] They include hypoglycemia, blood glucose level less than 50 mg/100 ml, and relief of the symptoms following ingestion of glucose. These three manifestations are known in the literature as Whipple's triad.

Insulinomas are the commonest islet cell tumors of the pancreas, or at least as common as pancreatic gastrinomas.[4] Most of them are benign—adenomas—in character. Islet cell carcinomas are estimated to occur in less than 1 per 100,000 population.[12,13,20] Among the carcinomas, functioning tumors with hormonal production comprise 79% of the total, whereas the remaining 21% are hormonally inactive.[1]

The tumors can be seen at any age, from the very young to the sixth or seventh decade of life.[3,17,18] The average age of the patient with pancreatic insulinoma is approximately 42 years.[5] Howard et al.[9] reviewed the literature on the subject and found no difference in incidence between males and females.

PATHOLOGY

Howard et al.[9] in 1950 and Stefanini et al.[21] in 1974 reviewed the literature and summarized the pathological characteristics of insulinomas. With regard to size, 87% of the insulinomas measure from 0.5 to 5.0 cm in diameter. Similarly, the majority of them, 83%, are single in character. They are firm in consistency and yellowish in color. Histologically, they are composed of beta cells that are arranged in cords or nests. The malignant lesions may display anaplasia. However, this is not an overwhelming feature and actually it is the clinical behavior rather than the histological pattern that determines the nature of the tumor. The only indisputable criterion of malignancy is the demonstration of metastases. Approximately 15% of the lesions that were thought to be histologically benign pursued a malignant course in the series by Howard et al.[9] In the same series approximately 10% of all insulinomas were malignant.

There is an even distribution of the lesions with regard to the head, body, and tail of the pancreas, each of which contains 30–34% of the neoplasms.[21] The coexistence of islet cell tumors with other endocrinopathies (multiple endocrine adenomatosis) has been established. This incidence is in the range of 5–10%. Abnormalities relating to the parathyroids, pituitary, adrenal, cortex, and thyroid gland have been reported.[7,22]

CLINICAL

The clinical symptoms and signs associated with severe hypoglycemia are common for adenomas and insulin-producing carcinomas. There is a severe drop of the levels of blood glucose during the night and for this reason the clinical manifestations are very pronounced in the early morning hours. Headaches and in severe cases confusion, drowsiness, and silly behavior occur. In more serious situations convulsions or coma follow. This is similar to insulin-produced shock. The bizarre emotional and psychological behavior is followed by amnesia. Under such circumstances, fasting blood sugar level may be well below 35 mg/100 ml.

It is important to associate the fasting hypoglycemia with inappropriately elevated plasma insulin levels in order to establish the diagnosis. Fasting hypoglycemia alone may occur in other conditions, such as nonpancreatic tumors, in patients with liver disease, and in those with hyperfunctioning anterior pituitary or hypofunctioning adrenal cortex. In infants and children idiopathic hypoglycemia should also be ruled out.[3,7]

When a rapid fall of the blood sugar takes place, it is manifested clinically by acute hunger, sweating, tachycardia, and weakness. Diplopia and ataxia, which may also exist, have at times been confused with alcohol intoxication. Administration of glucose relieves the hypoglycemic attack and this, of course, is part of the so-called "Whipple's triad."[3]

The diagnosis is based on the elevated insulin levels, which fail to decrease in view of the great hypoglycemia. This is a distinct feature of the insulinoma patient. Oral administration of diazoxide is accompanied by a rise of the blood glucose levels. Diazoxide is an insulin inhibitor and therefore this test is of diagnostic importance.

An essential examination at the present time in arriving at the correct diagnosis is the radioimmunoassay evaluation of the plasma insulin.[25] There is also a significant elevation of proinsulin. Proinsulin is present within the beta cells and is converted by proteolysis into insulin and C-peptide, or connecting peptide. It has been shown that malignant islet cell tumors have a higher value of proinsulin compared to benign adenomas.[18] Biochemical investigation may include other tests, such as glucose tolerance, tolbutamide tolerance, glucagon administration, and leucine administration.

Radiographically Olsson[15] was the first to report on the angiographic findings of insulinoma. The tumors are quite vascular, producing a homogeneous blush following celiac catheterization and contrast medium injection. In patients with large tumors or especially when metastatic extensions in the vicinity have taken place, displacement of the vessels is also seen. The overall accuracy in diagnosing insulinomas by means of arteriography is, according to Fulton, et al.[6] 91%. In the series by other authors the success rate is in the range of 70–80%.[15,21]

When pancreatic islet cell tumors are hormonally inactive, they present as abdominal masses that create biliary tract obstruction and jaundice or they are incidental findings during laparotomy for other causes[18,19] (Fig. 101-1).

Patients with islet cell carcinomas have in addition to their hormonal problems a malignancy to deal with, which eventually will produce metastases. The common metastatic sites are the regional lymph nodes and the liver.[7]

TREATMENT AND RESULT

The appropriate form of therapy is surgical resection. This presents relatively small difficulties, provided that preoperative arteriograms have demonstrated the tumor, that the tumor is solitary, and that no metastatic disease is present. Under these circumstances, the results are excel-

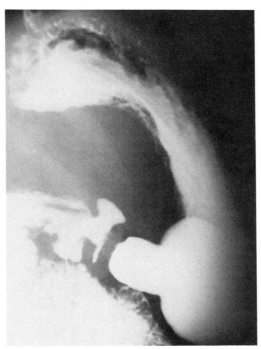

FIG. 101-1. Malignant islet cell tumor. Lateral view
shows anterior displacement of the stomach.

lent. Fonkalsrud et al.[5] reported no major
problems under these conditions in patients followed for periods ranging from
two to five years.

When the tumors are multiple or when
demonstration by means of arteriography
has been impossible or when pancreatic
adenomatosis prevails, the management is
more difficult. Under these circumstances,
it is recommended that 50–80% of the
pancreas be resected.[7] At times, a second
or third operation has been necessary in
order to correct the patient's symptoms.[21]
For these patients, blind pancreatic resection is the only form of definitive therapy,
and obviously this carries a considerable
risk.[7]

The surgical treatment applies to both
benign and malignant insulinomas. For
malignant insulinomas that appear to be
unresectable or those that have intraabdominal metastases at the time of the exploration, chemotherapy is the alternative

form of management. Diazoxide causes
direct insulin inhibition but possesses no
antitumor effect, therefore the neoplasm
continues to grow and metastasize at its
own pace. L-Asparaginase depresses the
plasma insulin, resulting in rise of
the blood sugar levels; however, the
drug itself is hepatotoxic. The main
chemotherapeutic agent employed is
streptozotocin. It has been shown in animals that it selectively destroys the pancreatic beta cells. Broder and Carter[1,2] reported on 52 patients with pancreatic islet
cell carcinomas treated with streptozotocin. Among them, there were four with
pure insulinomas. Of these, two showed
good response and two responded poorly.
The drug was administered intravenously
or intraarterially. Kraybill et al.[11] reported
on a patient with malignant insulinoma
metastatic to the liver who was originally
treated with 5-fluorouracil without success. Streptozotocin was administered
thereafter, which produced a definite decrease in liver size; however, subsequent
liver tumor became refractory to the drug.
Following a trial with tubercidin, which
also failed, the patient was placed on
Adriamycin infusion in conjunction with
diazoxide. Although his disease continued to progress, he was surviving
seven years from the time of the diagnosis.

Herbai and Lundin[8] reviewed the literature and reported a case of their own with
regard to the effectiveness of streptozotocin therapy. They obtained a 22-month
survival on a patient with demonstrable
metastatic liver deposits. Recently, Moertel et al.[14] reviewed the effectiveness
of streptozotocin alone compared to
streptozotocin in combination with
5-fluorouracil in the treatment of advanced islet cell carcinomas. In a group
study that included 84 patients there were
15 with malignant insulinomas. Although
satisfactory or excellent response was obtained in three of eight patients treated
with streptozotocin alone, good responses

were obtained in six of seven among those treated with streptozotocin and 5-fluorouracil. The authors considered a favorable response to be a reduction of the tumor mass by more than 50% or decrease in the laboratory values by more than 50%. Complete response was considered the disappearance of all clinical and laboratory signs. The superior results of the combined therapy were obtained uniformly for the entire islet cell carcinoma group and not for malignant insulinomas specifically.[14]

PROGNOSIS AND SURVIVAL

Although the prognosis of benign insulinomas is excellent provided the tumors have been resected completely, patients with malignant insulinomas in general eventually die of their tumor. Howard et al.[9] in their extensive literature review found only one apparent survivor among 37 patients considered to have malignant insulinoma. In spite of the eventual poor outcome metastatic islet cell carcinomas are slowly growing neoplasms and they afford a lengthy survival. Broder and Carter[2] note that patients who responded well to chemotherapy have had longer survival than those who did not. The average survival of the former was in the range of 42 months as opposed to 17 months for the latter.

Moertel et al.[14] found the median survival of patients with advanced islet cell carcinomas treated by streptozotocin and 5-fluorouracil to be 26 months. The survival of patients similarly staged who were treated by streptozotocin alone was 16 months. The same authors note that the survival curves are identical for both functioning and nonfunctioning islet cell carcinomas.

REFERENCES

1. Broder, L.E., and Carter, S.K.: Pancreatic islet cell carcinoma. I. Clinical features of 52 patients. *Ann Intern Med* **79**:101, 1973.

2. Broder, L.E., and Carter, S.K.: Pancreatic islet cell carcinoma. II. Results of therapy with streptozotocin in 52 patients. *Ann Intern Med* **79**:108, 1973.

3. Dahms, B.B., Lippe, B.M., Dakake, C., Fonkalsrud, E.W., and Mirra, J.M.: The occurrence in a neonate of a pancreatic adenoma with nesidioblastosis in the tumor. *Am J Clin Pathol* **65**:462, 1976.

4. Ellison, E.H., and Wilson, S.D.: The Zollinger-Ellison syndrome updated. *Surg Clin North Am* **47**:1115, 1967.

5. Fonkalsrud, E.W., Dilley, R.B., and Longmire, W.P.: Insulin secreting tumors of the pancreas. *Ann Surg* **159**:730, 1964.

6. Fulton, R.E., Sheedy, P.F., McIlrath, D.C., and Ferris, D.O.: Preoperative angiographic localization of insulin-producing tumors of the pancreas. *AJR* **123**:367, 1975.

7. Harrison, T.S., Child, C.G., 3rd, Fry, W.J., Floyd, J.C., Jr., and Fajans, S.S.: Current surgical management of functioning islet cell tumors of the pancreas. *Ann Surg* **178**:485, 1973.

8. Herbai, G., and Lundin, Å.: Treatment of malignant metastatic pancreatic insulinoma with streptozotocin. Review of 21 cases described in detail in the literature and report of complete remission of a new case. *Acta Med Scand* **200**:447, 1976.

9. Howard, J.M., Moss, N.H., and Rhoads, J.E.: Hyperinsulinism and islet cell tumors of the pancreas. *Int Abstr Surg* **90**:417, 1950.

10. Howland G., Campbell, W.R., Maltby, E.J., and Robinson, W.L.: Dysinsulinism: Convulsions and coma due to islet cell tumor of the pancreas with operation and cure. *JAMA* **93**:674, 1929.

11. Kraybill, W.G., Jr., Anderson, D.D., Lindell, T.D., and Fletcher, W.S.: Islet cell carcinoma of the pancreas: Effective therapy with 5-fluorouracil, streptozotocin, and tubercidin. *Am Surg* **42**:467, 1976.

12. Lopez-Kruger, R., and Dockerty, M.D.: Tumors of the islets of Langerhans. *Surg Gynecol Obstet* **85**:495, 1947.

13. Moldow, R.E., and Connelly, R.R.: Epidemiology of pancreatic cancer in Connecticut. *Gastroenterology* **55**:677, 1968.

14. Moertel, C.G., Hanley, J.A., and Johnson, L.A.: Streptozotocin alone compared with streptozotocin plus fluorouracil in the treatment of advanced islet-cell carcinoma. *N Engl J Med* **303**:1189, 1980.

15. Olsson, O.: Angiographic diagnosis of an islet cell tumor of the pancreas. *Acta Chir Scand* **126**:346, 1963.

16. Pearse, A.G.E.: Common cytochemical and ultrastructural characteristics of cells producing polypeptide hormones (the APUD series) and their relevance to thyroid and ultimobranchial C

cells and calcitonin. *Proc R Soc Lond [Biol]* **170**:71, 1968.

17. Rickham, P.P.: Islet cell tumors in childhood. *J Pediatr Surg* **10**:83, 1975.

18. Schein, P.S.: Islet cell tumors: Current concepts and management. *Ann Intern Med* **79**:239, 1973.

19. Shield, C.F., Haff, R.C., and Murray, H.M.: Islet cell tumors of the pancreas. *Am J Surg* **128**:709, 1974.

20. Spencer, H.: Pancreatic islet-cell adenomata. *J Pathol Bacteriol* **69**:259, 1955.

21. Stefanini, P., Caboni, M., Patrassi, N., De Bernardinis, G., Negro, P., and Blandamura, V.: The value of arteriography in the diagnosis and treatment of insulinomas. *Am J Surg* **131**:352, 1975.

22. Welbourn, R.B.: Current status of apudomas. *Ann Surg* **185**:1, 1977.

23. Whipple, A.O.: Hyperinsulinism in relation to pancreatic tumors. *Surgery* **16**:289, 1944.

24. Wilder, R.M., Allan, F.N., Power, W.H., and Robertson, H.E.: Carcinoma of the islands of the pancreas: Hyperinsulinism and hypoglycemia. *JAMA* **89**:348, 1927.

25. Yalow, R.S., and Berson, S.A.: Immunoassay of endogenous plasma insulin in man. *J Clin Invest* **39**:1157, 1960.

102

Pancreatic Gastrinoma
(Zollinger-Ellison Syndrome)

ZOLLINGER AND ELLISON[14] in 1955 described a syndrome characterized by the following triad of symptoms: 1) overwhelming peptic ulcer diathesis with several recurrences in spite of repeated operations, 2) gastric hypersecretion, and 3) the presence of nonbeta islet cell tumors of the pancreas. Gregory *et al.*[3] in 1960 demonstrated that the ulcerogenic syndrome was due to an excessive secretion of gastrin by the pancreatic tumors and their metastases. Gastrin is a potent secretagogue, under the influence of which high volumes of acid gastric juice are secreted. Gastrin also leads to hyperplasia of the gastric mucosa and to a lesser extent it promotes pepsin secretion.[16] In addition, it increases the contractions of the stomach, stimulates the flow of the bile, relaxes the sphincter of Oddi, stimulates water and enzyme secretion by the pancreas, and releases insulin.[4] Normally, gastrin activity is most prominent in the region of the gastric antrum; however, the duodenum, jejunum, and ileum exhibit small, but definite, gastrin activity.[6]

As all islet cell tumors, gastrinomas of the pancreas are APUD cell tumors, or apudomas. They belong to the paraendocrine group because they produce a hormone normally not found in the pancreas. It is now known that gastrinomas may arise from the gastrin-producing cells (G cells) of the stomach or the duodenum in the form of hyperplasia or as carcinomas. These latter gastrinomas are classified as orthoendocrine apudomas.[11]

The exact incidence of the Zollinger-Ellison syndrome (ZES) among the population suffering from peptic ulcer disease has not been defined. It is suspected that several cases of minor severity remain diagnosed as ordinary ulcer disease. It is estimated that ZES accounts for less than 1% of peptic ulcer disease.[5]

Most patients present during the third through the fifth decades of life; however, the syndrome has been seen in patients younger than the age of 20 years. There is possibly a slight male predominance.[2,5]

PATHOLOGY

In general, gastrinomas are tumors of small size and they may be difficult to locate.[9] In only 50% of the 249 cases reviewed by Ellison and Wilson,[2] were the tumors solitary, located mainly in the head and the tail of the pancreas. Multiple lesions were seen in 29% and microadenomatosis involving the entire gland in 19%. Malignant tumors composed 61% of the clinical material and the remaining 39% were benign. Regional lymph node metastasis to the paraduodenal and parapancreatic groups or to the nodes of the stomach was found in 53% of the malignant cases. In addition local extension was present in 48% of the tumors, and metastases to the liver were found in 48%.[2]

Microscopically, benign and malignant gastrinomas may have the same appearance. The only certain way to establish malignancy is the demonstration of metastasis. The cells are usually well differentiated and are arranged in trabecular patterns, or in sheets or nests.[5] Extraction of gastrinoma produces gastrin, which can be measured by bioassay or by radioimmunoassay techniques.[7,8]

CLINICAL

The typical ulcerogenic tumor syndrome presents with a fulminating ulcer diathesis, diarrhea, or steatorrhea. There is gross gastric hypersecretion and elevation of the serum gastrin levels.[15] The intensity of the symptoms, as well as their relative predominance, vary from patient to patient, and in this manner smaller clinical subgroups may be identified.[15] Pain as a result of the ulcer is the commonest symptom, seen in 74% of the cases followed by diarrhea in 36%. Acute perforation, melena, and hematemesis occur in approximately 20% of the cases.[2] Steatorrhea has been reported in many patients, but the exact incidence has not been determined.[5] A common presentation of the syndrome is pain recurring a few days or a few weeks after ulcer surgery, with new radiographic signs. There is gastric hypersecretion relieved only by continuous nasogastric suction.[5]

The disease is often associated with other endocrine abnormalities, which manifest themselves as carcinomas, adenomas, or as diffuse hyperplasias of the involved glands. The commonest such condition is hyperparathyroidism. Less frequently, pituitary, thyroid, adrenal, and ovarian tumors have been encountered.[10] A familial tendency for these multiple endocrine gland neoplasias has been described.[12]

Radiographic examination of the upper gastrointestinal tract plays an important role in the diagnosis. In 75% of the patients an ulcer is present in the duodenal bulb or in the immediate postbulbar region.[5] The finding of an ulcer crater beyond the ligament of Treitz is considered to be a pathognomonic sign.[16] The rugal folds of the stomach are hypertrophic and there is a large amount of fluid present. These are the results of gastrin stimulation. The small bowel may be normal or it may give the impression of nontropical sprue.[5]

Arteriography with selective pancreatic angiograms yields a tumor recognition in 30–50% of the cases.[5]

Evaluation of the gastric acid hypersecretion and of the serum gastrin level are the laboratory means of establishing the diagnosis. Fasting serum gastrin levels, with or without calcium and secretin stimulation are generally higher than in normal individuals. Although a number of cases show borderline values, patients with the typical ulcerogenic syndrome have gastrin concentrations 10 times that of normal. Bioassay and the much more accurate radioimmunoassay techniques are used in gastrin determinations.[5]

TREATMENT AND RESULTS

The treatment of the ZES is surgical and it entails removal of the target organ, namely, the stomach. The patient and his family are preoperatively presented with the facts of the disease and with the surgical plan. Those patients whose gastrin is definitely elevated should undergo no other procedure than total gastrectomy. In rare occasions when pancreatic or duodenal gastrinomas are evident during exploration (10%), simple excision of the tumor may be performed, as a "wait and see" policy.[5,15] Blind pancreatic resections or total pancreatectomy are no longer practiced. In addition to thorough palpation of the duodenum in order to locate duodenal gastrinomas, the lymph nodes in the gastroduodenal ligament should be excised and examined for evidence of metastases and if other metastatic sites are to be found they should be resected, provided the procedure does not endanger the patient's life. Their removal decreases the level of the circulating gastrin. Palpation of the duodenum up to the ligament of Treitz is also necessary in order to determine the presence of ulcers.[15] It is obvious that the surgical procedure does not aim primarily at the reduction of gastrin but at the removal of the organ the hormone acts upon. The lethal potential of the syndrome is not due to local tumor growth or to overwhelming metastases from gastrinoma but to the severe and repeated peptic ulcers and the associated complications. Young children should also undergo total gastrectomy if they are to survive their fulminating disease.[15] For reconstruction the Roux-en-Y type of anastomosis has been performed.

The preoperative measures should include treatment with no calcium-containing antacids and anticholinergics; even low-dose, 2000 rad, radiotherapy to the stomach might be considered in an effort to reduce the acidity.

A recurrence rate of at least 50% is to be expected among patients whose treatment has been less than total gastrectomy, because in patients with ZES the parietal cell mass is sixfold the normal.

In the postoperative period the patient's weight and caloric intake should be monitored. Injection of vitamin B_{12} should be given monthly. Nutritional difficulties due to narrowing at the anastomosis also may develop, another reason that follow-up radiographic examinations of the upper gastrointestinal tract are needed.

In those situations in which liver or lymph node metastases are found during exploration, gastrectomy is not contraindicated. The tumor growth is usually very slow and the main imminent danger is the severe ulcer diathesis. It is obvious that

gastrin levels remain high in all patients whose treatment has been only gastrectomy.

Patients with metastatic inoperable gastrinomas may respond to streptozotocin.[1] The liver is the commonest site, where the metastases tend to be multiple. For this reason, liver scans are recommended as part of the follow-up of these patients.[15] Patients with malignant gastrinomas who have been treated by gastrectomy usually die of extensive metastatic disease to the liver.[5]

PROGNOSIS AND SURVIVAL

Wilson and Ellison[2,13] analyzed the survival rates according to the type of surgical resection the patients had. The extent of the gastric resection greatly influences the survival. At the time of the studies, only 25% of the patients who had no stomach resection were alive. There were 50% survivors among patients who had had subtotal gastrectomy, whereas 70% of those who were treated by total gastrectomy were living. The best survival was found among those patients who had total gastrectomy as the initial form of therapy.[2,13]

Data from the Zollinger-Ellison tumor registry indicate that of 265 patients treated by total gastrectomy, 81 subsequently died. This represents a mortality rate of 30%. The cause of death was postoperative complications in 60% of the cases, advancing malignancy in 20%, and other medical diseases in 20%.[5]

The five-year survival of patients with malignant gastrinoma and treated by total grastectomy is 40%, approximately. The growth rate of malignant gastrinomas is very slow.[15]

REFERENCES

1. Cryer, P.E., and Hill, G.J., II.: Pancreatic islet cell carcinoma with hypercalcemia and hypergastrinemia. Response to streptozotocin. *Cancer* **38:**2217, 1976.

2. Ellison, E.D., and Wilson, S.D.: The Zollinger-Ellison syndrome: Re-appraisal and evaluation of 260 registered cases. *Ann Surg* **160:**512, 1964.

3. Gregory, R.A., Tracy, H.J., French, J.M., and Sircus, W.: Extraction of a gastrin-like substance from pancreatic tumor in case of Zollinger-Ellison syndrome. *Lancet* **1:**1049, 1960.

4. Grossman, M.I.: Gastrin and its activities. *Nature* **228:**1147, 1970.

5. Isenberg, J.I., Walsh, J.H., and Grossman, M.I.: Zollinger-Ellison syndrome. *Gastroenterology* **65:**140, 1973.

6. Lai, K.S.: Studies on gastrin, Part II. Quantitative study of the distribution of gastrin-like activity along the gut. *Gut* **5:**334, 1964.

7. McGuigan, J.E., and Trudeau, W.L.: Studies with antibodies to gastrin. Radioimmunoassay in human serum and physiological studies. *Gastroenterology* **58:**139, 1970.

8. Moore, F.T., Murat, J.E., Endahl, G.L., Baker, J.L., and Zollinger, R.M.: Diagnosis of ulcerogenic tumor of the pancreas by bioassay. *Am J Surg* **113:**735, 1967.

9. Ptak, T., and Kirsner, J.B.: The Zollinger-Ellison syndrome, polyendocrine adenomatosis and other endocrine associations with peptic ulcer. *Adv Intern Med* **16:**213, 1970.

10. Walsh, J.H., and Sleisenger, M.H.: Clinical syndromes associated with tumors of the pancreas. *DM* 1–30, June, 1967.

11. Welbourn, R.B.: Current status of the apudomas. *Ann Surg* **185:**1, 1977.

12. Wermer, P.: Endocrine adenomatosis and peptic ulcer in a large kindred: Inherited multiple tumors and mosaic pleiotropism in man. *Am J Med* **35:**205, 1963.

13. Wilson, S.D., and Ellison, E.H.: Survival in patients with the Zollinger-Ellison syndrome treated by total gastrectomy. *Am J Surg* **111:**787, 1966.

14. Zollinger, R.M., and Ellison, E.H.: Primary peptic ulcerations of the jejunum associated with islet cell tumors of the pancreas. *Ann Surg* **142:**709, 1955.

15. Zollinger, R.M.: Islet cell tumors of the pancreas and the alimentary tract. *Am J Surg* **129:**102, 1975.

16. Zollinger, R.M.: Islet cell tumors and the alimentary tract. *AJR* **126:**933, 1976.

103

WDHA Syndrome
(Watery Diarrhea, Hypokalemia, Achlorhydria Syndrome)
(Pancreatic Cholera Syndrome)

VERNER AND MORRISON[9] in 1958 described two patients with non-B islet cell pancreatic tumors who presented with profuse watery diarrhea. Unlike the patients with Zollinger-Ellison syndrome (ZES), the gastric acid secretion was low and peptic ulcers were absent. Subsequently, Bloom *et al.*[2] demonstrated elevated plasma levels and the presence within these tumors of a vasoactive peptide (vasoactive intestinal peptide, VIP) which is responsible for the main clinical and biochemical changes of the syndrome. The peptide stimulates the flow of the small bowel juice, producing watery diarrheas with potassium loss, and it inhibits the secretion of the gastric acid.[1] The severe diarrhea is similar in character to that produced by the *Vibrio cholerae*, whose enterotoxin affects the metabolism of the intestinal mucosa cells.[4]

As with the rest of the islet cell tumors, VIP-producing tumors are APUD cell tumors. Welbourn[11] classifies them into the paraendocrine group because the hormone produced does not represent a normal pancreatic hormone. Vasoactive intestinal polypeptide is normally secreted by the small and the large intestine.

There is a preponderance of male patients among the cases reported thus far, the ratio of male to female being 3:1.[10] The median average age of the reported patients has been 45 years, approximately.

PATHOLOGY

The tumors, when discrete, are easily identified during the surgical exploration, most of them located in the body and the tail of the pancreas. Approximately 80% of them have been found in these regions.[8]

Verner and Morrison[10] reviewed 55 reported cases of patients with WDHA syndrome. Of them 37% had malignant tumors, 43% benign, and in the remaining 20% the growth was in the form of benign hyperplasia.

Greider *et al.*[5] performed a comparative histological examination of the pancreatic islet cell tumors. It was their conclusion that no differential morphological features could be found between those that metastasized and those that did not. Moreover, the histological criteria alone were considered unreliable in distinguishing with certainty the islet cell tumors from each other. Morphologically, diarrheogenic tumors as well as those of ZES do resemble each other in that they may exhibit glandular formations, a feature not seen in alpha or beta cell neoplasms[5] (Fig. 103-1). Histochemical, ultrastructural, and biochemical studies are required in order to label the cell of origin. Obviously, the clinical symptoms carry considerable weight in this process.

CLINICAL

Severe watery diarrhea is the main clinical symptom, the duration of which varies from a few weeks to several years prior to the diagnosis. Usually, it is more than one year in duration.[10] It is accompanied by great potassium loss, with an average excretion of 300 mEq of potassium in the stools per day. During the acute exacerbations, the daily fluid loss could be as high as 5 liters.[8] Severe metabolic acidosis may also occur as a result of bicarbonate loss in the stool.

The inhibitory action of the VIP upon the histamine stimulation of the gastric mucosa results in hypo- or achlorhydria. This occurs despite the fact that biopsies indicate that the gastric mucosa is within normal limits.[8,11]

Hypercalcemia has often been seen in these patients, actually with higher frequency than in patients with ZES. The mechanism is unclear.

Other clinical signs and symptoms include skin flushing, cardiomyopathy due to the strong cardiac inotropic action of the VIP, and hypertension. There is eventually renal failure in the form of vacuolar nephropathy, resulting from severe and repeated episodes of electrolyte and fluid imbalance. This is a life-threatening development and most patients with uncontrollable tumors have died from it.[12]

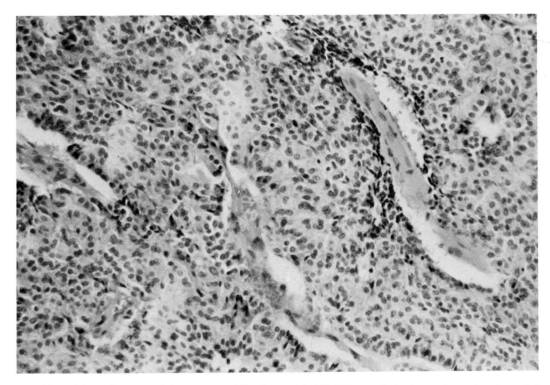

FIG. 103-1.   Islet cell tumor of the pancreas (diarrheogenic). Highly vascularized neoplasm showing solid sheets of small orderly cells with attempts at glandular formation in a 74-year-old male.

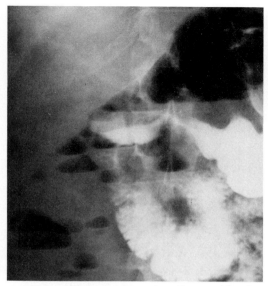

FIG. 103-2.   WDHA syndrome in a 45-year-old male. Severe watery diarrhea of six months' duration. Erect view of the abdomen demonstrates several air-fluid levels resulting from the excessive amount of fluids in both the small and the large bowel. (Courtesy R.P. Gold *et al. AJR* **127**:397, 1976.)

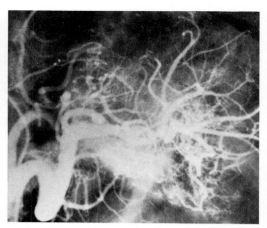

FIG. 103-3.   WDHA syndrome. Same patient as in Figure 103-2. The tumor occupied the tail of the pancreas and invaded the spleen. It was supplied primarily by the splenic artery, as this selective arteriogram shows. The mass was extremely vascular. (Courtesy R.P. Gold *et al. AJR* **127**:397, 1976.)

Radiographically, nonbeta islet cell tumors producing the WDHA syndrome appear on arteriography as vascular lesions, with large feeding vessels and dense capillary stain[3] (Figs. 103-2, 103-3, 103-4). Gold *et al.*[3] in reviewing the subject recommend transaxial computerized tomography when a pancreatic tumor is suspected clinically. A dilated nonobstructed gallbladder is present in several of the patients with WDHA syndrome.[12]

Indirect immunofluorescence techniques employing VIP antiserum provide positive results when reacting with sera obtained from patients. The high VIP levels in the plasma may also be assessed by radioimmunoassay techniques.[2]

TREATMENT AND RESULTS

Multiple hospitalizations are needed during the course of the disease in order to bring about a correction in the continuously deranged electrolyte balance and to rectify the dehydration and hypovolemia.

Because of the constant loss, however, this is a difficult task, even after vigorous intravenous fluid administration and potassium replacements.

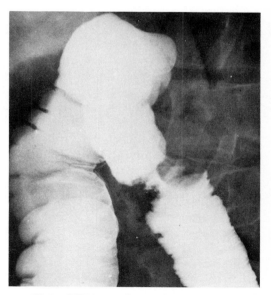

FIG. 103-4.   WDHA syndrome. Same patient as in Figure 103-2. Following extensive resection, the tumor recurred in 14 months. Barium enema shows involvement of the splenic flexure. In addition there was disease in retroperitoneal region, the mesenteric lymph nodes, and the omentum. (Courtesy R.P. Gold *et al. AJR* **127**:397, 1976.)

The basic therapy is surgical removal of the tumor responsible for the syndrome. The preoperative preparation may take several days, during which the water and electrolyte balance are corrected to the extent possible. Temporary symptom relief at this time can be obtained by steroid administration.[12] Following arteriographic examination, surgical extirpation of the tumors has often been feasible. The lesions are in these cases well circumscribed, often large in size.[8,12] In case of a normal pancreas, the procedure to be performed during the first operation is subtotal pancreatectomy. If this does not result in cure and if microscopic examination reveals diffuse hyperplasia of the nonbeta cells in the submitted specimen, a total pancreatectomy is necessary for complete cure.[10] In the postoperative period, there is a dramatic relief from the symptoms and potassium replacement is no longer needed. The achlorhydria of the stomach ceases as free hydrochloric acid appears. The elevated serum calcium levels return to normal.[12]

If resection is not possible, as in cases of far-advanced metastatic disease, palliative measures may be considered. Adrenal cortical steroids, as previously mentioned, may bring temporary symptomatic relief. Partial resection of the tumor brings about a decrease in the severity of the symptoms. Following this type of therapy, Kahn et al.[6] inserted catheters into the hepatic arteries of two patients, both of whom had extensive liver metastases. Streptozotocin, in doses of 1.5 g/M² was infused intraarterially at intervals of five to seven days. After a treatment course of three to five doses, one patient was symptom-free 12 months later and the other died of unrelated cause 13 months after the initiation of the therapy, with only moderate diarrhea present.

Moore et al.[7] reported on a 32-year-old female patient with a large unresectable diarrheogenic tumor treated by radiation therapy, receiving approximately 4000 rad

tumor dose. The mass decreased in size and the diarrhea subsided over the ensuing two months. The patient remained well for four years. The symptoms at that point returned and the mass reappeared. Partial resection gave considerable symptom relief of over a year's duration. This was a malignant variant, metastasizing to the regional lymph nodes.

PROGNOSIS AND SURVIVAL

Should the operation be successful and the tumor benign in character, dramatic symptom relief takes place and permanent cure occurs.[12] In contrast, patients with the malignant form who were operated upon had a mean survival time of 14 months.[3]

Verner and Morrison[10] in their literature review found that 13% of all cases were diagnosed at autopsy. All of them had benign, potentially curable tumors. Eight of 11 patients who had diffuse nonbeta cell hyperplasia were cured surgically.

REFERENCES

1. Barbezat, G.O., and Grossman, M.I.: Cholera-like diarrhoea induced by glucagon plus gastrin. Lancet 1:1025, 1971.
2. Bloom, S.R., Polak, J.M., and Pearse, A.G.E.: Vasoactive intestinal peptide and watery-diarrhoea syndrome. Lancet 2:14, 1973.
3. Gold, R.P., Black, T.J., Rotterdam, H., and Casarella, W.J.: Radiologic and pathologic characteristics of the WDHA syndrome. AJR 127:397, 1976.
4. Graham, D.Y., Johnson, C.D., Bentlif, P.S., and Kelsey, J.R., Jr.: Islet cell carcinoma, pancreatic cholera, and vasoactive intestinal peptide. Ann Intern Med 83:782, 1975.
5. Greider, M.H., Rosai, J., and McGuigan, J.E.: The human pancreatic islet cells and their tumors. II. Ulcerogenic and diarrheogenic. Cancer 33:1423, 1974.
6. Kahn, R., Levy, A.G., Gardner, J.D., Miller, J.V., Gorden, P., and Schein, P.S.: Pancreatic cholera: Beneficial effects of treatment with streptozotocin. N Engl J Med 292:941, 1975.
7. Moore, F.T., Nadler, S.H., Radefeld, D.A., and Zollinger, R.M.: Prolonged remission of diarrhea

due to nonbeta islet cell tumor of the pancreas by radiotherapy. *Am J Surg* **115:**854, 1968.

8. Schein, P.S., DeLellis, R.A., Kahn, C.R., Gorden, P., and Kraft, A.R.: Islet cell tumors: Current concepts and management. *Ann Intern Med* **79:**239, 1973.

9. Verner, J.V., and Morrison, A.B.: Islet cell tumor and a syndrome of refractory watery diarrhea and hypokalemia. *Am J Med* **25:**374, 1958.

10. Verner, J.V., and Morrison, A.B.: Endocrine pancreatic islet disease with diarrhea. Report of a case due to diffuse hyperplasia of nonbeta islet tissue with a review of 54 additional cases. *Arch Intern Med* **133:**492, 1974.

11. Welbourn, R.B.: Current status of apudomas. *Ann Surg* **185:**1, 1977.

12. Zollinger, R.M.: Islet cell tumors of the pancreas and the alimentary tract. *Am J Surg* **129:**102, 1975.

104

Pancreatic Glucagonoma

PANCREATIC GLUCAGONOMAS arise from the alpha cells of the islets of Langerhans. These cells normally secrete glucagon; therefore the tumors are considered to be orthoendocrine apudomas.[11] Glucagon is a polypeptide that maintains the hepatic glucose production needed for energy requirements. Whenever the cerebral glucose level is diminished either by insufficient exogenous glucose intake or because of excessive glucose utilization, or because of abnormalities in the cerebral blood flow, the level of the glucagon rises in relationship to insulin. This increases the hepatic glucose production initially by glycogenolysis, and later through increased synthesis of new glucose. The interaction between the glucagon and insulin and the rise of one relative to the other determines whether glucose is added to or removed from the extracellular compartment and whether amino acids are used for protein synthesis, or for glyconeogenesis. Basically, glucagon is the biological antagonist of insulin.[9]

Glucagonomas have been recognized recently and, although their overall incidence is not clear, certainly they represent a rare tumor. The first reported case was by McGavran et al.[6] in 1966. Since that time, a number of case reports have appeared in the literature. It was Mallinson et al.[5] who in 1974 reported nine cases and formulated the so-called "glucagonoma syndrome."

Review of the literature revealed an average age of 54 years among 16 reported patients. Twelve were female and four were male.

PATHOLOGY

The histological appearance of glucagonomas is very similar to those of all islet cell tumors. The tumors are well vascularized and made up of sheets and trabeculae of cells with large nuclei and single large nucleoli.[1,4] The tumors may exhibit features of benign adenoma or histological characteristics of a carcinoma. The malignant lesions appear to be more common. Six of 8 cases in which the histology was available, reported by Mallinson et al.,[5] were malignant in character. So were the cases described by Scully and McNeely,[7] by Danforth et al.,[1] by Lightman and Bloom,[4] by Ingemansson,[2] by Leichter et al.,[3] and by Tiengo et al.,[8] as was the very first case described by McGavran et al.[6] Electron microscopy reveals that they are composed of cells that carry the characteristics of the alpha cells. They contain dense secretory granules and radioimmunoassay reveals high glucagon concentration. The metastatic malignant glucagonoma carries similar features.[5]

CLINICAL

Skin lesions are a characteristic of these tumors. Rash develops, which usually is widespread, more prominent in the lower abdomen, perineum, thighs, buttocks, and the upper extremities. The skin lesions occur also in the face. They are erythematous in character and later on they become elevated with a central blistering. The blisters eventually rupture and healing takes place with discoloration of the involved skin. In areas of friction, however, such as in the groin or the perineum, a weeping surface remains open. This cycle, from the appearance of the lesions to their healing process, takes one to two weeks. Simultaneous presence of lesions at various stages of development is often the case. Minor traumas contribute greatly to the production of the skin eruptions. Histologically, the change involves the epidermis, where bullous disruption of the stratum of malpighii is present.[5] A normocytic, normochromic anemia is often to be found. There is a pronounced weight loss and diabetes is present in most of these patients. The symptoms usually have been noted for more than a year prior to the establishment of the diagnosis.

In recent years radioimmunoassays for pancreatic glucagon provide specific information as to the levels of the pancreatic glucagon. In patients with glucagonoma the plasma glucagon may reach 10 to 30 times that of the normal level.[3,5] Selective catheterization of the pancreatic vein for hormonal assay has shown similarly very high glucagon concentrations.[2] Because the majority of glucagonomas are malignant in character and because the liver is the primary target organ for metastatic disease, liver scans should be included in the diagnostic work-up. This has been helpful often in establishing the diagnosis of metastatic deposits[6,7] (Fig. 104-1). In advanced cases metastases to the abdominal lymph nodes may be found.[3]

High as they are, glucagon plasma concentrations are modest by comparison to the huge size some of these neoplasms attain. It appears that most activity is due to proglucagon elevation, a weaker biosynthetic precursor.[1,7]

The primary tumors and their metastases grow slowly over a period of several years, affording a long survival. If, following surgery, recurrence develops, there is a parallel elevation of the glucagon level in the plasma.

Glucagonomas may coexist with other APUD system tumors of the pancreatic islands. In these cases other hormones, such as insulin, gastrin, or ACTH, are produced in addition to glucagon.[1,8]

TREATMENT AND RESULTS

The treatment of choice is surgical removal of the tumor. Lightman and Bloom[4] described a patient whose entire glucagonoma syndrome promptly subsided following surgical resection. There was an immediate postoperative decrease in the insulin requirements and the levels of the plasma glucagon showed a dramatic decrease. Warin[10] described a case in which the entire syndrome disappeared 48 hours following excision of the pancreatic tumor. Danforth et al.[1] reported a patient who underwent resection of a large pancreatic tumor and remained asymptomatic for four years prior to his developing recurrent symptoms.

For recurrent or metastatic disease, treatment with streptozotocin has been the first choice. Scully and McNeely[7] in a case presentation reported improvement of the skin lesions, normalization of the glucose tolerance test, and a decrease of the metastatic liver deposits as determined by arteriography, following such therapy. Danforth et al.[1] experienced a 10-month palliative period following a six week course of streptozotocin in a dose of 1.5 g/M[2].

The presence of diabetes requires increasing amounts of insulin and adjustment of the diet prior to the establishment of the diagnosis or in case of uncontrolled disease. A very difficult problem, particularly in malignant tumors, has been the

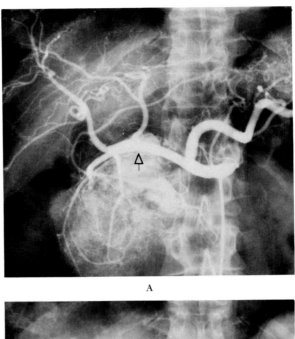

A

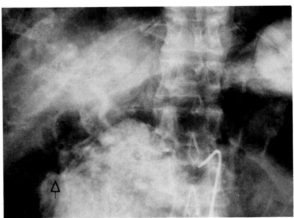

B

weight loss. The medical management of these patients includes the treatment of frequent thrombotic episodes from the venous system and psychiatric consultation because of the occasionally severe personality changes.

The skin lesions have been found to be responsive to oral tetracycline or to systemic steroids. Diiodohydroxyquinoline at a dose of 650 mg three times daily has also been effective in improving the skin changes.[5]

PROGNOSIS AND SURVIVAL

In most patients the lesion is carcinoma rather than adenoma. Because of this, the prospects for ultimate cure are very small; however, due to the slow growth of these tumors, survival in terms of years may be achieved. Surgical resection, even incomplete, chemotherapy, and supportive measures are all helpful to that effect.

Reviewing the literature, we encountered eight patients who were eligible for

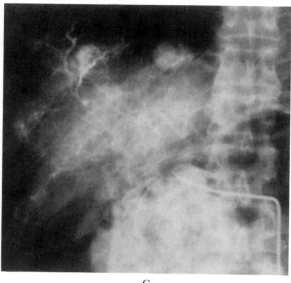

C

FIG. 104-1. Glucagonoma of the pancreas in a 64-year-old
male. (A): The arterial phase of the celiac arteriogram demonstrates a large hypervascular mass in the region of the head of
the pancreas. Several pathological vessels are present. (B): In
the parenchymal phase a dense tumor stain is seen. (C): Hepatic angiogram demonstrates several discrete hypervascular
metastatic tumor nodules. (Courtesy K. J. Cho, *AJR* **129**:159,
1977.)

a five-year follow-up. Of these, five were
alive at that time and three had succumbed to their disease. Of the living,
however, two eventually died because of
their tumor at 7 and 13 years, respectively,
from the time of the diagnosis.[1,4,6,10]

REFERENCES

1. Danforth, D.N., Jr., Triche, T., Doppman, J.L.,
   Beazley, R.M., Perrino, P.V., and Recant, L.:
   Elevated plasma proglucagon-like component
   with a glucagon-secreting tumor. Effect of streptozotocin. *N Engl J Med* **295**:242, 1976.
2. Ingemansson, S., Lunderquist, A., and Holst, J.:
   Selective catheterization of the pancreatic vein
   for radioimmunoassay in glucagon-secreting carcinoma of the pancreas. *Radiology* **119**:555, 1976.
3. Leichter, S.B., Pagliara, A.S., Greider, M.H.,
   Pohl, S., Rosai, J., and Kipnis, D.M.: Uncontrolled diabetes mellitus and hyperglucagonemia
   associated with an islet cell carcinoma. *Am J Med*
   58:285, 1975.
4. Lightman, S.L., and Bloom, S.R.: Cure of

insulin-dependent diabetes mellitus by removal
of a glucagonoma. *Br Med J* **1**:367, 1974.
5. Mallinson, C.N., Bloom, S.R., Warin, A.P., Sal-
   mon, P.R., and Cox, B.: A glucagonoma syndrome. *Lancet* **2**:1, 1974.
6. McGavran, M.H., Unger, R.H., Recant, L., Polk,
   H.C., Kilo, C., and Levin M.E.: A glucagon secreting alpha-cell carcinoma of the pancreas. *N
   Engl J Med* **274**:1408, 1966.
7. Scully, R.E., and McNeely, B.U.: Case records of
   the Massachusetts general hospital. *N Engl J Med*
   292:1117, 1975.
8. Tiengo, A., Fedele, D., Marchiori, E., Nosadini,
   R., and Muggeo, M.: Suppression and stimulation mechanisms controlling glucagon secretion
   in a case of islet-cell tumor producing glucagon,
   insulin, and gastrin. *Diabetes* **25**:408, 1976.
9. Unger, R.H.: Alpha- and beta-cell interrelation-
   ships in health and disease. *Metabolism* **23**:581,
   1974.
10. Warin, A.P.: Necrolytic migratory erythema with
    glucagon-secreting tumor of the pancreas. *Proc R
    Soc Med* **67**:1008, 1974.
11. Welbourn, R.B.: Current status of the apudomas.
    Ann Surg **185**:1, 1977.

105

Cystadenocarcinoma of the Pancreas

CYSTADENOCARCINOMA OF THE pancreas is rare. Many years may elapse before the individual surgeon or even the individual institution encounters such a case. The first case recorded in the United States was by Lichtenstein[6] in 1934, and his literature review revealed only one additional well-documented case, described by Kauffman in 1911. Cystadenoma of the pancreas, which is the benign counterpart, is also rare.[2]

Miller et al.[7] in an autopsy study of primary pancreatic cancer found one papillary cystadenocarcinoma among 202 cases. Cullen et al.[3] reported 17 cases of accepted cystadenocarcinomas of the pancreas from a study based on 2,400,000 admissions at the Mayo Clinic. During the same period of time, 44 cystadenomas were encountered. Becker et al.[2] found two cases among 2,182,427 admissions to the Charity Hospital in New Orleans. In 993 pancreatic operations performed at the Lahey Clinic Foundation during a 40-year period only 17 cystadenocarcinomas were found by Warren and Hardy.[8] This represents an incidence of approximately 1.7%, which coincides with that observed by Ilgren et al.[4] in a similar study.

Most patients are women. Actually there is a striking female predominence. Becker et al.[2] in a literature review found 76% of all reported tumors to have occurred in females. Pancreatic cystadenomas similarly exhibited female predominence. The median patient age at the time of the diagnosis was 45 years.

PATHOLOGY

Grossly, the tumor is cystic in appearance. There are, however, differences from the more common pancreatic cysts. It is surrounded by a thin capsule that contains several dilated veins. It is multiloculated and the surface has a honeycomb appearance. The cysts vary in size and they are filled with serous, mucinous, or sanguinous fluid. The tumor size is 10.0 cm, approximately.[1] According to Cullen et al.,[3] the malignant character of the lesion is determined by one of the following criteria: 1) local invasion, 2) regional lymph node involvement or distant metastases, 3) invasion of the cyst wall, and 4) histological dedifferentiation. The walls of the cyst are formed by fibrous connective tissue, which is penetrated by vascular structures. Connective tissue is also present in the septa between the cysts. Their lining is columnar epithelium, which exhibits papillary formations (Fig. 105-1). There is enough evidence to suggest seriously that some of the tumors represent malignant transformation of benign pancreatic cystadenomas.[2,3,8]

CLINICAL

The patients present with an upper abdominal mass accompanied by vague abdominal pain or discomfort. On physical examination, the mass can be felt in the left upper quadrant. In some cases it has been found in the midepigastrium or in

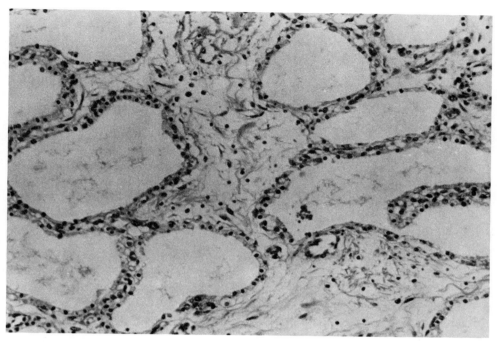

FIG. 105-1.   Pancreatic cystadenocarcinoma. Cystic irregular large structures lined by mucin-secreting cells and containing mucin.

the right upper quadrant. It is cystic, large, and nontender in character. The duration of its presence varies from a few months to several years.

Included in the clinical picture are nausea, vomiting, diarrhea, and jaundice.[3,4,8]

Plain radiographs of the abdomen may show curvilinear calcifications within the tumor. Barium studies reveal extrinsic pressure deformities on the stomach and duodenum or displacement of the transverse colon and the splenic flexure[1,5] (Fig. 105-2). Arteriography has shown the tumors to be profusely vascular, a feature not found in the common solid adenocarcinoma.[1]

The patients lack the laboratory findings of pancreatitis.[8] In addition the absence from the clinical history of alcoholism, drug addiction, trauma, cholelithiasis, or previous attacks of pancreatitis strongly supports the diagnosis of cystadenoma or cystadenocarcinoma versus pancreatic cyst.[8] The tumors are evenly distributed between all parts of the pancreas: the head, the body, and the tail.[5]

Metastases develop relatively late. They occur in the liver, regional lymph nodes, and the peritoneal surfaces.[5,8]

TREATMENT AND RESULTS

In spite of the small number of reported cases follow-up studies provide an insight as to the appropriate surgical procedure. Cystadenocarcinoma is more amenable to surgery than the common adenocarcinomas. It is necessary to perform a wide tumor resection with a rim of normal pancreatic tissue around it. This form of therapy is expected to achieve a 50% cure rate. Marsupialization, performed in earlier years, is now viewed only as a temporary step. It should be followed by a second procedure for a total tumor removal.[4,5] At the present time, there are no reports on the effects of systemic chemotherapy on the management of this disease. Radi-

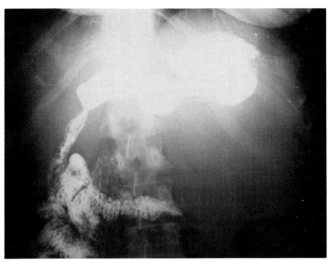

FIG. 105-2. Cystadenocarcinoma of the pancreas in a 46-year-old female. There is a large tumor mass originating in the pancreas which displaces the stomach upward and the jejunal loops downward. There is marked widening of the duodenal loop.

ation therapy has been referred to in passing.[8]

PROGNOSIS AND SURVIVAL

Early diagnosis and complete surgical removal should produce favorable results.[4] Certainly, the prognosis is far better and far more hopeful than that of pancreatic carcinoma.

Cullen et al.[3] reported survivals ranging from 1 to 17 years among 7 of 11 patients who underwent complete surgical excision. On the basis of the review by Becker et al.[2] the two-year-survival rate is 57%. The five-year survival, as derived from the same clinical data, is 45%, approximately.

REFERENCES

1. Barbee, C.L., DeMelo, F.B., and Grace, T.B.: Cystadenoma and cystadenocarcinoma of the pancreas. *J Surg Oncol* **8**:1, 1976.

2. Becker, W.F., Welsh, R.A., and Pratt, H.S.: Cystadenoma and cystadenocarcinoma of the pancreas. *Ann Surg* **161**:845, 1965.

3. Cullen, P.K., Jr., ReMine, W.H., and Dahlin, D.C.: A clinicopathological study of cystadenocarcinoma of the pancreas. *Surg Gynecol Obstet* **117**:189, 1963.

4. Ilgren, E., Tang, C.K., and Thorbjarnarson, B.: Cystadenocarcinoma of the pancreas. *NY State J Med* **76**:548, 1976.

5. Knight, E.L., Wengert, P.A., and Ricci, J.A.: Cystadenocarcinoma of the pancreas. A case report and review of the literature. *Pa Med* **78**:51, 1975.

6. Lichtenstein, L.: Papillary cystadenocarcinoma of pancreas: case report, with notes on classification of malignant cystic tumors of the pancreas. *Am J Cancer* **21**:542, 1934.

7. Miller, J.R., Baggenstoss, A.H., and Comfort, M.W.: Carcinoma of the pancreas; effect of histological type and grade of malignancy on its behavior. *Cancer* **4**:233, 1951.

8. Warren, K.W., and Hardy, K.J.: Cystadenocarcinoma of the pancreas. *Surg Gynecol Obstet* **127**:734, 1968.

106

Cystosarcoma Phyllodes

THIS RATHER UNCOMMON neoplasm of the breast was described by Müller in 1838.[7] He considered it to be a benign lesion and he stressed the fact that the name was given not to imply malignancy but simply to describe the fleshy appearance of the tumor. A reappraisal of the natural history of this disease during the last 40 years, however, has shown that the reference to "sarcoma" was not that inappropriate after all. Indeed, it is now known that approximately 25% of these neoplasms behave in a frankly malignant way and exhibit metastatic characteristics common with those of the soft tissue sarcomas.[5] Since the tumor is not rare, a number of significant publications have been devoted to this issue and they have dealt primarily with the differential diagnostic characteristics, both clinical and pathological, on the basis of which the benign or the malignant nature of the tumor should be determined and the appropriate therapy rendered.

The incidence of cystosarcoma phyllodes has been reported as ranging from 0.3–0.9% of all breast tumors.[5] Halverson and Hori-Rubaina[4] in reviewing the experience at the Ellis Fischel State Cancer Hospital with this tumor found 3182 cases of breast cancer seen from 1940 to 1971. Of these, 16 patients (0.5% incidence) had cystosarcoma phyllodes. There is a race difference in that Caucasians comprise approximately 85% of the entire group.[5]

The age range is very wide. The tumor has been reported in a 5-year-old child and in patients 80 or 90 years old. The median age at the time of the diagnosis is 58–60 years.[4,8,9]

PATHOLOGY

By most accounts, the tumors are solitary in character and large in size. In the experience of Hajdu et al.[3] the average measurement of a tumor with benign course was 4.0 cm, whereas that of malignant tumors was 16.0 cm. The median greatest diameter was found to be 15.0 cm in the material examined by Halverson and Hori-Rubaina[4] of 16 patients with cystosarcoma phyllodes. In general the neoplasms are sharply delineated and often lobulated.[6,11] The cut surface is composed of a pattern containing areas of necrosis and hemorrhage, areas of bulging pinkish-gray tissue, and areas softer and yellowish in color and gelatinous in consistency. The name has been derived from a cleft formation bordered by leaflike papillary processes. A gelatinouslike material is contained within cysts and is more often seen in larger tumors.[10]

Histologically, there is a basic similarity in the structure of cystosarcoma phyllodes as compared to that of fibroadenoma of the breast. This is due to the fact that both tumors are composed of epithelial and connective tissue elements in such a pattern that the connective tissue stroma encircles or distorts the epithelial lined spaces (Fig. 106-1). Treves and Sunderland[10] in 1951 presented histological crite-

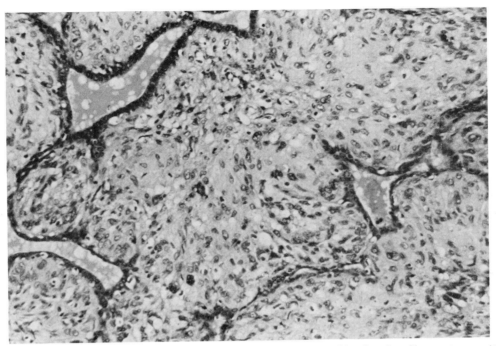

FIG. 106-1. Cystosarcoma phyllodes. Irregular breast ducts separated by abundant fibrous stroma with cells exhibiting variations in nuclear size and shape and an increased number of mitotic figures.

ria by which the benign, borderline, and malignant varieties of cystosarcoma phyllodes could be distinguished. The earliest microscopic indication of a malignant change was focal subepithelial stromal cellularity and anaplasia. The occurrence of bizarre giant cells in a benign-appearing stroma was not considered evidence of transformation. In a more recent work by Norris and Taylor[8] a retrospective analysis of the gross and microscopic findings was correlated with the clinical behavior of the disease. No single feature was found to be entirely reliable as a clear-cut finding in the malignant or the benign variety. In general the size of the tumor appears to be of importance. No tumor less than 4.0 cm in diameter having fewer than three mitotic figures per 10 high power fields examined in the areas of the greatest mitotic activity proved to be fatal.[8]

Basically, it is the stroma that is responsible for the malignant behavior whenever this takes place. Metastases are blood borne in character and generally the pattern is that of a malignant sarcoma. It is generally agreed upon that cellular atypism, increased number of mitotic figures, and infiltrative tumor margins should be considered suspiciously but not conclusively as indicators of a malignant course.[5,9] Metastasis to the axillary lymph nodes is conspicuously rare. Axillary adenopathy is due to reactive hyperplasia rather than metastasis.[9,10]

CLINICAL

The commonest presenting symptom is that of a rather large tumor in the breast, often of recent development. Dilated overlying veins may be found and usually the entire formation is painless.[4,9–11] The vascular prominence is due primarily to venous congestion. The tumors are solitary in character in most instances and as a rule they do not ulcerate, nor do they involve the skin. They have occurred in all quad-

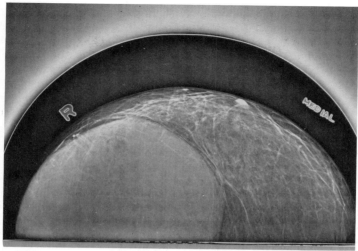

FIG. 106-2.   Cystosarcoma phyllodes in a 63-year-old female. Xeroradiography reveals an extremely large tumor mass occupying the lateral aspect of the breast.

rants of the breast, the majority of them (88%) being found in the outer one-half (Figs. 106-2, 106-3).

Local recurrence in the chest wall can be seen in both the benign and the malignant form. In the former it is due to incomplete removal of the tumor, whereas in the latter it can be part of generalized disease. In the experience of Hajdu *et al.* the majority of adequately resected cystosarcomas do not recur locally. This includes the malignant forms as well as the benign.[3]

Most of the benign lesions recur in close proximity to the previous excisional site, usually some years after the primary surgery. Malignant cystosarcomas tend to recur within the first year. The rate of recurrence for malignant cystosarcoma was found to be 8% and that of benign cystosarcoma is higher, approximately 18%. This is due primarily to the fact that benign cystosarcomas have been treated with limited local excisions.[3] The histology of the recurrent tumors is basically the same as the original ones.

Distant metastatic sites include, mainly, the lung (66%) and the skeletal system

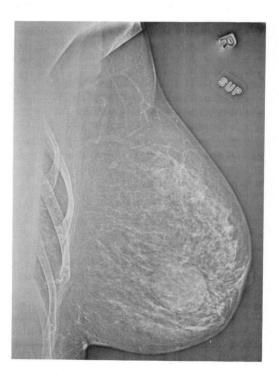

FIG. 106-3.   Cystosarcoma phyllodes in a 54-year-old female. Xeroradiography demonstrates a well-circumscribed tumor in the central aspect of the right breast.

(28%). The heart and the liver have also been implicated. To a lesser extent practically every organ and tissue have been reported as recipients of metastases.[6,8,10] These metastases are blood borne and the malignant metastasizing element appears to be a poorly differentiated mesenchymal cell. There is no evidence on light and electron microscopy to support the presence of epithelial cells participating in this process.[2]

TREATMENT AND RESULTS

It is generally agreed upon by all authors that surgery is the basic form of therapy. Radiation in the few cases that it has been applied as well as chemotherapy have been ineffective in terms of controlling the disease locally.[9] In view of the fact that axillary metastases are rare postoperative radiotherapy to the lymph nodes has not been given, as a rule.

There is considerable difference of opinion among the various authors as to the appropriate procedure. Proponents of local excision point out the incidence of local recurrence or distant metastases after simple mastectomy is the same, approximately, as in local excision.[1]

Most authors advocate simple mastectomy. Because axillary lymph node metastases are rare, no axillary node dissection is advocated.

Hajdu et al.[3] point out that local recurrence occurred in 4 of 49 patients with malignant cystosarcoma phyllodes and this represented 8% of the total number of patients with malignant cystosarcomas. Three of the four patients had surgery short of mastectomy. The same authors point to an incidence of 18% of benign cystosarcomas recurring following local excision and therefore accomplishing only partial removal of the primary. Halverson and Hori-Rubaina[4] on the basis of their experience advocate a simple mastectomy as the basic and adequate treatment for this neoplasm. The same opinion is expressed

by West et al.;[11] however, Oberman[9] recommends removal of the underlying pectoral muscles because frequently chest wall recurrence will extend to involve them.

Norris and Taylor[8] recommend that the treatment be individualized according to the clinical and histological signs. Possibly for small neoplasms wide local excision and for larger neoplasms a simple mastectomy, regardless of histological appearance, should be considered as adequate treatment. Excision of the pectoralis major muscle may be necessary if the fascia of the muscle is invaded. Low axillary node dissection should supplement the mastectomy for patients with enlarged axillary lymph nodes and for tumors with great mitotic activity.[8] Radical mastectomy has not prevented local recurrence and, of course, has no effect on disseminated disease should the course be that of a malignant lesion.[8,10]

PROGNOSIS AND SURVIVAL

The prognostic criteria on the basis of the gross clinical appearance and microscopic examination were put forth by Norris and Taylor[8] in 1967. In spite of some discussion generated by their views, it is generally accepted that their criteria serve a useful purpose as guidelines in terms of prognosticating a benign or malignant course. Tumors with well-circumscribed margins carry a better prognosis than those with an infiltrating, ill-defined outline. Their recurrence rate was 15% in the former compared with 38% in the latter. In terms of size of the lesion, small tumors less than 4.0 cm rarely metastasize, whereas the majority of metastasizing tumors were large at the time of the diagnosis. In terms of cellular atypia, those with minimal cytological atypism caused only 7% of the deaths. As atypism increases, so does the death rate.[8] These views are corroborated by the results of Hajdu et al.[3] who, reporting on recurrent cystosarcoma phyllodes, considered bulky tumors, long duration, and cellular atypia in the periductal areas as indicators of probable malignant course.

The actual survival rate after exclusion of deaths unrelated to the tumor was 80% at five years in the series by Norris and Taylor.[8] This was based on 94 patients with cystosarcoma phyllodes whose clinical and pathological findings were studied at the Armed Forces Institute of Pathology.

We have tabulated the survival rate on the basis of reports available in the literature dealing with patients who developed metastatic disease. The survival rate at the end of the two-year period was 40%, and at five years, 13% of the patients were alive.[2,3,5,6,9-11]

REFERENCES

1. Blichert-Toft, M., Hansen, J.P.H., Hansen, O.H., and Schiødt, T.: Clinical course of cystosarcoma phyllodes related to histologic appearance. *Surg Gynecol Obstet* **140**:929, 1975.
2. Fernandez, B.B., Hernandez, F.J., and Spindler, W.: Metastatic cystosarcoma phyllodes. A light and electron microscopic study. *Cancer* **37**:1737, 1976.
3. Hajdu, S.I., Espinosa, M.H., and Robbins, G.F.: Recurrent cystosarcoma phyllodes. A clinicopathologic study of 32 cases. *Cancer* **38**:1402, 1976.
4. Halverson, J.D., and Hori-Rubaina, J.M.: Cystosarcoma phyllodes of the breast. *Am Surg* **40**:295, 1974.
5. Kessinger, A., Foley, J.F., Lemon, H.M., and Miller, D.M.: Metastatic cystosarcoma phyllodes: A case report and review of the literature. *J Surg Oncol* **4**:131, 1972.
6. Lester, J., and Stout, A.P.: Cystosarcoma phyllodes. *Cancer* **7**:335, 1954.
7. Müller, J.: Ueber den feinern Ban und die Formen der krankhaften Geschwülste. Lfg. I. G. Retimer, Berlin, 1838.
8. Norris, H.J., and Taylor, H.B.: Relationship of histologic features to behavior of cystosarcoma phyllodes. Analysis of ninety-four cases. *Cancer* **20**:2090, 1967.
9. Oberman, H.A.: Cystosarcoma phyllodes. A clinicopathologic study of hypercellular periductal stromal neoplasms of breast. *Cancer* **18**:697, 1965.
10. Treves, N., and Sunderland, D.A.: Cystosarcoma phyllodes of the breast: A malignant and a benign tumor. A clinicopathological study of seventy-seven cases. *Cancer* **4**:1286, 1951.
11. West, T.L., Weiland, L.H., and Clagett, O.T.: Cystosarcoma phyllodes. *Ann Surg* **173**:520, 1971.

107

Granulosa Cell Tumor of the Ovary

GRANULOSA CELL tumor of the ovary was first described in 1855 by Rokitansky. Following the description of thecoma in 1932 by Loeffler and Priesel, the two entities were classified together under the term "feminizing tumors of the ovary." This definition was due to the fact that a substantial proportion of these growths are estrogen secreting with physiological, as expected, results.

Novak[10] proposed that the origin of granulosa-theca tumors is from undifferentiated cells within the ovarian stroma. This idea has been generally accepted and both neoplasms are now carried under the subdivision of gonadal stromal tumors.

The World Health Organization has classified ovarian tumors on the basis of their histology rather than on the basis of their function. Included under the subdivision of sex cord stromal tumors are granulosa cell tumor and the tumors of the thecoma-fibroma groups.[13]

Granulosa cell tumors have been reported comprising up to 4% of all ovarian neoplasms. However, it seems that their actual incidence is somewhat lower. Lusch et al.,[6] reporting on the clinical material from the Mayo Clinic, found them to constitute 1.63% of 3800 ovarian tumors studied. Anikwue et al.[2] found 30 granulosa cell tumors and 39 theca cell tumors among 9326 cases reviewed at the New York Hospital–Cornell Medical Center. The respective incidences were therefore 0.32 and 0.41%.

The age spectrum has been rather wide, ranging from early childhood through the seventh and eighth decades of life.[6,15] The mean and median average age at the time of the diagnosis by most authors is in the range of 50 years.[3,4] It follows therefore that more than 50% of the patients are postmenopausal at the time of the diagnosis.[2,16]

PATHOLOGY

The most frequent gross appearance of a granulosa cell tumor is that of a multicystic mass with hemorrhage into the cysts, but often the tumor is completely solid. Rarely, it forms a single large cyst.[12] The size varies from microscopic to that of several centimeters, on the average being in the range of 5–10 cm. in diameter.[2,12] Involvement of the opposite ovary is uncommon. This was seen in 4% of the cases reported by Sjöstedt and Wahlén.[15]

Histologically, the characteristic pattern is the formation of the so-called "Call-Exner bodies," which are made by granulosa cells as they surround small cystic areas containing cell debris. This is the so-called "microfollicular pattern" to be found in 60% of the cases (Fig. 107-1). Other patterns encountered are the macrofollicular, the watered-silk pattern, the trabecular, the solid, tubular, and diffuse or sarcomatoid.[2,16]

Due to the endocrine function of the tumors, endometrial hyperplasia is encountered in a large proportion of patients. Thus, in a review of recent publica-

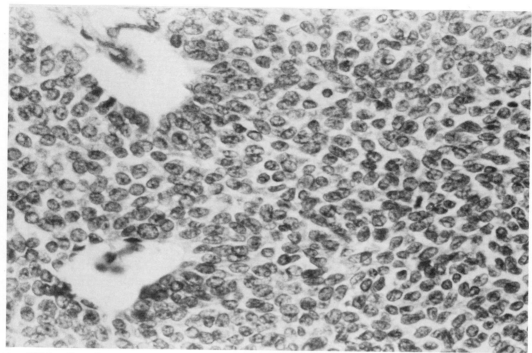

FIG. 107-1. Granulosa cell tumor of the ovary. Solid fields of granulosa cells with two Call-Exner bodies.

tions, adenomatous hyperplasia either alone or associated with polypoid formations was encountered in 70% of the cases. In addition 11% of the cases showed some form of endometrial proliferation consistent with estrogen activity. Atypical hyperplasia was encountered in 4% of the cases and frank adenocarcinoma either alone or associated with hyperplasia was seen in 4.2% The occurrence of adenocarcinoma in patients with granulosa cell tumor of the ovary and in patients with thecomas has been described by several authors. Finally, inactive endometrium was present in the remaining, approximately, 10% of the cases.[1–4,15,16]

CLINICAL

The commonest presenting symptom is abnormal uterine bleeding, the result of estrogen stimulation of the endometrium. Precocious puberty with progressive breast development and uterine bleeding occur in younger girls prior to puberty. Madden and MacDonald[7] reported on a 3.5-year-old patient whose granulosa-theca cell tumor was shown to produce and secrete directly estradiol 17β. In premenopausal patients menstrual dysfunctions in the form of menorrhagia or metrorrhagia are common. Occasionally, however, oligomenorrhea or amenorrhea are encountered. More than 50% of the postmenopausal patients have vaginal bleeding as the presenting sign.[1–4,16] Breast changes are encountered in 10–20% of all patients with granulosa cell tumors.[1,2] Very occasionally the patients exhibit mild masculinization effects, indicating androgenic activity of the tumor.[2,3,11]

The plasma estrogens in granulosa and theca cell tumors have not been completely evaluated. Very few patients with granulosa cell tumors reported in the literature had determination of their urinary estrogen output and of the plasma estrogen levels prior to their surgery. In the review by Anikwue et al.[2] the authors report that most of 12 such patients reported showed marked decrease of their 24-hour urinary estrogen output postoperatively.[2]

Abdominal enlargement and abdominal pain are the commonest nonhormonal symptoms reported by the patients.

On pelvic examination, the presence of an adnexal mass is detected in approximately 50% of the cases and an enlarged uterus can also be often identified.[2,3] A few patients have ascites present.

Staging, according to the Federation of Gynecology and Obstetrics classification at the time of surgery shows that the overwhelming majority of the patients are Stage I. Thus, in the series of 37 patients reported by Schwartz and Smith[11] from M.D. Anderson Hospital 24 were Stage Ia; one, Stage Ib; one, Stage Ic; two, Stage IIa; one Stage IIb, and eight, Stage III. There was no patient in the Stage IV group. In the series reported by Stenwig et al.[16] 78% of the patients were Stage I; 17.8%, Stage II; and 4.2%, Stage III.

Distant metastases are extremely rare. Recurrence is manifested by pelvic and abdominal dissemination along the peritoneal surfaces.

TREATMENT AND RESULTS

The treatment of pure thecomas should be different than that of granulosa cell tumors. For practical purposes, pure thecomas are benign and unilateral oophorectomy should suffice. Of course, in perimenopausal and postmenopausal women bilateral salpingo-oophorectomy (BSO) and hysterectomy may be performed as well, so that the potential of developing an endometrial tumor is eliminated at the same time.[4,9]

The treatment of granulosa cell tumors as reported in the literature includes a wide spectrum of procedures, ranging from simple hysterectomy to total abdominal hysterectomy (TAH) with BSO ac-companied by radiation therapy and chemotherapy. Most patients in most series underwent TAH and BSO.[3,4,11] The question posed is which is the optimal therapy. Sjöstedt and Wahlén evaluating the results of unilateral oophorectomy with or without postoperative radiotherapy in women younger than the age of 40 years found only one patient dying of the disease 19 years after the primary surgery. This patient was in the nonirradiated group. Excluding two patients dying from unrelated causes and one dying in the immediate postoperative period, all the remaining patients were followed for periods in excess of five years and no recurrences were noted. On this basis, the authors conclude that prognosis after a unilateral oophorectomy during the fertile age is good and, since no difference between the irradiated and nonirradiated group was shown, postoperative radiotherapy is not necessary. In the non-irradiated group 15 pregnancies occurred in the ensuing years.[15] Similar management as far as the young premenopausal patients is concerned is followed at the M.D. Anderson Hospital and reported by Schwartz and Smith.[11] Should the patient have a ruptured tumor, however, total abdominal irradiation plus irradiation boost to the pelvis should follow.

Patients older than the age of 40 years or those whose family has been completed undergo TAH and BSO. Postoperative radiotherapy in Stage I disease has been questioned by most authors. Actually, Stenwig et al.[16] comparing Stage I patients treated by surgery alone and those treated by surgery combined with postoperative radiotherapy found no statistical difference in terms of survival. Sjöstedt and Wahlén[15] found the five-year-cure rate of those patients who received surgical treatment alone to be 82.7%, against 85.6% for those patients who were treated by surgery and postoperative radiotherapy. Obviously, this is not an overwhelming difference. In the opinion of Norris and Chorlton[9] radiation therapy should be reserved for those situations in which the tumor is beyond the ovary and for symptomatic late recurrences. Indeed, due to the fact that radiotherapy has been effective in palliating the disease, the question of prophylactic postoperative radiotherapy in patients with more advanced stages at the time of surgery is quite valid in our view. Goldston et al.[4] reported on three premenopausal patients with Stage III disease who were treated by TAH, BSO, and low-dosage radiotherapy in the range of 2000 to 2500 rad to the pelvis. All patients were surviving without signs of tumor at 15, 21, and 26 years after therapy. Simmons and Sciarra[14] reported on a series of patients with late recurrent granulosa cell tumors who were managed by combinations of debulking procedures and radiotherapy. This program afforded the patients long survivals in terms of several years from the time of their recurrence. Stenwig et al.[16] recommend external radiotherapy to all patients in Stage II or higher. Removal of as much bulk as possible during surgery is recommended by all authors. With the advent of chemotherapy, consideration to this form of management may be given should the residual tumor aggregates following surgery be greater than 2.0 cm in diameter. Alkeran alone produced no complete response in nine patients with recurrent carcinoma, according to Schwartz and Smith,[11] although partial response for seven months was observed in one patient. Lusch et al.[6] reported on a 58-year-old patient with recurrent tumor 18 years following the original therapy. Following a partial debulking procedure, the patient was placed on monthly courses of Alkeran at a dose of 0.7 mg/kg (48/50 mg. each month in divided doses over four days) for 19 monthly courses. The patient was surviving at the time of the report without clinical symptoms. Malkasian et al.[8] reported objective tumor response in 3 of 12 patients treated with cyclophosphamide receiving a total of 1500 mg in divided doses over three days and repeated monthly.[8] Combination chemotherapy appears to be more promising. Actinomycin D, 5-fluorouracil, and cyclophosphamide was administered to two patients with Stage III granulosa cell tumors. The first patient had metastatic disease in the omentum and the anterior peritoneum and small bowel mesentery at the time of the surgery and received 12 monthly courses that were followed by a second-look procedure. There were no signs of tumor present and she was reported alive 35 months from the time of the initial surgery. The second patient had omental metastases and received three courses of systemic chemotherapy with this program. She was reported alive 27 months following the initial diagnosis with no evidence of disease.[11]

We have participated in the management of eight patients with granulosa cell carcinoma. Of four patients with Stage I and II disease, one received postoperative pelvic irradiation and is alive and well at six years. The remaining three developed pelvic and abdominal recurrences following TAH and BSO. Radiation therapy was given at that point. One patient is surviving at 13 years and the other two have died of their disease at 3 and 5.5 years.

Two patients with Stage III disease received pelvic and abdominal irradiation postoperatively and they are both alive and well at five and six years. Two patients with Stage IV disease were treated by a combination of surgery, radiotherapy, and chemotherapy, dying at three years of their disease.

In our limited experience therefore postoperative radiotherapy should be given consideration for Stages I, II, and III.

PROGNOSIS AND SURVIVAL

From the clinical point of view, it is a safe policy to consider all granulosa cell ovarian tumors as potentially malignant. The difficulty lies with the correct *a priori* prognostication of the individual case. This is not an easy task and actually there are several differences to be found among the various reports in the literature. More specifically, the rate of local recurrence and the mortality rate as well as the survival have been variously reported by individual institutions and investigators. Thus, Fox *et al.*[3] found at the time of their survey that approximately 30% of their 92 patients had either died because of their ovarian tumor or were alive with metastatic or recurrent disease. Six of 37 patients reported by Schwartz and Smith[11] (16.2%) developed recurrence postoperatively. Of these, two had intraperitoneal gold instillation due to tumor rupture and a third patient had a total abdominal irradiation postoperatively. Anikwue *et al.*[2] encountered a 30% recurrent rate in granulosa cell tumors. Stenwig *et al.*[16] reviewing 118 cases of granulosa cell tumor of the ovary found the recurrence rate to be 21%, and Norris and Chorlton[9] state that in their material recurrences occurred only in 7% of the patients with granulosa elements.[9,16] It is stressed by all authors that recurrences may occur very late in the course of the disease—10–15 years after the diagnosis—and several such patients have been reported.[14–16]

The five-year-survival rate in the series reported by Sjöstedt and Wahlén[15] was 84.1%; the 10-year rate, 75%; the survival at 15 years, 62.7% and at 20 years, 58.3%. This is an uncorrected rate and among the patients dying are included those with active tumor and those with intercurrent disease. In the series reported by Stenwig *et al.* the five-year survival for Stage I disease was 91.8%; for Stage II, 75.9%; and for Stage III, 22.5%. These represent relative survival rates corrected for intercurrent deaths. Although for Stage I disease no significant changes in survival were seen at 10 and 15 years, there was a considerable drop to 60.9 and 27.2%, respec-

tively, for patients with Stage II disease.[16] Fox *et al.*[3] calculated the corrected survival rates for all patients in their series with granulosa cell tumor of the ovary to be 68% at five years, 59% at 10 years, and 51% at 20 years. Finally, on a more pessimistic note, Kalavathi[5] reported 47.8% five-year survival and 21.7% survival at 10 years.

Norris and Chorlton[9] summed up the reasons for the reported differences as follows: 1) a mistaken inclusion of metastatic and primary adenocarcinomas in the category of granulosa tumors will decrease the survival rates, 2) deaths due to intercurrent disease are not properly accounted for, and 3) an admixture of granulosa cell tumors and thecomas will affect the survival rates. Series with a high number of thecomas will have higher survival rates.

Undoubtedly certain factors effect the prognosis. Of these the stage of the disease at the time of the diagnosis, the tumor size, and the degree of cellular atypia have been shown to be of importance. On the other hand, the mode of therapy, the particular histological pattern, and the presence of absence of ascites at the time of the surgery have little, if any, effect on prognosis.[3,16]

The concensus as reflected in the more recent literature is that granulosa cell tumor represents a potentially malignant neoplasm whose degree of malignancy needs to be individually evaluated and considered.

REFERENCES

1. Anderson, W.R., Levine, A.J., and MacMillan, D.: Granulosa-theca cell tumors: Clinical and pathologic study. *Am J Obstet Gynecol* **110:**32, 1971.
2. Anikwue, C., Dawood, M.Y., and Kramer, E.: Granulosa and theca cell tumors. *Obstet Gynecol* **51:**214, 1978.
3. Fox, H., Agrawal, K., and Langley, F.A.: A clinicopathologic study of 92 cases of granulosa

cell tumor of the ovary with special reference to the factors influencing prognosis. *Cancer* **35**:231, 1975.

4. Goldston, W.R., Johnston, W.W., Fetter, B.F., Parker, R.T., and Wilbanks, G.D.: Clinicopathologic studies in feminizing tumors of the ovary. 1. Some aspects of the pathology and therapy of granulosa cell tumors. *Am J Obstet Gynecol* **112**:422, 1972.

5. Kalavathi, N.: Granulosa cell tumour—hormonal aspects and radiosensitivity. *Clin Radiol* **22**:524, 1971.

6. Lusch, C.J., Mercurio, T.M., and Runyeon, W.K.: Delayed recurrence and chemotherapy of a granulosa cell tumor. *Obstet Gynecol* **51**:505, 1978.

7. Madden, J.D., and Mac Donald, P.C.: Origin of estrogen in isosexual precocious pseudopuberty due to a granulosa-theca cell tumor. *Obstet Gynecol* **51**:210, 1978.

8. Malkasian, G.D., Jr., Webb, M.J., and Jorgensen, E.O.: Observations on chemotherapy of granulosa cell carcinomas and malignant ovarian teratomas. *Obstet Gynecol* **44**:885, 1974.

9. Norris, H.J., and Chorlton, I.: Functioning tumors of the ovary. *Clin Obstet Gynecol* **17**:189, 1974.

10. Novak, E.: *Gynecologic and Obstetric Pathology with Clinical and Endocrine Relations*. W.B. Saunders, Philadelphia, 1958.

11. Schwartz, P.E., and Smith, J.P.: Treatment of ovarian stromal tumors. *Am J Obstet Gynecol* **125**:402, 1976.

12. Scully, R.E.: Ovarian tumors. A review. *Am J Pathol* **87**:686, 1977.

13. Serov, S.F., and Scully, R.E.: Histological typing of ovarian tumours. In *International Histological Classifications of Tumors*. World Health Organization, Geneva, 1973.

14. Simmons, R.L., and Sciarra, J.J.: Treatment of late recurrent granulosa cell tumors of the ovary. *Surg Gynecol Obstet* **124**:65, 1967.

15. Sjöstedt, S., and Wahlén, T.: Prognosis of granulosa cell tumours. *Acta Obstet Gynecol Scand (Suppl 6)* **40**: 1961.

16. Stenwig, J.T., Hazekamp, J.T., and Beecham, J.B.: Granulosa cell tumors of the ovary. A clinicopathological study of 118 cases with long-term follow-up. *Gynecol Oncol* **7**:136, 1979.

108

Dysgerminoma of the Ovary

THE TUMOR WAS histologically identified by Chenot in 1911 and subsequently described in greater detail by Meyer in 1930, who named the neoplasm "disgerminoma" in order to indicate that it arises from neutral cells. The name was changed to dysgerminoma later and it is now thought that the neoplasms arise from primitive germ cells existing in their early stage of gonadal genesis, representing counterparts of the seminomas.[8]

It is an uncommon tumor, accounting approximately for 1–2% of all primary ovarian neoplasms.[5,7] It favors the young age group. Thus, in the series by Talerman et al.[7] 80% of the patients were less than 30 years of age at the time of the diagnosis, and in the series by Asadourian and Taylor[2] the median age was 22 years, with a range from 6 to 56. All nine cases reported by Afridi et al.[1] were less than 30 years old and all 17 patients reported by Koller and Gjønnaess[6] were premenopausal. In the series by Thoeny et al.[9] from the Mayo Clinic, 48% of the tumors occurred in women who were 20 years or younger and 85% of all dysgerminomas were seen in patients younger than 30 years. The age range in that particular series of 27 cases was between 12 and 54 years.

PATHOLOGY

In most patients the neoplasms involve one ovary at the time of the surgery; however in approximately 10% of the cases bilateral ovarian involvement is encountered.[2] In the series by Talerman et al.[7] bilateral tumors were present in 6 of 22 reported cases. Extension beyond the ovaries, representing either direct extension into the pelvis or involvement of the pelvic and periaortic lymph nodes, is present in 20–30% of the cases.[2,7]

The tumor is solid, roughly spherical or lobulated in shape, the diameter ranging from a few to 40 or 50 cm. The average diameter was 15–20 cm.[1,2] The surface is smooth and the consistency rather firm.

Histologically, the neoplasm infiltrates the ovary and only occasionally a small part of the organ remains uninvolved as a recognizable structure. Although the actual pattern varies from lesion to lesion, the individual dysgerminoma cells are quite uniform and distinct. They are large and polygonal with distinct cell borders, a rather clear or granular cytoplasm, and rounded or ovoid nuclei. Irregular clumps of chromatin and prominent nucleoli are to be found. Areas of necrosis and hemorrhage are frequent. Lymphocytic infiltration is present in the majority of the lesions and it is rather marked in 15–20% of the cases.[2] This infiltration is interstitial in the connective tissue among the tumor cells that arrange themselves in alveolar, columnar, or "mosaic" patterns (Fig. 108-1). Mitoses can frequently be observed.[2,9]

Admixtures of tumor elements other than dysgerminoma may exist. They constitute other types of malignant germ cell tumors, such as embryonal carcinoma,

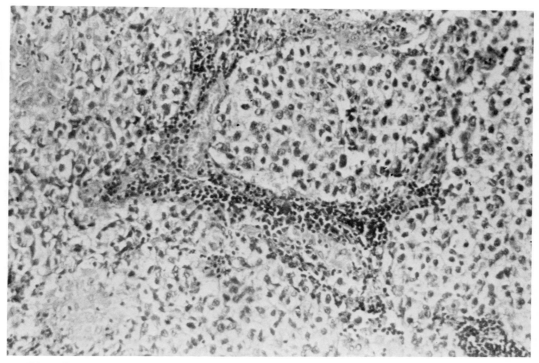

FIG. 108-1. Dysgerminoma of the ovary. Germinal cells are seen within a connective tissue network. The network is infiltrated by lymphocytes.

teratocarcinoma, and choriocarcinoma, which have been found in approximately 10% of the cases; however, such tumors have been excluded in the more recent literature reports because their prognosis varies from that of pure dysgerminoma.[2,6,9]

CLINICAL

The two main clinical symptoms reported by all authors reviewing this subject are: the presence of an abdominal mass or abdominal enlargement and the presence of abdominal or pelvic pain. These two clinical symptoms are encountered with practically the same frequency and often accompany each other.[7,9] Menstrual irregularity, primarily in the form of menorrhagia occurred in 15% of the patients reported by Asadourian and Taylor.[2] From the same series, 10% of the patients were asymptomatic and the tumor was diagnosed during a routine pelvic examination.

The duration of the symptoms has varied from a few weeks up to one or two years; however, in the majority of the cases, the average waiting period is five to six months.

A familial history has been uncovered in a small number of the reported cases.[5,7] The early impression that dysgerminoma was associated often with gonadal dysgenesis is somewhat exaggerated. A few of the patients, however, have been found to have uterine hypoplasia and masculine habitus.[2,7,9]

On pelvic examination a mass is palpable, a physical finding encountered in most but not all the patients.

Following exploratory laparotomy and subsequent resection, the pathological staging of dysgerminoma at presentation has shown that in most cases the disease is Stage I. Thus, involvement of one ovary was seen in 68% of the patients, according to a composite review we performed on this subject, and bilateral ovarian involvement was seen in 8%. Therefore 76% of dysgerminomas were Stage I, 13% were Stage II, with disease extending into the pelvis, 9% were Stage III, with primary involvement of the retroperitoneal lymph nodes, and a few patients presenting with extraabdominal metastases, primarily to the supraclavicular lymph nodes, comprised the remaining 2% with Stage IV disease.[1,2,6,7,9]

The mode of extension is local infiltration into the adjacent pelvic organs but primarily lymphatic in character, metastasizing to the regional retroperitoneal lymph nodes and then in continuity to the supraclavicular nodal stations. In this respect, as in many others, it resembles testicular seminoma.

TREATMENT AND RESULTS

Due to the fact that most cases are Stage I disease at the time of the diagnosis, unilateral oophorectomy has been the commonest form of primary therapy. Although there is no controversy in terms of managing more advanced stages by means of total abdominal hysterectomy and postoperative radiotherapy, a difference of opinion exists as to the appropriate management of Stage I disease. Due to the fact that most patients are young, the question has been raised by some authors as to the advisability of bilateral oophorectomy and postoperative radiotherapy for this particular group. Because dysgerminoma is radiosensitive, it is suggested by some authors that radiation can always be called upon to salvage recurrent disease following limited surgery. These authors feel that unilateral oophorectomy is a justifiable procedure for the treatment of unilateral dysgerminomas when preservation of the ovarian function is desired.[2] There is evidence, however, that not all recurrent cases are salvagable by

radiotherapy. In the opinion of most authors the risk of recurrence and that of distant metastasis is considerable and in spite of the high rate of curability it is difficult to conceive that deaths will not occur should the tumor be allowed to spread rapidly. Therefore postoperative radiotherapy to the pelvis and the periaortic lymph nodes is recommended by Thoeny et al.[9] Jackson,[5] Koller and Gjønnaess,[6] Afridi et al.,[1] and Talerman et al.[7] For those patients with Stage IA disease who are young and wish to have children, the unilateral salpingo-oophorectomy should be accompanied by biopsy from the other ovary and careful palpation and possible biopsy of the periaortic lymph nodes. In our institution lymphangiography following the establishment of the diagnosis of ovarian dysgerminoma has been performed.

For Stage II disease, pelvic irradiation and irradiation of the periaortic lymph nodes following surgical resection of the tumor to the extent possible is at the present time the established form of therapy. Should the periaortic lymph nodes be positive, either clinically or on radiographic grounds, irradiation to the mediastinum and both supraclavicular fossae is to follow at the completion of the periaortic lymph node therapy. When given prophylactically, 3000 rad in three to four weeks is the recommended dosage; however, when disease is present 4000–4500 rad is a more appropriate dose.

Following unilateral salpingo-oophorectomy, recurrence to the opposite ovary occurred in two of four cases among the patients reported by Koller and Gjønnaess[6] in nine months and three years following the original surgery. The third patient developed retroperitoneal lymph node recurrence three years after her original surgery. Finally, the fourth patient had the remaining ovary removed for what proved to be a simple cyst four months later after her primary operation. None of the five patients subjected to unilateral salpingo-oophorectomy and post-operative radiotherapy to the pelvis and the periaortic lymph nodes developed recurrence. Of 6 cases in which bilateral salpingo-oophorectomy was performed one did not receive postoperative radiotherapy and died 10 years later with abdominal recurrence, the remaining five were postoperatively irradiated and remained well two to four years after therapy.[6]

Fourteen of the patients reported by Thoeny et al.[9] were treated by unilateral salpingo-oophorectomy without post-operative radiotherapy, the so-called "conservative approach." Of them, six, or 43%, developed recurrence. In the series by Jackson[5] all eight patients who were treated postoperatively were surviving without evidence of disease, six of them in excess of five years and two for one and two years postoperatively. In the same series four patients were treated for recurrent disease whose original therapy had been surgery alone. Asadourian and Taylor,[2] reviewing their experience at the Armed Forces Institute of Pathology, found tumor recurrence to occur in 10 of 46 patients treated with unilateral oophorectomy (22%). Six of the 10 patients were subsequently successfully managed; however, four died of their disease. Afridi et al.[1] stated that of seven patients with Stage IIA disease or less who underwent complete surgical resection of their tumor at the time of the initial operation, five developed recurrence. Of these, two had postoperative pelvic irradiation and significantly enough developed recurrences above the level of the pelvis. The other three did not receive postoperative radiotherapy and had recurrences both in the pelvis and above the pelvis. Further irradiation resulted in four of the five patients being alive and well at the time of the report. It is therefore the author's recommendation that in Stages IB and IIA postoperative radiotherapy to the level of 3000 rad be delivered to the pelvis

and periaortic lymph nodes and, if the periaortic lymph nodes are positive at laparotomy, then the mediastinum and supraclavicular fossa on the left side be treated at 2500 rad. For Stages IC, IIB, III and some of Stage IV, the whole abdomen should be treated at the level of 3000 rad in six weeks, followed by a booster dose of 1000 to 1500 rad in two weeks to the pelvis and the periaortic lymph nodes. Finally, in some of the Stage IA patients who are young and wish to have children, conservative unilateral salpingo-oophorectomy may be carried out while the other ovary is bivalved and biopsied. Careful palpation and biopsy of the periaortic nodes during this time is necessary as well. Peritoneal washings could be obtained for cytology.[1] Patients with extensive abdominal disease (Stage III) are salvagable with a combination of bilateral salpingo-oophorectomy and partial resection of the masses followed by abdominal irradiation. Five of seven such patients reported by Jackson[5] were alive 3, 6, 10, and 15 years following their postoperative radiotherapy. Others have had similar experiences as well.[1,6]

Recent reports on the effectiveness of chemotherapy, indicate excellent responses and prolonged remissions in patients with metastatic ovarian dysgerminoma. Boyes et al.[3] treated two patients who developed metastases several years following their initial treatment with cyclophosphamide. Both patients were alive and well seven years later. Cohen and Goldsmith[4] reported on a 17-year-old patient with Stage II dysgerminoma. Following unilateral salpingo-oophorectomy the patient received radiotherapy to the entire abdomen at the level of 3100 rad. The kidneys were shielded at the 2000 rad level. The patient presented with multiple abdominal masses and with a large liver, which showed multiple metastases on a liver scan. A program of cyclophosphamide, 200 mg daily for four days, and actinomycin D, 0.5 mg daily for five days, was initiated. There was partial response;

however, abdominal recurrence promptly returned two months later and at this point a program consisting of vincristine, 1 mg on day 1 and 0.5 mg on day 4, bleomycin, 15 units on day 1 and 30 units intravenously on days 2, 3 and 4, was started. Subsequently the program was changed to vincristine and methotrexate intravenously and it was continued for 18 months. The therapy was discontinued approximately three years from the time of the initiation. During the ensuing two years after the cessation of all therapy, the patient had no evidence of recurrent disease. The authors recommend that consideration to bleomycin and *Vinca* alkaloids should be given by the clinician when confronted with advanced metastatic ovarian dysgerminoma.[4]

PROGNOSIS AND SURVIVAL

The overall prognosis is good. The tumor presents at an early stage, being amenable to surgical resection, metastasizes in an orderly fashion, if it does, and is sensitive to radiation and to combination chemotherapy.

Indeed there is some difference in the survival of earlier reports, reflecting primarily incorrect histological classification, since several patients included in those studies had dysgerminoma in admixture with other germ cell tumors. Certainly, inadequacy of therapy could also be considered a cause of poorer results.[1] A histological feature of prognostic significance has been the degree of lymphocytic or granulomatous stromal infiltration. In the series recorded from the Armed Forces Institute of Pathology 54 patients whose tumors had complete absence or only a minimal amount of lymphocytes present showed a mortality rate

of 20%, whereas of 15 patients with marked lymphocytic or granulomatous reaction only one (6.7%) died.[2] No other factor seems to effect the prognosis.

The actuarial survival rate at five years was 86% in the series of 105 patients reported by Asadourian and Taylor.[2] Similarly, the corrected five-year survival was 91% in the series reported by Boyes et al.[3] These figures contrast, for the reasons just stated, to earlier survival rates reported in the range of 60–75%.[9] Obviously, the stage of the disease at the time of the diagnosis is an important factor.[9]

REFERENCES

1. Afridi, M.A., Vongtama, V., Tsukada, Y., and Piver, M.S.: Dysgerminoma of the ovary: Radiation therapy for recurrence and metastases. *Am J Obstet Gynecol* **15**:190, 1976.
2. Asadourian, L.A., and Taylor, H.B.: Dysgerminoma. An analysis of 105 cases. *Obstet Gynecol* **33**:370, 1969.
3. Boyes, D.A., Pankratz, E., Galliford, B.W., White, G.W., and Fairey, R.N.: Experience with dysgerminomas at the Cancer Control Agency of British Columbia. *Gynecol Oncol* **6**:123, 1978.
4. Cohen, S.M., and Goldsmith, M.A.: Prolonged chemotherapeutic remission of metastatic ovarian dysgerminoma. Report of a case. *Gynecol Oncol* **5**:299, 1977.
5. Jackson, S.M.: Ovarian dysgerminoma. *Br J Radiol* **40**:459, 1967.
6. Koller, O., and Gjønnaess, H.: Dysgerminoma of the ovary. A clinical report of 20 cases. *Acta Obstet Gynecol Scand* **43**:268, 1964.
7. Talerman, A., Huyzinga, W.T., and Kuipers, T.: Dysgerminoma. Clinicopathologic study of 22 cases. *Obstet Gynecol* **41**:137, 1973.
8. Teilum, G.: *Special Tumors of Ovary and Testis and Related Extragonadal Lesions. Comparative Pathology and Histological Identification.* J.B. Lippincott, Philadelphia, 1976.
9. Thoeny, R.H., Dockerty, M.B., Hunt, A.B., and Childs, D.S., Jr.: A study of ovarian dysgerminoma with emphasis on the role of radiation therapy. *Surg Gynecol Obstet* **113**:692, 1961.

109

Endodermal Sinus Tumor of the Ovary
(Yolk Sac Tumor)

SCHILLER[11] IN 1939 presented the histological features of a group of neoplasms that he considered to be of mesonephric origin. Teilum[8-10] performed comparative studies between the so-called "mesonephric" tumors described by Schiller and rat placentas. Through this work, he was able to identify within the "mesonephric" tumors, patterns reminiscent of the yolk sac and the allantois of the placenta. In this way he separated a group of malignant gonadal neoplasms and he reclassified them.

These are highly malignant tumors occurring in young patients. They are to be distinguished from mesonephric carcinoma of the ovary. The pure mesonephric ovarian carcinoma is a disease appearing in the older age group and has a relatively good prognosis. The prognosis of yolk sac tumor, a disease of germ cell origin, is extremely poor.

Due to the fact that identification of endodermal sinus tumor is relatively recent, literature from earlier years should not be utilized for data collection. Up to this point, there have been more than 200 cases of well-defined yolk sac tumors reported.[2-4]

The average age of the patients in the series reported by Jimerson and Woodruff[3] was 18 years with a range from 1.5 to 40 years. Kurman and Norris,[4] reporting on 71 patients, found the average to be 19 years, with individual ages ranging from 14 months to 45 years.

The tumor comprises 8.5 of all ovarian neoplasms seen in patients younger than the age of 20 years.[4,7]

PATHOLOGY

The gross appearance is somewhat deceptive. It is a well-encapsulated neoplasm whose average diameter at laparotomy is in the range of 15–20 cm. In most cases there is a unilateral ovarian involvement without evidence of intraperitoneal dissemination. For this reason, it can be perceived as a relatively benign growth.[3,4]

On cut surface large areas of hemorrhage and necrosis are present. Cysts varying in size from a few millimeters to 2 cm can be seen scattered diffusely throughout the tissue, giving it a honeycomb appearance.[4]

Schiller regarded the tumor to be of mesonephric origin because he identified "glomerulus-like" structures. It is now believed that these formations represent the endodermal sinuses of the placenta. They are diverticular formations of the yolk sac endoderm as it expands and dissects around the branches of the allantoic vessels.[8] The origin of germ cell tumors is the germ cell, a totipotential cell seen in the very early days of fetal development. It is from this cell that an embryonal pathway develops forming the embryo, and another extraembryonal pathway gives rise to tissues related to placenta, cord, membranes, and yolk sac. Tumors like germinomas and teratomas are germ cell in origin arising from the embryonal pathway. Yolk sac tumors are germ cell in origin arising from the extraembryonal pathway.[3] The tumors mimic histologically the extraembryonic membranes as seen during the early gestation days.[8–10]

There are four predominant patterns. The reticular pattern is the most common, characterized by a formation of spaces and channels. These areas are lined by flat or cuboidal cells, each having indistinct borders and scanty cytoplasm. The pseudopapillary pattern is comprised of cells arranged around blood vessels with large cuboidal shape, clear cytoplasm, and hyperchromatic nuclei. The polyvesicular vitelline pattern is characterized by a dense spindle cell stroma containing cysts. The cysts are lined by mucinous, columnar, cuboidal, or flattened cells (Fig. 109-1). Finally, a mixture of these patterns may be present.[4] The pseudopapillary pattern contains the so-called "Schiller-Duval bodies," representing basically concentric cell configurations. Hyaline droplets are another hallmark of the endodermal sinus tumors. It is within this substance that alphafetoprotein has been identified (Fig. 109-2). Monitoring of alpha fetoprotein has been useful in correlating tumor progression or tumor regression.[6,12]

CLINICAL

Abdominal pain is the commonest presenting symptom. This occurred in 77% of the cases reported by Kurman and Norris[4] and in 66% of the cases reported by Jimerson and Woodruff.[3] Less often, the presenting signs are those of an enlarging abdomen or of a pelvic mass. This is seen in 20–30% of the cases. Usually there are no irregularities of the period.[3,4]

There is a very rapid tumor growth.

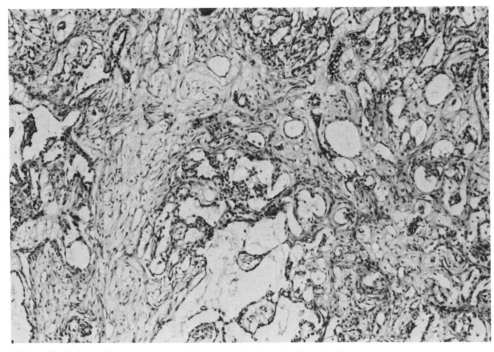

FIG. 109-1.   Endodermal sinus tumor of the ovary. Polyvesicullar vitelline pattern.

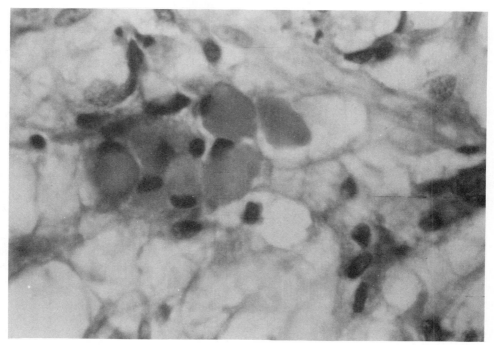

FIG. 109-2.   Endodermal sinus tumor of the ovary. Globules of periodic acid-Schiff-positive material corresponding to alpha fetoprotein.

Therefore the duration of the symptoms is quite brief. Two-thirds of the patients reported awareness of the disease for two or less weeks prior to their examination.

Fever has been encountered in 24% of the cases and when associated with an abdominal mass, particularly involving the right ovary, the diagnosis of acute appendicitis can be made.[4]

Staging the disease on the basis of the Federation of Gynecology and Obstetrics classification shows the majority of endodermal sinus tumors (72–75%) to be Stage Ia at the time of the diagnosis. From the remaining patients, approximately 6% are Stage II; 15–20%, Stage III; and very few, Stage IV.[3]

Ascites is not common. Only 16% of the patients with Stage I disease had fluid at the time of the diagnosis.[4]

TREATMENT AND RESULTS

Following physical examination and admission, exploratory laparotomy has been undertaken in practically all cases. Because the majority of the tumors are localized and are benign-looking neoplasms and because of the young age of the patients, the commonest procedure has been unilateral salpingo-oophorectomy. All but 3 of 18 patients with Stage I disease who underwent unilateral salpingo-oophorectomy died of their tumor, as reported by Kurman and Norris.[4] Similarly, 17 of 19 patients died in the series reported by Jimerson and Woodruff.[3] Would bilateral salpingo-oophorectomy and hysterectomy improve the prognosis and survival? There is no evidence to that effect. Of 14 patients treated in this manner, there were only two long-term survivors.[3,4]

Pelvic radiotherapy has been ineffective in controlling the disease, in the experience of others and ours.

Chemotherapy has a definite role to play in the management of this tumor. Single agent therapy utilizing triethylenemelamine has provided a 13-month survival in a reported case.[3] Single agent therapy utilizing chlorambucil has also been successful.[1] The mainstay of therapy, however, is combination chemotherapy. Multiple drug treatments utilizing actinomycin D and cyclophosphamide with 5-fluorouracil or vincristine have been successful in maintaining survivals in excess of two years.[2,4,7] Among the treated patients, there are many long survivors, attesting to the effectiveness of such a therapy. In a disease whose mean survival time from surgery to death is only seven months we now have several patients apparently cured of their tumor.

PROGNOSIS AND SURVIVAL

At the present time, it is somewhat difficult to state the survival rate precisely. It is known that the overall actuarial survival at three years without chemotherapy is in the range of 13%. The tumors disseminate rapidly intraabdominally, bringing about a quick demise. At this time, it is believed that several patients can be cured from their tumor following the application of postoperative chemotherapy with the agents already described. Although recurrences can still occur following such a program, it is unquestionable that the survival even of these patients has been extended significantly.[1,4,7]

REFERENCES

1. Ettinger, D.S., Parmley, T.H., Owellen, R.J., and Davis, T.E.: Endodermal sinus tumor. Report of a case with remission following chemotherapy. *Obstet Gynecol* **49(Suppl):**53s, 1977.
2. Forney, J.P., Di Saia, P.J., and Morrow, C.P.: Endodermal sinus tumor. A report of two sustained remissions treated postoperatively with a combination of actinomycin D, 5-fluorouracil and cyclophosphamide. *Obstet Gynecol* **45:**186, 1975.
3. Jimerson, G.K., and Woodruff, J.C.: Ovarian extraembryonal teratoma. I. Endodermal sinus tumor. *Am J Obstet Gynecol* **127:**73, 1977.
4. Kurman, R.J., and Norris, H.J.: Endodermal sinus tumor of the ovary. A clinical and pathologic analysis of 71 cases. *Cancer* **38:**2404, 1976.
5. Norris, H.J., and Jensen, R.D.: Relative frequency of ovarian neoplasms in children and adolescents. *Cancer* **30:**713, 1972.
6. Sell, A., Sogaard, H., and Norgaard-Pedersen, B.: Serum alpha-fetoprotein as a marker for the effect of post-operative radiation therapy and/or chemotherapy in eight cases of ovarian endodermal sinus tumour. *Int J Cancer* **18:**574, 1976.
7. Smith, J.P., and Rutledge, F.: Advances in chemotherapy for gynecologic cancer. *Cancer* **36:**669, 1975.
8. Teilum, G.: Endodermal sinus tumors of the ovary and testis. Comparative morphogenesis of the so-called mesonephroma ovarii (Schiller) and extraembryonic (yolk sac-allantoic) structures of the rat's placenta. *Cancer* **12:**1092, 1959.
9. Teilum, G.: Classification of endodermal sinus tumour (mesoblastoma vitellinum) and so-called "embryonal carcinoma" of the ovary. *Acta Pathol Microbiol Scand* **64:**407, 1965.
10. Teilum, G.: *Special Tumors of Ovary and Testis and Related Extragonadal Lesions. Comparative Pathology and Histological Identification.* J.B. Lippincott, Philadelphia, 1976.
11. Schiller, W.: Mesonephroma ovarii. *Am J Cancer* **35:**1, 1939.
12. Wilkinson, E.J., Friedrich, E.G., and Hosty, T.A.: Alpha-fetoprotein and endodermal sinus tumor of the ovary. *Am J Obstet Gynecol* **116:**711, 1973.

110

Endodermal Sinus Tumor in Other Locations

THE ORIGIN OF the primordial sex cell presumably lies within the endoderm of the yolk sac from which the cells migrate to the gonadal sites. It is from these cells that germ cell tumors arise. Deviation from the path during migration, however, leads to the occurrence of extragonadal germ cell tumors.

Thiele *et al.*[2] reported on a 14-month-old child with such a neoplasm occupying the right pelvis. The patient was treated with actinomycin D, vincristine, and radiation therapy with a dramatic initial response. Rapidly, however, chest metastasis developed and further chemotherapy was administered. Death occurred in four months.

Allyn *et al.*[1] reported on an 11-month-old female infant with endodermal sinus tumor of the vagina. Following radical surgery, which included bilateral pelvic node dissection and radiotherapy, multiple courses of actinomycin D were administered. The patient was without evidence of disease seven years later. The authors reviewed endodermal sinus tumors of the vagina. Thirteen cases, including their own, were to be found. The five-year-survival rate was less than 10%.[1] All reported cases have been treated prior to the current knowledge regarding the effectiveness of systemic chemotherapy.

REFERENCES

1. Allyn, D.L., Silverberg, S.G., and Salzberg, A.M.: Endodermal sinus tumor of the vagina. Report of a case with 7-year survival and literature review of so-called "mesonephromas." *Cancer* **27:**1231, 1970.
2. Thiele, J., Castro, S., and Lee, K.D.: Extragonadal endodermal sinus tumor (yolk sac tumor) of the pelvis. *Cancer* **27:**391, 1971.

111

Brenner Tumor of the Ovary

BRENNER IN 1907 described under the title "oophoroma folliculare" an uncommon and distinct ovarian neoplasm. Meyer[7] in 1932 presented an extensive review on the subject and he introduced the term "Brenner's tumor."

Brenner tumors comprise 1.7–2.6% of all ovarian tumors.[2] They were considered uniformly benign in nature until 1945 when von Numers[12] reported on two patients who died of their tumor within one year from the diagnosis. Histologically, cellular atypism and numerous mitoses were present. Uncommon as Brenner tumors are, their malignant variants are even more uncommon. It is estimated that less than 1% of all Brenner tumors of the ovary show malignant behavior.[9]

The average age of the patients is in the range of 50 years.[2,6] For this reason, several of them are postmenopausal at the time of the diagnosis. Idelson[5] in a comprehensive review of malignant Brenner tumors found the average age to be 60.3 years. Miles and Norris[8] found the median age of what they called proliferative Brenner tumors to be 50 years, whereas the age of patients with the clearly malignant variants was 68 years. The authors suggested that this difference in age may indicate a gradual progression from one group to the other.

PATHOLOGY

The histogenesis of Brenner tumor has been discussed considerably. They are now considered to be of epithelial origin and they are classified as such.[8] They may develop from several different epithelial structures. Sternberg[11] has pointed out that the most characteristic feature is a close relationship between a transitional and a mucinous columnar epithelium.

The tumors vary in size from microscopic lesions to those measuring several centimeters. The proliferative and the malignant Brenner tumors have average diameters in the range of 15–16 cm.[5,8] The masses are solid, mostly firm; however, cystic areas may be present. Their surface is smooth or partially lobulated, covered by a smooth serosal lining. Bilateral ovarian involvement occurs in 7–7.5% of the cases.[2,6]

Histologically, epithelial cells resembling transitional epithelium of the urinary tract are to be found embedded in a connective tissue stroma. The cells vary in size and shape and usually are distinct from the stromal component. At times, they form a central lumen, the cells of which show metaplasia to a mucinous glandular epithelium. The stroma appears to be predominantly fibrous in some tumors, whereas in others it resembles the theca externa (Fig. 111-1). Some tumors have approximately equal amounts of these two types of stroma. Furthermore, some Brenner tumors consist mostly of epithelial cells and others consist mostly of stroma with relatively few epithelial nests. Occasionally, luteinization of the stroma is present.[2] The malignant form of Bren-

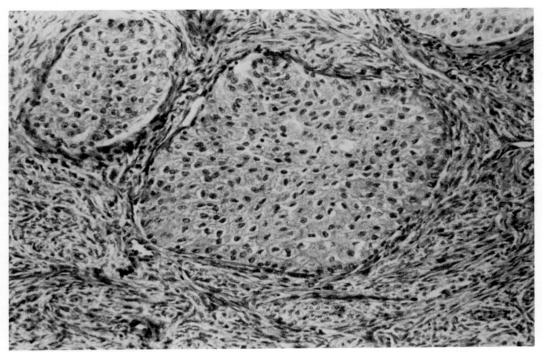

FIG. 111-1.   Brenner tumor of the ovary. Islands of transitional cells against a background of fibrous stroma.

ner's tumor is being addressed with increasing frequency.[1,8–10] Histologically, a definite transition from the benign Brenner epithelium to the malignant portion is to be seen.[4] The appearance is that of a transitional cell carcinoma with numerous mitoses and nuclear atypia. Stromal invasion is demonstrated.[9] In addition to the benign and the malignant forms of Brenner tumor, Miles and Norris[8] identified the so-called "proliferative" type. Such types exhibit numerous areas where epithelium resembling that of the urinary bladder—urothelium—is abundantly proliferates. This transitional cell epithelium, however, lacks the characteristics of an overt carcinoma.[8]

CLINICAL

The most common presenting symptoms include abdominal discomfort or pain, a feeling of swelling or fullness, and abdominal enlargement. These symptoms are similar to those found in ovarian tumors in general, and there are no differing signs between the benign and the malignant forms.[2,5,6]

In addition, patients with hormonally active Brenner tumors present with menstrual irregularities. Thus, intermenstrual bleeding or postmenopausal bleeding is encountered in 35–40% of the patients. The high incidence of bleeding abnormalities reflects the incidence of hormonally active tumors. Hormone production can be seen in both the benign and the malignant forms and it is associated with endometrial hyperplasia, the result of estrogen stimulation.[2,3,5,6]

In the malignant variant, the average symptom duration prior to the diagnosis has been about four months.[8] On pelvic examination, large adnexal masses are found, extending at times into the lower abdomen.[1,3,4,8]

Pathological staging during laparotomy has shown that the majority of the malignant Brenner's tumors are Stage I. Reviewing the literature, we found that 80% of the lesions were confined to one or both ovaries at the time of the diagnosis. The remaining were Stage II and Stage III, equally divided. Ascitic fluid is occasionally present.

TREATMENT AND RESULTS

Abdominal hysterectomy and bilateral salpingo-oophorectomy has been performed on most patients. Occasionally, radiation therapy has been given postoperatively.[5,9]

Malignant Brenner tumors have a rapid course. Their recurrences are similar to those of other ovarian tumors, being primarily pelvic and abdominal in character. They occur within few months following surgery, and eventually metastases to the periaortic lymph nodes and the liver take place. Distant metastases to the lungs and the bones have been described.[4,5,10]

PROGNOSIS AND SURVIVAL

For the majority of patients with Brenner tumor, resection of the involved ovary or ovaries amounts to cure.

The malignant variant, on the other hand, appears to have a rather serious prognosis. In reviewing the literature, we have tabulated the survival of these patients. At the end of the first year, the actuarial survival was 50%. At the end of the second year, it decreased to 33%; at the end of the third year, it was 15%; and at five years, 5%. This indeed is a virulent neoplasm. It is possible that with the advent of modern chemotherapy the survival rates will be improving.

It is important for prognostic purposes to differentiate the proliferative group, as described by Miles and Norris.[8] These tumors have decidedly a good prognosis. Seven such cases reported by the authors were alive and well for periods ranging from 2.5 to 13.5 years.

REFERENCES

1. Beck, H., Raahave, D., and Boiesen, P.: A malignant Brenner tumour of the ovary with subcutaneous metastases. *Acta Pathol Microbiol Scand [A]* **85**:859, 1977.
2. Ehrlich, C.E., and Roth, L.M.: The Brenner tumor. A clinicopathologic study of 57 cases. *Cancer* **27**:332, 1971.
3. Foda, M.S., and Shafeek, M.A.: Malignant Brenner tumor. *Obstet Gynecol* **13**:226, 1959.
4. Hull, M.G.R., and Campbell, G.R.: The malignant Brenner tumor. *Obstet Gynecol* **42**:527, 1973.
5. Idelson, M.G.: Malignancy in Brenner tumors of the ovary, with comments on histogenesis and possible estrogen production. *Obstet Gynecol Surv* **18**:246, 1963.
6. Jorgensen, E.O., Dockerty, M.B., Wilson, R.B., and Welch, J.S.: Clinicopathologic study of 53 cases of Brenner's tumors of the ovary. *Am J Obstet Gynecol* **108**:122, 1970.
7. Meyer, R.: Der tumor ovarii Brenner. *Zentralbl Gynaekol* **65**:770, 1932.
8. Miles, P.A., and Norris, H.J.: Proliferative and malignant Brenner tumors of the ovary. *Cancer* **30**:174, 1972.
9. Pratt-Thomas, H.R., Kreutner, A., Jr., Underwood, P.B., and Dowdeswell, R.H.: Proliferative and malignant Brenner tumors of ovary. Report of two cases, one with Meigs' syndrome, review of literature, and ultrastructural comparisons. *Gynecol Oncol* **4**:176, 1976.
10. Shafeek, M.A., Osman, M.I., and Hussein, M.A.: Malignant Brenner tumor of the ovary. *Gynecol Oncol* **6**:282, 1978.
11. Sternberg, W.H.: Nonfunctioning ovarian tumors. In *The Ovary*, Grady, H.G., and Smith, D.E., Eds. Williams & Wilkins, Baltimore, 1963.
12. von Numers, C.: Contribution to the case knowledge and histology of the Brenner tumor: Do malignant forms of the Brenner tumor also occur? *Acta Obstet Gynecol Scand (Suppl 2)* **25**:114, 1945.

112

Androblastoma of the Ovary (Sertoli-Leydig Cell Tumors)

IN THE CLASSIFICATION of the ovarian tumors, as published by the World Health Organization, androblastomas (Sertoli-Leydig cell tumors) are categorized as sex cord stromal tumors.[15] Due to their endocrine function and the spectacular clinical manifestations they can produce, there is an abundance of individual case reports in the literature, as well as of large series. The reader is apt to encounter a multitude of synonyms, overlapping terms, and conflicting histogenetic theories.[1–5,7–9,11,17,18]

In the present review we will describe those particular aspects of androblastomas which relate primarily to their malignant potentiality. The majority of these tumors are benign in character. Information with regard to clinical, endocrinological, and histopathological features can be obtained by referring to recent publications on the subject. As such, the articles by Sternberg and Dhurandhar,[16] Norris and Chorlton,[8] Ireland and Woodruff,[4] and Scully[14] are recommended.

Androblastomas (Sertoli-Leydig cell tumors, arrhenoblastomas) are seen primarily in young patients. The majority of patients in the series reported by Pedowitz and O'Brien[11] were between 10 and 40 years of age. The median age of 31 patients reported by O'Hern an Neubecker[9] at time of the treatment, was 34 years.

These are uncommon tumors, since they constitute less than 1% of all ovarian neoplasms. They are encountered only one-fifth to one-tenth as often as granulosa cell tumors.[8]

PATHOLOGY

For working purposes, the original description of what Meyer called "arrhenoblastoma" remains the most practical and the most applicable with regard to what is termed at this time "androblastoma" or "Leydig-Sertoli cell tumor."[7]

The various histological presentations can be classified into three types. Type I is composed of Sertoli cells, which form the main bulk of the lesion. They are arranged in well-differentiated tubular structures and they are uniform, cuboid, or columnar in appearance. In the interstitial tissue small clusters of Leydig cells, polyhedral in character, are to be seen. Crystalloids of Reinke have been found only in a few cases within the Leydig cells. Type II tumors are composed of Sertoli cells, smaller and slightly spindle shaped or round in character, forming more rudimentary tubular structures, whereas the Leydig cells are randomly scattered in small clumps and may be indistinct. This variety, the intermediate form, is probably the single most common variety of androblastoma. Type III lesions are poorly differentiated, composed of small spindle-shaped cells with frequent mitoses. Leydig cells are usually present; however, a thorough search is necessary in order to identify them. This form resembles fibrosarcoma and has been at times labeled as sarcomatoid.[6,7,9,11,14]

The gross appearance of the tumors is similar to that of granulosa-thecal tumors. They are basically solid neoplasms, soft or rubbery in consistency, and cystic areas may be present. The cut surface is yellow and areas of hemorrhage and necrosis are frequently observed.[8] The majority are 6.0–15.0 cm in diameter. Involvement of the opposite ovary is to be found in less than 5% of the cases.

CLINICAL

The spectacular clinical changes produced by the endocrine activity of androblastoma overshadow the local pelvic symptoms that are common to all ovarian tumors. It must, however, be said at the onset that not all clinically masculinizing tumors belong to the androblastoma group and that, conversely, not all androblastomas are masculinizing. As pointed out by most authors, virilization is most frequently associated with the less differentiated forms, those forms that contain a considerable component of stromal cells.[17] In the review by O'Hern and Neubecker[9] virilizing changes were seen in 50% of the well-differentiated tumors Type I, about 70% of the intermediate type Type II, and in all cases with Type III histology.

The endocrine manifestations develop over a prolonged period of time and the average patient has observed the changes for more than a year prior to the diagnosis. Actually, several patients have had symptoms for many years. The early manifestations are menstruation-related, with oligomenorrhea and amenorrhea being the commonest symptoms. The defeminization continues with sterility, atrophy of the breast tissues, and loss of the female figure. Gradually, male characteristics, hir-

sutism, recession of the hairline, hypertrichosis of the rest of the body, deepening of the voice, and enlargement of the clitoris.[1,2,4,5,7,8,10,11,13,17,18]

A palpable mass was found in 74% of the patients, but only 39% had abdominal complaints in the series reported by Ireland and Woodruff.[4]

Pregnancy may coexist with androblastoma if the neoplasm is hormonally inactive or if conception takes place prior to the appearance of the neoplasm. Galle et al.[3] reviewed 15 cases of androblastoma (arrhenoblastoma) complicating pregnancy and reported a case of their own.

Electron microscopic studies have shown that the steroid production is primarily a function of the Leydig cells and of Leydig-like cells that are to be found in the stroma.[8] The level of the urinary 17-ketosteroid excretion, more often than not, is within normal limits, in spite the marked virilization changes the patients exhibit.[2,4,9,11] This is due to the fact that the tumors produce androsterone and testosterone, both substances accounting for very mild elevations of the urinary 17-ketosteroids.[1,11,12]

The incidence of malignancy among patients with androblastoma has been variously reported in the literature. Javert and Finn[5] conducted a retrospective analysis of 80 previously reported cases. Using as criteria for malignancy gross evidence of local extension during surgery or recurrence and death from metastases, they found 24 patients with malignant tumors.

Pedowitz and O'Brien[11] estimated the incidence of malignancy to be 21.3%. The authors reviewed the literature and found that of 240 cases earlier reported, 51 had pursued a malignant course. More specifically, 42 patients were dead from their tumor and nine were living with active disease present. Of those dying, 37 did so during the first five years, the remaining succumbing 10–15 years after the diagnosis. The highest recurrence rate was noted among patients with Type III tumors

(42%) and the lowest recurrence rate (12.8%) was seen among patients with Type I.

O'Hern and Neubecker[9] examined the material and evaluated the data of 31 patients with arrhenoblastoma. Follow-up data for an average period of 5.5 years were available in 29 patients. Of these, 25 were living and well at the time of the report, four had died of other causes, and only one patient, with Type III disease, was dead due to her tumor. The low incidence of malignancy (3%) is attributed by the authors to their strict criteria for diagnosing arrhenoblastomas. They point out that adenocarcinomas may appear with somewhat similar histological patterns and, should they be included in any series, the percentage of malignant cases will obviously increase. This remark has been made by others as well.[4,8,9]

Ireland and Woodruff[4] reviewed the Emil Novack Ovarian Tumor Registry. Of 67 cases, there were five recurrences with subsequent deaths. They account for an incidence of malignancy of 7%. The same authors classified separately under the title "Sertoli-Leydig cell tumors" a well-differentiated group of masculinizing neoplasms. There was one recurrence with subsequent tumor-related death among them (4%).

Apparently, during pregnancy the tumors exhibit a more malignant course. Among 16 cases of arrhenoblastoma during pregnancy, as evaluated by Galle *et al.*,[3] seven showed malignant behavior, either metastasizing or locally recurring.

TREATMENT AND RESULTS

The treatment is surgical. Removal of the involved ovary is the recommended procedure. The majority of the patients are of child-bearing age; therefore the opposite ovary, if uninvolved, should be left intact. At times, the opposite ovary may have a polycystic appearance, as a result of high androgen levels. This is not to be confused with tumor involvement. A wedge resection can be performed for confirmation.

If the patient is in the older age group, bilateral salpingo-oophorectomy can be performed.

In case of clinical evidence of malignancy, the procedure should be similar to that for all ovarian cancers, namely, total abdominal hysterectomy, bilateral salpingo-oophorectomy, and omentectomy.[1,2,4,5,11,13]

Following surgery, normal menstruation is reestablished in one to three months. Several patients have subsequently become pregnant, delivering normal children. It takes several months for the defeminization process to reverse. There is a gradual enlargement of the breasts and reappearance of the female habitus. There is an improvement in the voice and a decrease in the size of the clitoris. Although the hair growth slows down, as a rule the already developed hypertrichosis persists.[1,2,9,11]

The role of radiation therapy and particularly that of systemic chemotherapy in the management of the malignant variants remains to be evaluated. The Gynecologic Oncology Group currently accrues data.

PROGNOSIS AND SURVIVAL

There is general agreement that Meyer's Type III tumors or corresponding tumors differently labeled in subsequent classifications carry a serious prognosis because they are potentially malignant.[2,4,7,11]

As a rule, by the time the malignant nature of the neoplasm is manifested, the local recurrence is beyond control and so is, of course, the development of distant disease. Therefore, with a few exceptions, all patients with malignant androblastomas (arrhenoblastomas) have died of their tumor.[3,4,5,11]

REFERENCES

1. Cruikshank, D.P., and Chapler, F.K.: Arrheno-blastomas and associated ovarian pathology. *Obstet Gynecol* **43**:539, 1974.
2. Cruikshank, D.P., Yannone, M.E., and Chapler, F.K.: Arrhenoblastoma associated with adrenal androgenic hyperfunction. *Obstet Gynecol* **43**:535, 1974.
3. Galle, P.C., McCool, J.A., and Elsner, C.W.: Arrhenoblastoma during pregnancy. *Obstet Gynecol* **51**:359, 1978.
4. Ireland, K., and Woodruff, J.D.: Masculinizing ovarian tumors. *Obstet Gynecol Surv* **31**:83, 1976.
5. Javert, C.T., and Finn, W.F.: Arrhenoblastoma. The incidence of malignancy and the relationship to pregnancy, to sterility and to treatment. *Cancer* **4**:60, 1951.
6. Kraus, F.T.: *Gynecologic Pathology.* C.V. Mosby, St. Louis, 1967.
7. Meyer, R.: Pathology of some special ovarian tumors and their relation to sex characteristics. *Am J Obstet Gynecol* **22**:697, 1931.
8. Norris, H.J., and Chorlton, I.: Functioning tumors of the ovary. *Clin Obstet Gynecol* **17**:189, 1974.
9. O'Hern, T.M., and Neubecker, R.D.: Arrhenoblastoma. *Obstet Gynecol* **19**:758, 1962.
10. Pedowitz, P., and Pomerance, W.: Adrenal-like tumors of the ovary; review of the literature and report of two new cases. *Obstet Gynecol* **19**:183, 1962.
11. Pedowitz, P., and O'Brien, F.B.: Arrhenoblastoma of the ovary. Review of the literature and report of 2 cases. *Obstet Gynecol* **16**:62, 1960.
12. Personen, S., and Mikkonen, R.: Observations on the significance of dehydroepiandrosterone, androsterone and etiocholanolone determinations in the differential diagnosis of certain adrenal and ovarian diseases. *Acta Endocrinol* **27**:170, 1958.
13. Ramzy, I., and Bos, C.: Sertoli cell tumors of ovary. Light microscopic and ultrastructural study with histogenetic considerations. *Cancer* **38**:2447, 1976.
14. Scully, R.E.: Ovarian tumors. A review. *Am J Pathol* **87**:686, 1977.
15. Serov, S.F., Scully, R.E., and Sobin, L.H.: Histological typing of ovarian tumors. In *International Histological Classification of Tumors*, No. 9. World Health Organization, Geneva, 1973.
16. Sternberg, W.H., and Dhurandhar, H.N.: Functional ovarian tumors of stromal and sex cord origin. *Hum Pathol* **8**:565, 1977.
17. Teilum, G.: Estrogen-producing Steroli cell tumors (androblastoma tubulare lipoides) of human testis and ovary; homologous ovarian and testicular tumors. III. *J Clin Endocrinol* **9**:301, 1949.
18. Teilum, G.: *Special Tumors of Ovary and Testis and Related Extragonadal Lesions. Comparative Pathology and Histological Identification.* J. B. Lippincott, Philadelphia, 1976.

113

Gonadoblastoma

THE TUMOR WAS described by Scully in 1953. In a subsequent review he defined as gonadoblastoma a neoplasm that contains a mixture of germ cells and elements resembling immature granulosa or Sertoli cells. Leydig cells or luteintype cells may or may not be present. It is grouped under the gonadal tumors and it is by itself benign, having, however, the capacity to produce malignant neoplasms. It is found in patients with abnormal sexual development. The majority of the reported patients are females. Both the female and male patients exhibit sex abnormalities, such as virilization in the former and cryptorchidism, hypospadias, and female internal sex organs in the latter. Karyogram examinations shows the presence of a Y chromosome in almost 90% of the cases.[4,6]

The patients are young, the age ranging from 10 to 38 years at the time of the diagnosis, with many patients being younger than 15.[1,2,4–6]

PATHOLOGY

The tumor arises in the ovary or in a gonadal streak. Grossly, it is a soft fleshy growth but it can also be firm and cartilaginous. Actually, the presence of calcifications with this cartilage casts a characteristic radiographic shadow. The size varies from very small to neoplasms of 8 cm or larger. When a germinoma develops within the pure gonadoblastoma, much larger sizes can be attained.[1,4,6]

Histologically, germ cells and small epithelial cells resembling immature Sertoli and granulosa cells are necessary in order to establish the diagnosis, according to Scully.[4] The germ cells exhibit considerable mitotic activity. Within the pure gonadoblastoma, hyalinization, calcification, and the development of a secondary germinoma can take place (Figs. 113-1, 113-2). Thus, dysgerminomas, embryonal teratomas, embryonal carcinomas, endodermal sinus tumors, and choriocarcinomas have been reported developing in gonadoblastomas. Gonadoblastoma itself does not metastasize; however, these secondary germinomas determine the prognosis of the individual patient.[1,4,5]

CLINICAL

The individual patients on whom gonadoblastomas occur can be subdivided into three groups: nonvirilized phenotypic females, virilized phenotypic females, and phenotypic males. Amenorrhea is a common symptom in all phenotypic females and is practically universal. On pelvic examination masses can be felt corresponding to the neoplasm; however, this is not always possible because the tumor may occur higher in the pelvis or in the retroperitoneal space arising from a gonadal streak.

The external genitalia are often poorly developed. At operation in the majority of

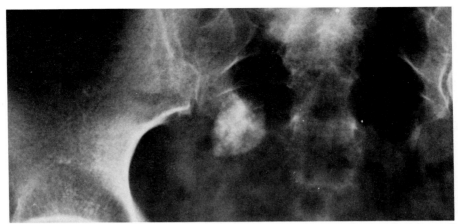

FIG. 113-1. Gonadoblastoma in a 31-year-old female. There is a mottled, well-circumscribed calcification in the right gonadal region. Spina bifida occulta is present from S1 and below. (Courtesy E. Q. Seymour. *AJR* **127**:1001, 1976.)

the patients a uterus and ovarian tubes can be found. In virilized phenotypic females and in phenotypic males secondary sex organ of the male, such as prostate, epididymis, and vas deferans may be identified.[2,4]

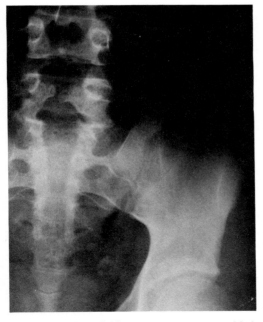

FIG. 113-2. Gonadoblastoma in a 14-year-old female. Faint calcification is seen in the left gonadal area. Spina bifida occulta, often coexisting, is present from L1 and below. (Courtesy E. Q. Seymour. *AJR* **127**:1001, 1976.)

TREATMENT AND PROGNOSIS

Resection of the tumor is all that is needed in order to control pure gonadoblastomas. If the karyogram shows Y chromosomes present, it is concluded that the remaining gonad represents a testicle; therefore it should be removed as well. In a patient with a normal karyogram, however, the opposite ovary should be only biopsied and if it is free of disease it should be left untouched.[3] It is necessary to remove the tumor prior to its malignant transformation. When secondary germ cell tumors develop, the prognosis depends on the individual histology. In general patients with dysgerminomas have done well and have been successfully managed by surgery and postoperative radiotherapy.[6] On the other hand, all patients whose gonadoblastomas transformed into embryonal carcinomas and endodermal sinus tumors or choriocarcinomas have died of their disease. The average survival time is approximately 18 months.[5]

REFERENCES

1. Garvin, A.J., Pratt-Thomas, H.R., Spector, M., Spicer, S.S., and Williamson, H.O.: Gonadoblastoma: Histologic, ultrastructural, and histochemical observations in five cases. *Am J Obstet Gynecol* **125**:459, 1976.

2. Saunders, D.M., Barratt, J., and Grudzinskas, G.: Feminization in gonadal dysgenesis associated with ovarian gonadoblastoma. *Obstet Gynecol* **46:**93, 1975.
3. Schellas, H.F.: Malignant potential of the dysgenetic gonad. *Obstet Gynecol* **44:**455, 1974.
4. Scully, R.E.: Gonadoblastoma. A review of 74 cases. *Cancer* **25:**1340, 1970.
5. Talerman, A.: Gonadoblastoma associated with embryonal carcinoma. *Obstet Gynecol* **43:**138, 1974.
6. Williamson, H.O., Underwood, P.B., Jr., Kreutner, A., Jr., Robergs, J.F., Mathur, R.S., and Pratt-Thomas, H.R.: Gonadoblastoma: Clinico-pathologic correlation in six patients. *Am J Obstet Gynecol* **216:**579, 1976.

114

Sertoli Cell Tumor of the Testis

SERTOLI CELL TUMORS belong to the gonadal stromal group of neoplasms arising from the Sertoli cells of the testis, cells that normally perform a supportive action. They are uncommon neoplasms accounting for less than 1% of all testicular tumors. Collins and Symington[1] found six Sertoli cell tumors among 995 testicular neoplasms when reviewing the material of the British Testicular Tumor Panel. It is of interest to note that Sertoli cell tumor is the commonest testicular neoplasm in dogs, comprizing approximately 40% of all testicular tumors seen in these animals.[2] In human beings the majority of the neoplasms are benign in character and only a small percentage, approximately 10%, pursue a malignant course. They can be seen in all ages, from the very young to octogenarians.[3,6]

PATHOLOGY

The tumor exhibits a preference for the left testis, which is twice as often involved as the right. They are firm in consistency but they may contain cystic areas. They are well encapsulated and necrosis and hemorrhage are rare.[4]

Microscopically, there is more than one form. The well-differentiated tumors are composed of tubular structures resembling seminiferous tubules. They are made of hexagonal or tall columnar cells with large round nuclei. They are easily recognizable and they are the commonest form (Fig. 114-1). Mitotic figures are usually not present. Other patterns in addition to the tubular are the diffuse stromal and the mixed or intermediate pattern, according to Teilum.[7] The diffuse stromal pattern is composed of spindle-shaped cells with little cytoplasm, resembling the primitive gonadal stroma.[4] It is necessary, however, that in some part of the tumor tubules be identified with or without lumen lined by cells resembling normal Sertoli cells.[7]

In judging the malignant nature of a Sertoli cell tumor microscopically, invasion of the paratesticular structures appears to be a reliable sign, as well as the large size of the tumor. Increased mitotic activity and poor differentiation with sparse tubular formation are microscopic signs indicating that possibly the lesion is malignant. However, since these criteria have not been well established, it is only the presence of metastases distally that establishes the diagnosis of a malignant Sertoli cell tumor.[4,7]

CLINICAL

The presenting symptom is that of a testicular mass or of a nodule or just swelling. Pain may or may not be present. As the mass enlarges, it is apt to be more painful. At times, only slight discomfort may be present in spite of a large tumor.[3,5,6] On physical examination, the enlarged testis will be found. Decreased libido and gynecomastia have been encountered in some patients.[4] Testicular atrophy of the

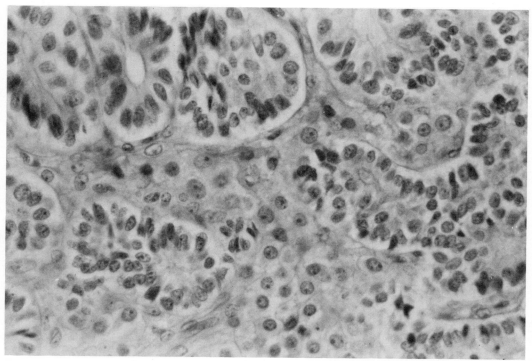

FIG. 114-1. Sertoli cell tumor of the testis. Tubular structures formed and lined by Sertoli cells. The intervening tissue consists of Leydig cells.

remaining testicle or depressed spermatogenesis have been reported.[4]

TREATMENT AND RESULTS

The tumors are usually benign; therefore inguinal orchiectomy will be the therapy for the majority of the patients. Due to the fact that the histological criteria of malignant Sertoli cell tumor have not been definitely established, cases of malignant Sertoli cell tumor found in the literature deal only with those patients who have developed metastatic disease. Morin and Loening[3] reported a case of malignant Sertoli cell tumor and reviewed the literature on the subject. Of 67 cases of Sertoli cell tumor, seven were shown to have metastatic disease developing.

The malignant variant may occur in all ages, from the very young to the old. Metastatic disease develops primarily in the lymph nodes and it involves not only the retroperitoneal but also the pelvic and inguinal groups. Metastasis to the bone and local recurrence in the skin of the region have been reported as well.[3] The survival of patients with malignant Sertoli cell tumor is difficult to tabulate due to fragmented information. Four patients were dead within a year from the time of diagnosis.[3] Talerman[6] reported one patient who was doing well eight months following the diagnosis of retroperitoneal lymph node involvement. The patient had received radiation therapy (3000 rad over four weeks).[6] Two additional patients had survived more than 18 months.[3] At this time, no statement as to the effectiveness of any particular chemotherapeutic agent is available.

REFERENCES

1. Collins, D.H., and Symington, T.: Sertoli cell tumour. *Br J Urol (Suppl)* **36:**52, 1964.
2. Cotchin, E.: Testicular neoplasms in dogs. *J Comp Pathol Therap* **70:**232, 1960.
3. Morin, L.J., and Loening, S.: Malignant androblastoma (Sertoli cell tumor) of the testis. A case report with a review of the literature. *J Urol* **114:**476, 1975.
4. Mostofi, F.K., and Price, E.B., Jr.: *Tumors of the Male Genital System.* Armed Forces Institute of Pathology, Washington, D.C., 1973.
5. Siller, J.J., and Farah, R.N.: Androblastoma (Sertoli-cell tumor). *J Urol* **106:**565, 1971.
6. Talerman, A.: Malignant Sertoli cell tumor of the testis. *Cancer* **28:**446, 1971.
7. Teilum, G.: *Special Tumors of Ovary and Testis and Related Extragonadal Lesions. Comparative Pathology and Histological Identification.* J. B. Lippincott, Philadelphia, 1976.

115

Interstitial (Leydig) Cell Tumor of the Testis

INTERSTITIAL CELL tumors of the testis belong, under the current nomenclature, to the so-called "gonadal stromal tumors," or sex cord tumors, of the testis.[7] The histology of the normal testis is composed of germinal cells and of supportive Sertoli and Leydig (interstitial cells). The Leydig cells in response to luteinizing hormone are the main source of testosterone production. The World Health Organization has adopted the term "sex cord," or stromal tumors, into which are included the Leydig cell tumors and the Sertoli cell tumors of the testis.[7] Both the Leydig and the Sertoli cells originate from the primitive gonadal stroma.[5]

Leydig cell tumors represent 3% of all testicular neoplasms.[5] The majority of the cases pursue a benign course and approximately only 10% of the Leydig cell tumors are malignant.[2,5] They occur in all age groups with 25% of the neoplasms seen in boys younger than the age of 15 years.[2]

PATHOLOGY

The gross appearance of interstitial cell tumors is that of a spherical solid and rather well-circumscribed mass with a homogeneous cut surface. In the experience of Teilum[9] areas of necrosis or hemorrhages are never seen. Diffuse testicular enlargement at times or one or more nodules may be found.[5]

Histologically, the cells resemble the interstitial cells of the testis; however, some degree of anaplasia and some mitotic ac-

tivity may be observed.[9] Mostofi and Price[5] distinguish four types of cells on histological examination. The most common are medium-sized hexagonal cells with indistinct cell membrane and a round or oval vesicular nucleus. Occasional large, binucleated, or multinucleated cells are present. The cells arrange themselves in nests, cords, or islands. The stroma shows varying degrees of hyalinization.[5]

The presence of the so-called "Reinke crystals" is considered a pathognomonic feature by the same authors. However, Teilum[9] calls the finding inconstant and not necessary. Criteria for malignant Leydig cell tumor include increased mitotic activity and extension to the adjacent testicular structures, as well as evidence of vascular invasion. These findings, however, although suspicious, are not absolute and it is only the presence of distant metastasis that will confirm the diagnosis of malignancy.[5]

CLINICAL

Leydig cell tumors developing in children produce precocious puberty. When seen in adults they produce gynecomastia in approximately 20–25% of the cases. These feminizing manifestations are due to increased production of estrogen as detected in both urinary excretion and in the plasma. The majority of adults, however, have no endocrine manifestations. The main presenting symptom is testicular enlargement with or without pain. The endocrine symptoms gradually disappear following orchiectomy.[3]

Mahon et al.[4] in a literature review on malignant interstitial cell testicular tumors found that the malignant variant occurs only in adults. The authors reviewed 12 cases from the literature and added one of their own. The average age of the patients with malignant Leydig cell tumors was 60 years at the time of the diagnosis. All patients with the exception of one presented with a testicular mass. By definition, malignant interstitial cell tumor is one that metastasizes, all patients eventually developing metastatic disease and dying of it. The retroperitoneal nodes, the liver, and the lung were the commonest metastatic sites. Other areas of metastasis included the skeletal system, the abdominal cavity, and the inguinal and pelvic lymph nodes.[4]

The recommended treatment should the tumor present histological features indicative of malignancy is radical orchiectomy. Radiation therapy can be used for palliation purposes in terms of pain relief.[10] Of the chemotherapeutic agents ortho, para'-DDD has been shown to be effective in the management of metastatic disease. Liver metastases and metastases to supraclavicular nodes have decreased in size with the use of this agent.[4,8]

As far as the survival of patients with benign interstitial cell tumor is concerned, it should not be affected following the removal of the neoplasia. A gradual reversal of the hormonal manifestations is expected, particularly among the patients who have developed feminizing symptoms. The return to normalcy is accompanied by regain of the lost libido. The average median survival of patients with

malignant interstitial cell tumor has been approximately three years. In some patients the disease pursues a rapid course with death occurring in a few months, whereas in others it pursues a chronic slow course. One patient is reported cured of his disease following resection of a solitary lung metastasis. He died eight years postthoracotomy and autopsy revealed no evidence of other metastases.[6]

REFERENCES

1. Abelson, D., Bulaschenko, H., Trommer, P.R., and Valdes-Dapena, A.: Malignant interstitial-cell tumor of the testis treated with o, p'-DDD. Metabolism 15:242, 1966.
2. Dalgaard, J.B., and Hesselberg, F.: Interstitial tumors of the testes. Two cases and survey. Acta Pathol Microbiol Scand 41:219, 1957.
3. Gambrilove, J.L., Nicolis, G.L., Mitty, H.A., and Sohval, A.R.: Feminizing interstitial cell tumor of the testis: Personal observations and a review of the literature. Cancer 35:1184, 1975.
4. Mahon, F.B., Jr., Gosset, F., Trinity, R.G., and Madsen, P.O.: Malignant interstitial cell testicular tumor. Cancer 31:1208, 1973.
5. Mostofi, F.K., and Price, E.B., Jr.: Tumors of the Male Genital System. Armed Forces Institute of Pathology, Washington, D.C., 1973.
6. Parker, R.G.: Treatment of apparent solitary pulmonary metastases. J Thorac Cardiovasc Surg 36:81, 1958.
7. Serov, S.F., Scully, R.E., and Sobin, L.H.: Histological Typing of Ovarian Tumors. World Health Organization, Geneva, 1973.
8. Tamoney, H.J., and Noriega, A.: Malignant interstitial cell tumor of the testis. Cancer 24:547, 1969.
9. Teilum, G.: Special Tumors of Ovary and Testis and Related Extragonadal Lesions. Comparative Pathology and Histological Identification. J. B. Lippincott, Philadelphia, 1976.
10. Ward, J.A., Krantz, S., Mendeloff, J., and Haltiwanger, E.: Interstitial-cell tumor of the testis. Report of 2 cases. J Clin Endocrinol 20:1622, 1960.

116

Cloacogenic Carcinoma of the Anorectal Junction

THE PRESENCE OF transitional epithelium in the region of the pectinate line of the rectem was first described by Hermann and Desfosses in 1880. Grinvalsky and Helwig[1] again drew attention to this region in 1956 when they discussed the histology and the embryological derivation of this segment. It was their conclusion that the mucosa that is interposed between the anus and the rectum has structural characteristics similar to those of the cloacal entoderm. This mucosa is similar to that lining the urinary tract, both in appearance and in histochemical characteristics. From this segment originate the anal ducts that lead to the perianal glands, usually in a caudad direction but occasionally cephalad as well.[1] Because of its embryonic origin, the segment is capable of giving rise to neoplasms with a variety of histological patterns. These have been summarily named "transitional cloacogenic carcinomas." Following the recognition of this tumor group by Grinvalsky and Helwig, several cases of comparable histology were reported in the literature. Klotz *et al.*[3] in 1967 analyzed on the basis of 373 cases the clinical and pathological aspects of these tumors.

Transitional carcinomas represent approximately 2.5% of all anal and rectal neoplasms.[3,4] There is a female predominance, the sex ratio between women and men being 2:1. The age range is primarily between 50 and 70 years, although the tumor has been seen in a patient as young as 29 years of age.[3,4]

PATHOLOGY

On gross inspection, the tumors are indistinguishable from the usual adenocarcinomas of the region. They present as exophytic masses in most cases; however, a smaller number develop practically submucosally as intramural indurations (Fig. 116-1). An even smaller number of them appear as anal fissures.

At the anorectal junction, the columnar bowel epithelium changes into cuboidal. This latter epithelium covers the internal hemorrhoidal plexus and subsequently the 8–12 mucosal folds, the so-called "columns of Morgagnii." Distal to the cuboidal epithelium and interposed between it and the stratified squamous epithelium of the anal canal lies transitional cell epithelium. The width of the transitional zone is 3–12.0 mm. The anal glands originate here, each having its own orifice (Fig. 116-2). The cloacogenic carcinomas arise from this transitional epithelium and the associated glands.[1,4]

The basic histological pattern is that of a transitional cell carcinoma, like those seen in the urinary tract. This pattern is seen in approximately two-thirds of the cases and it is composed of circumscribed clusters of relative uniform cells with spherical or ovoid nuclei and infrequent mitoses.[4] The

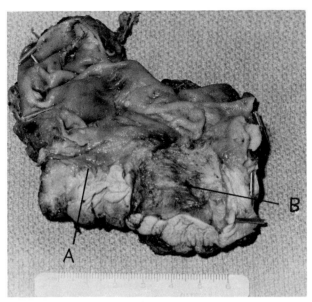

FIG. 116-1.   Cloacogenic carcinoma of the anorectal junction.
(A): Pectinate line. (B): Ulcerating tumor.

second pattern encountered is composed of nests of small cells with greater polymorphism and with hyperchromatic nuclei. Thin bands of stroma separate the cell groups and the peripheral cell layers exhibit the so-called "pallisading" arrangement. The overall appearance is reminiscent of basal cell carcinoma; therefore the term "basaloid" has been applied to this histological variety[2] (Fig. 116-3). Many variations of these two basic patterns have been reported. The tumors may resemble squamous cell, mucoepidermoid, or adenocystic carcinomas, and in the very anaplastic form it may resemble an oat cell carcinoma.[3] Tumors arising specifically from the anal ducts have shown a male preponderance at a ratio of 2:1. Nielsen

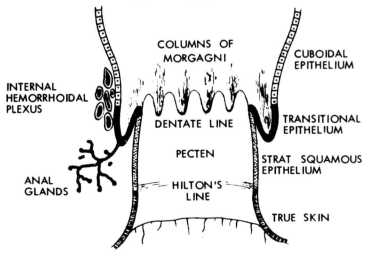

FIG. 116-2.   Detailed schematic drawing of the anorectal junction. (Courtesy S. Kheir et al. Arch Surg 104:47, 1972.)

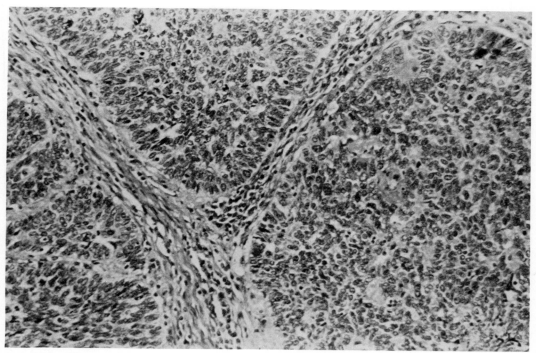

FIG. 116-3. Cloacogenic carcinoma of the rectum. Islands of poorly differentiated basaloid cells exhibiting peripheral palisading and infiltrating adjacent connective tissue.

and Koch[5] reviewed 123 cases of such tumors. Their histology was as follows: adenocarcinoma, 52% (64 patients); mucoepidermoid carcinoma, 10% (8 patients); and transitional cell carcinoma, 40% (49 patients).[5]

CLINICAL

Rectal bleeding associated with rectal pain or perineal discomfort is the common presentation. The symptoms have been present usually three to four months prior to the diagnosis. Actually, the range of symptom duration extends from 1 to 24 months. Other signs are constipation and change in the character of the bowel movements.[3,4]

Most of the tumors are located in the anterior rectal wall (37.2%). From this location, they extend to involve the rectovaginal septum. Vaginal involvement at the time of the diagnosis is present in

20.4% of the female patients. Prostatic extension was noted in 5%. As the disease advances, bladder, urethra, and sacrum, may all be infiltrated.[3,4]

Regional lymph node metastasis was present in 34% of the cases, according to Klotz et al.[3] In the series by Kheir et al.[4] the inguinal nodes were found to be particularly susceptible, showing metastatic disease in 50% of the cases.

Distant metastases to the liver, lungs, bones, and peritoneum have been reported. They developed in 19% of the cases.[3]

TREATMENT AND RESULTS

The treatment is definitive surgery. The selection of the appropriate procedure should be based on the tumor extent and on the presence or absence of lymph node involvement. These parameters together with the histological pattern are important factors in determining the success of the procedure. The most common procedure applied has been radical abdominal perineal resection, an operation done in more than 50% of the patients. The surgery has been extended to include posterior vaginectomy and inguinal node dissection in 15% of the reported cases. A small number of patients had local excision for submucosal tumors as their initial therapy. Radiotherapy has occasionally supplemented the surgical procedure, mostly in a postoperative fashion.

The natural history of the disease provides an insight as to the choice of therapy. It is known that local recurrences develop in 26% of the cases. The recurrences involve primarily the perineum, the rectum, the pelvis, and the vagina.[3] The posterior vaginal wall was the commonest site of extension in the series by Kheir et al.,[4] seen in one-third of the female patients. Inguinal lymph node involvement, if not present originally, will develop later and it should be anticipated as a tumor extension site in 50% of all patients.[4] It is therefore recommended that the abdominal perineal resection be supplemented by bilateral inguinal, femoral, and iliac lymph node dissection if there is a clinical suspicion of lymph node involvement and if the tumor is large. In addition posterior vaginectomy is recommended in women whose tumor is located on the anterior rectal wall.

We have participated in the management of six patients with transitional cloacogenic carcinoma of the anorectal junction. There were four female and two male patients, the average age of the group being 53 years. Diarrhea was the predominant symptom in three patients, diarrhea with rectal bleeding in one patient, pain with rectal bleeding in one, and rectal bleeding as the sole symptom in one.

Histologically, four of the lesions exhibited the basaloid type with areas of squamoid differentiation and two were transitional cell carcinomas. Two patients were treated palliatively because of extensive pelvic and abdominal metastases. They survived 3 and 11 months. Definitive therapy was administered in four patients. Abdominal perineal resection was performed in three patients, one of whom received 5000 rad in five weeks to the pelvis preoperatively. The fourth patient underwent a wide local excision, which was supplemented by external beam radiotherapy to the level of 5000 rad in five weeks and by an iridium-198 implant, delivering 2370 rad. Only this last patient remains alive and free of disease at the present time, 30 months following the completion of therapy. The other three died from recurrent pelvic tumor associated with metastases to the iliac and inguinal lymph nodes. The tumor is radioresponsive in our experience. Palliative therapy usually provides a long-lasting response. Radiation should also be considered as adjuvant therapy.

PROGNOSIS AND SURVIVAL

Tumors of the well-differentiated non-keratinizing transitional cell histology are reported to have a relatively good prognosis, averaging 70% five-year survival. Those with less differentiated elements or those in which squamoid differentiation is present approach 40% five-year-survival levels. Finally, it is agreed upon by all authors that the small cell basaloid tumors of the oat cell variety invariably have a fatal course.[2]

The prognosis is influenced by the size of the tumor and the status of the lymph nodes. In the absence of nodal metastases the cure rate was 51.7%. The salvage rate decreased to 14.3% for patients with lymphatic and venous permeation.[3] In the review of a large number of patients performed by Klotz et al.[3] the overall cure rate was 46.7%. Patients dying from their disease had an average survival of 27.8

months. Kheir *et al.*[4] similarly reported a five-year-survival rate of 50%.

REFERENCES

1. Grinvalsky, H.T., and Helwig, E.B.: Carcinoma of the anorectal junction. I. Histological considerations. *Cancer* **9**:480, 1956.
2. Grodsky, L.: Current concepts on cloacogenic transitional cell anorectal cancers. *JAMA* **207**:2057, 1969.
3. Klotz, R.G., Jr., Pamukcoglu, T., and Souilliard, D.H.: Transitional cloacogenic carcinoma of the anal canal. Clinicopathologic study of three hundred seventy-three cases. *Cancer* **20**:1727, 1967.
4. Kheir, S., Hickey, R.C., Martin, R.G., MacKay, B., and Gallager, H.S.: Cloacogenic carcinoma of the anal canal. *Arch Surg* **104**:407, 1972.
5. Nielsen, O.V., and Koch, F.: Carcinomas of the anorectal region of extramucosal origin with special reference to the anal ducts. *Acta Chir Scand* **139**:299, 1973.

INDEX